GW00363784

Correction to text on p. 223;

In 1968, the Institute of Obstetricians and Gynaecologists was established. Eight years later, two Faculties were established: the Faculty of Community Medicine (the name later changed to the Faculty of Public Health Medicine) and the Faculty of Occupational Medicine.

In 1981 the Faculty of Pathology was founded, followed, in 1982, by the Faculty of Paediatrics.

The Faculties and Institute play a central role within RCPI, as the training and professional bodies for doctors practising in the specialities they represent. Over many years, the Deans of the Faculties and the Chair of the Institute have served on the Council of RCPI, as senior executive members of the Council, and as President, Vice-President and Treasurer.

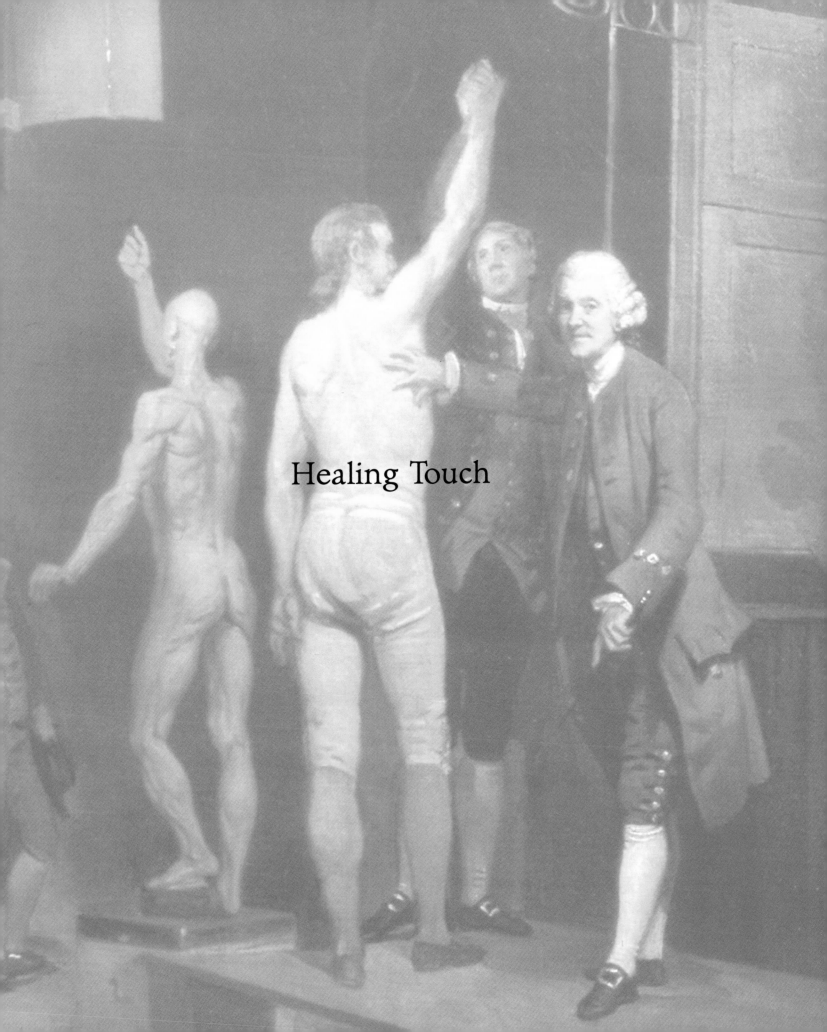

Healing Touch

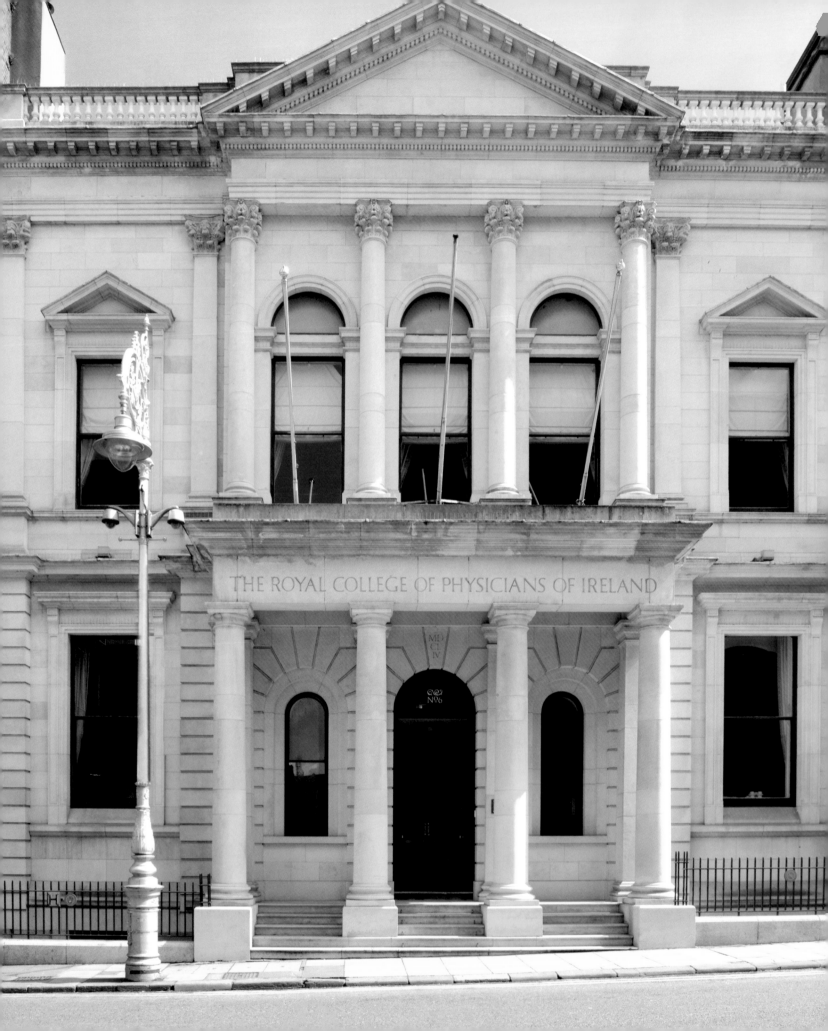

Healing Touch

An illustrated history of
the Royal College of Physicians of Ireland

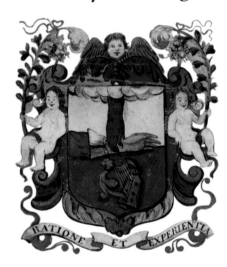

Alf McCreary

DESIGN AND PICTURE EDITOR
WENDY DUNBAR

THE ROYAL COLLEGE OF PHYSICIANS OF IRELAND

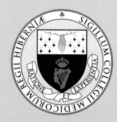

PAGE 1: Detail from Dr William Hunter
lecturing at the Royal Academy, c. 1772.
Painting by Johann Zoffany
ROYAL COLLEGE OF PHYSICIANS, LONDON

FRONTISPIECE: The Royal College of Physicians
of Ireland, No 6 Kildare Street, Dublin
PHOTOGRAPH BY DERMOTT DUNBAR

OPPOSITE: Drawing of the College Mace by
Sir Frederic William Burton, RHA
RCPI

First published in 2015 by
The Royal College of Physicians of Ireland

Text: Alf McCreary
Design: Wendy Dunbar, Dunbar Design
Copy-editor: Susan Feldstein
Indexer: Eileen O'Neill
Printed by Nicholson & Bass Ltd

ISBN 978-0-9559351-3-8

www.rcpi.ie

Contents

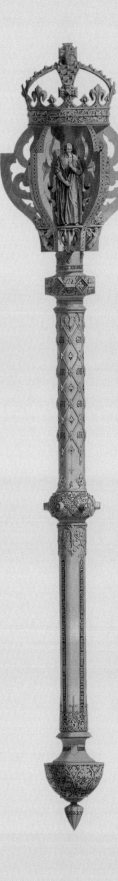

For over 360 years the Royal College of Physicians of Ireland
has had the principal aim of promoting and maintaining professional
standards in medicine. Over this period the name of the institution
has changed on a number of occasions.

1654 The Fraternity of Physicians of Trinity Hall was founded by
Dr John Stearne

1667 Name changed by Royal Charter to the College of Physicians in
Dublin

1692 Renamed by Royal Charter the King and Queen's College of
Physicians in Ireland

1890 Name changed by supplemental Charter to the Royal College of
Physicians of Ireland

Throughout this text, the term 'the College' will be used to refer to what is
now the Royal College of Physicians of Ireland. This is done to avoid
confusion which might arise from the various changes of name.

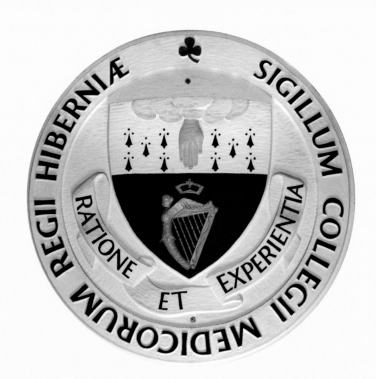

Foreword

When I agreed to write the story of the Royal College of Physicians of Ireland, I had little idea of the literary and historical adventure that lay ahead of me.

A few medical histories of the College had been produced a long time ago, but I decided early on that this account of RCPI would also set its story clearly in the context of the turbulent political and social developments in Ireland, and further afield, since 1654.

I also felt that it was important to provide more details of the personal, as well as the professional, lives of the medical figures whose dedication and vision helped to shape the College of Physicians through the challenges and turbulence of Irish history over more than 360 years.

The extensive archive of the College contains material of historical significance, and the inclusion of so many beautiful images, and facsimiles of key historical documents, has added greatly to the text.

I would like to pay a special tribute to my esteemed colleague, the book-designer and picture editor Wendy Dunbar, who has produced a magnificently-compiled visual dimension to the colourful story of the College, and its people.

This was a considerable professional challenge for both of us. It was rather like setting out to complete a huge jig-saw puzzle, with the added difficulty that many of the 'elusive' or 'missing' pieces were not even in the same box, but scattered far and wide in libraries, galleries and art collections at home and abroad.

It is my hope, therefore, that all the main pieces are now in their proper place, and that the reader will learn something new from the important story of the Royal College of Physicians of Ireland, and also about the history of these islands in a period of significant developments in medicine, politics, and major social issues.

ALF McCREARY
26 SEPTEMBER 2015

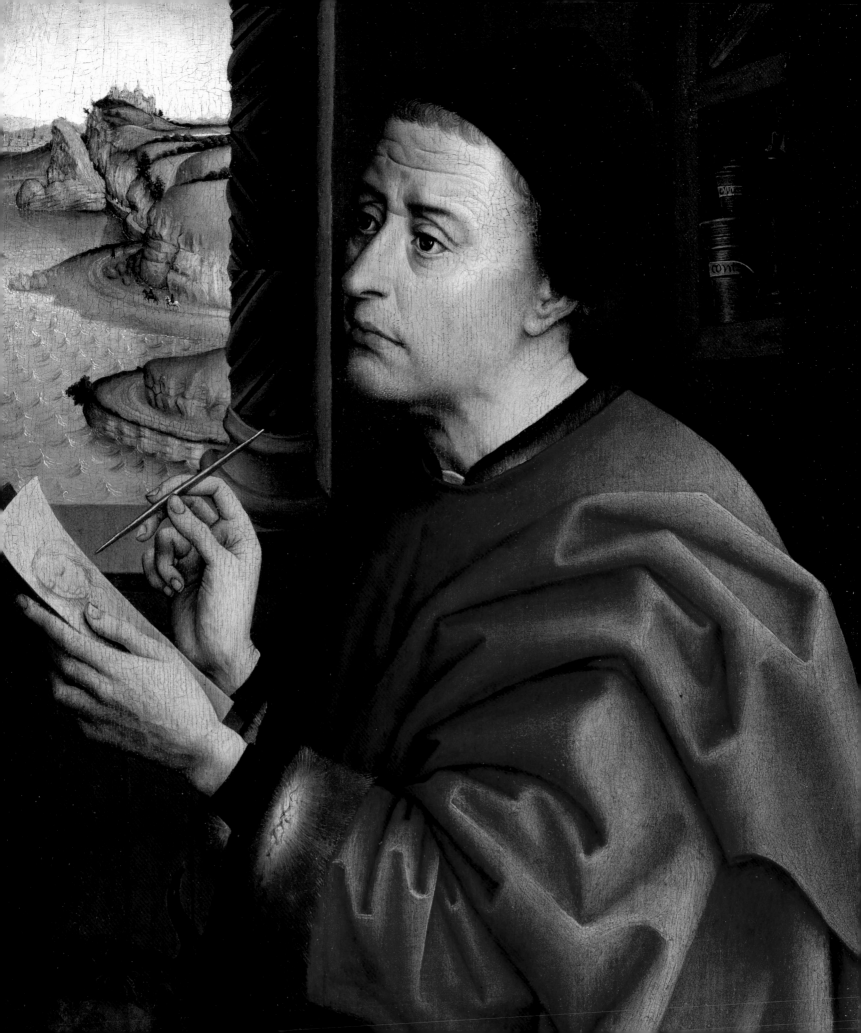

Arts and Science
Where Poetry and Medicine meet

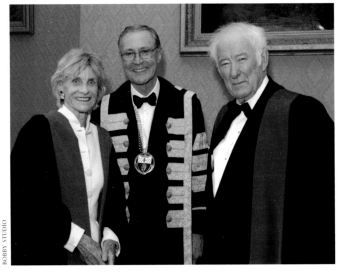

In June 2011 the Irish poet and Nobel Laureate Seamus Heaney received an Honorary Fellowship from the Royal College of Physicians of Ireland at their historic Kildare Street home in Dublin.

Dr John Donohoe, President of the Royal College of Physicians of Ireland, with Seamus Heaney and Jean Kennedy Smith who received Honorary Fellowships in 2011.

RCPI

BOBBY STUDIO

During an impressive ceremony, Dr Padraic Mac Mathuna, a Fellow of the College, paid a warm personal and official tribute to Heaney who, by that stage, was the most popular and acclaimed poet writing in the English language.

Jean Kennedy Smith, who served as US Ambassador to Ireland from 1993–98, also received an Honorary Fellowship at the ceremony in 2011.

Admission to Honorary Fellowship is one of the highest honours that the College can bestow. It is reserved for world leaders in medical science, and for exceptional contributors to the welfare of people and communities, both nationally and internationally.

Since 1728, when Honorary Fellowships were introduced at the College, the long list of distinguished recipients reads like a *Who's Who*, not only of medicine in Ireland and overseas, but also of some of the most influential figures in the broader political, social and cultural life of the nation and indeed a number of other countries. Those thus honoured include national Presidents, professors, politicians, inventors, visionaries, pragmatists and others from many different backgrounds, including the world of the Arts: all of them have made an important contribution to society through their work in their own particular area of influence.

Seamus Heaney was exceptionally gifted in the field of literature, and is widely regarded as the greatest Irish poet since W.B. Yeats. He was also a modest and unassuming person who carried his literary genius lightly, and the warmth of the citation for his Honorary Fellowship mirrored the affection of all those present, and indeed of the entire nation, for this remarkable poet and Irishman.

In his comprehensive tribute, Dr Mac Mathuna outlined Heaney's distinguished career, noting in particular his award of the Nobel Prize in

OPPOSITE:
St Luke, drawing the Virgin Mary. Painting after Rogier van der Weyden *c.* 1399–1464

The painters guild, along with doctors and anatomists, was held under the protection of St Luke, 'the beloved physician' and painter. .
The St Luke's Meeting and Dinner of the College is held annually on St Luke's Day, 18 October.

NATIONAL GALLERY OF IRELAND

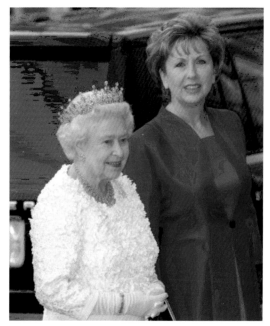

Literature in 1995 for 'works of lyrical beauty and ethical depth, which exalt everyday miracles and the living past'. He also stressed the sense in which, in this Honorary Fellowship ceremony, the worlds of art and science had come together to honour 'a great Irishman'.

In his citation, Dr Mac Mathuna highlighted the important parallels between the work of the poet and the work of the medical scientist. Alluding to one of Heaney's most celebrated poems, 'Digging', he cited the Nobel Laureate's own description of a poet as someone, 'who will dig, but with a pen, uncovering layers of both personal memory and history': a search for meaning which reflects the scientist's own quest for answers and new connections. Dr Mac Mathuna also quoted Albert Einstein, another Nobel Laureate, who once remarked: 'The most beautiful experience we can have is the mysterious. It is the source of all true art and science.'

The interaction between the worlds of art and medical science, and the central element of mystery in each to which Dr Mac Mathuna referred, is wonderfully captured in another of Seamus Heaney's poems, 'Out of the Bag', in which he recalls his childhood memories of Dr Joseph Philip Kerlin, the family physician from Magherafelt, who delivered the Heaney children into the world.[1]

The poet graphically describes the arrival of Dr Kerlin at the family's farmhouse to perform a home delivery – a widespread practice in Ireland during the first part of the twentieth century. In this vividly descriptive poem, Heaney recreates for the reader his childhood impression that, 'All of us came in Dr Kerlin's bag'. He carefully notes the tools of the doctor's trade:

> a whiff
> Of disinfectant, a Dutch interior gleam
> Of waistcoat satin and highlights on the forceps.

The crucial moment of delivery takes place behind closed doors and for the young Heaney, is steeped in secrecy and strange ritual. Finally Dr Kerlin places all his instruments back in his bag, 'the colour of a spaniel's inside lug', and he walks away from the family home,

> Until the next time came and in he'd come
> In his fur-lined collar that was also spaniel-coloured.

As a poet who immortalised the figure of the family physician in rural Ireland as no other has done, it is perhaps particularly apt that Seamus Heaney became an Honorary Fellow of the Royal College of Physicians of Ireland, some two years before his tragic death in 2013. The institution's recognition of the contribution of Heaney's literary genius is also a testament in itself to the special place held by the College in the cultural and social life of the Irish nation, above and beyond its central purpose of upholding and maintaining professional standards in the practice of medicine.

Heaney's name is recorded for posterity in a long list of Honorary Fellows, which dates back to 1728, when the first recipients were Sir Thomas Molyneux and Edward Wetenhall. Initially, the Honorary Fellowships were awarded to those who had resigned their Fellowship because of retirement, or because they were appointed to University Chairs or King's Professorships, but as time went on, the remit was broadened to include key individuals from all areas of activity. Significantly, the Royal Charter granted by King Charles II on 28 June 1667 named the first fourteen Fellows, and confirmed Dr John Stearne, who had founded the original Fraternity of Physicians of Trinity Hall in 1654, as the President for Life.

The long and fascinating story of the College has many twists and turns, and it begins in the Ireland of 1654, where the future of the island and of medicine itself was by no means predictable, or capable of receiving any reliable prognosis, medical or otherwise, during those highly turbulent days of Irish history.

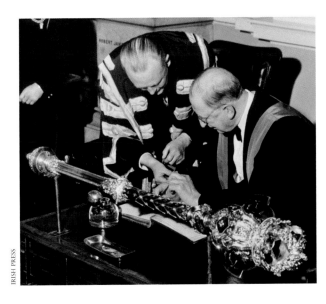

IRISH PRESS

President Eamon de Valera, 1882–1975, was made an Honorary Fellow of the College on St Luke's Day, 1967. To de Valera's right is President of the Royal College of Physicians of Ireland, Alan H Thompson.
RCPI

The Early Days

The Fraternity of Physicians of Trinity Hall,
founded in 1654 by Dr John Stearne, was the
forerunner of the Royal College of Physicians
of Ireland.

The Fraternity's main aim was to improve the widely varying practice of
medicine throughout the island, which itself was undergoing fundamental
political and social changes.

As one writer noted, much later, the history of Ireland in the first half of the
seventeenth century was 'rich in event, and perhaps bewildering in the number
and complexity of the interests involved'.

> The Irish, the old English, the new English, the royalists, the
> parliamentarians and the Scots – each of them played their separate parts in
> the confusion of events. But what happened at that time can be summarised
> in a single brief sentence: the land of Ireland changed hands.[1]

This crucial period included the execution of King Charles I in 1649, Oliver
Cromwell's invasion of Ireland that same year, with such bloody and far-
reaching consequences, and the Restoration of Charles II in 1660. In the years
following the 1641 Rebellion, many thousands of lives were lost in Ireland. The
dramatic changes continued throughout the rest of the century, culminating in
the Williamite Wars which secured the English throne for Protestantism and
consolidated the Protestant Ascendancy.

The seventeenth century was pivotal in the history of Ireland, and the
outcome of the various confrontations over land, as well as the competing
demands of religion and culture, continue to leave their mark on the island
today, especially in the North, where religion is now used largely as a tribal
label in a struggle over political control and territory.

It was against this daunting background of political uncertainty and
fundamental change that Dr John Stearne and his contemporaries worked hard
to bring discipline to the practice of medicine in Ireland in the first half of the
seventeenth century .

This ran the gamut from home cures to faith healing, and the intervention of
all kinds of quacks, barber-surgeons, and self-appointed healers, to the practice
of a small number of qualified physicians who were consulted by the better-off
customers in the medical marketplace.

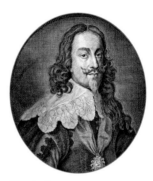

Charles I
RCPI

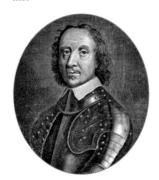

Oliver Cromwell
RCB LIBRARY

OPPOSITE: Dr John Stearne, the first
President of the College.
Painting by Stephen Catterson
Smith the elder, a copy of a portrait
in Trinity attributed to Hugh
Howard.
RCPI

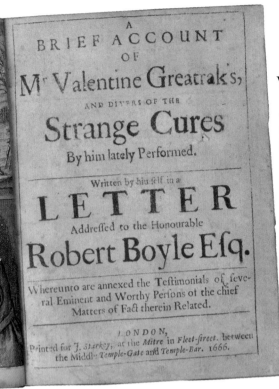

Title page from *A brief account of Mr Valentine Greatrak's and divers of the Strange Cures by him lately performed.*
RCPI

As one social and medical historian has noted, the state of Irish and Western medicine in the 1650s, when the Fraternity was founded,

> … had barely moved away from magic, and the ancient classical theories of Galen and Hippocrates. Diseases, and especially epidemics, were generally interpreted as buffets from the hand of God. An outbreak of plague that terrifyingly had killed one-third of Dubliners was within living memory.[2]

Primitive Medicine

Dublin was prone to outbreaks of plague, including a major epidemic in 1575 and another in 1604–5, and the lack of adequate facilities for treatment helped to underline the then primitive state of Irish medicine.

The standard of medicine in the early seventeenth century was so poor that in 1619, Dermot O'Meara an Oxford graduate, and a Catholic from a Tipperary dynasty of physicians to the influential Butlers of Ormonde, complained strongly to Sir Oliver St John, the Lord Deputy of Ireland. He wrote, in Latin:

> There are certainly more persons in Dublin at the present day practising the Art of Medicine than any other art, yet there are very few of them who have the six qualifications which Hippocrates requires in a medical doctor.
>
> Here, not only cursed mountebanks, ignorant barbers, and shameless quack compounders, but also persons of every other craft whatsoever, loose women, and those of the dregs of humanity who are either tired of their proper art and craft, or inflamed with an unbridled passion for making money – all have free leave to profane the holy temple of Aesculapius.[3]

Here might one not justly exclaim, in the words of the poet:

> Here are those
> Who, groping in the dark, are licensed still
> To rack the sick, and murder men at will.[3]

Thomas Arthur, a medical colleague of O'Meara who became one of the best-connected and most affluent physicians in Ireland, had similar views, and he was appalled at the damage and suffering caused by quack doctors and botched treatments.

Arthur noted, for example, that when he visited a Sir Basil Brooke, who had a blockage at the neck of his bladder, the patient had a fever, and was suffering from great pain which had been caused 'by a certain reckless physician who had prescribed beetles to be eaten'. All that Thomas Arthur could do was to advise the patient

> … to look out for the safety of his soul and have regard as quickly as possible for the disposal of his affairs.[4]

King Worried

Even the English Monarch himself was worried. King Charles I expressed concern about 'untrained' medical practitioners. He stated in a letter to Viscount Falkland, the Lord-Lieutenant of Ireland, that:

> ... the practice of physic is daily abused, in that our kingdom by wandering ignorant mountebanks and empirics, who, for want of restraint, do much abound, in the daily impairing of the healths, and hazarding the lives in general of our good subjects ... in Ireland.[5]

The King backed his words with actions, and he decreed that an Irish college of physicians should be established in Dublin, with the same articles and privileges as their colleagues in the London College of Physicians, which had received its first Charter from Henry VIII in 1518 and was re-incorporated by James I in 1617. Accordingly, a group of Irish doctors asked the London College to send them details of their establishment, statutes and charters.

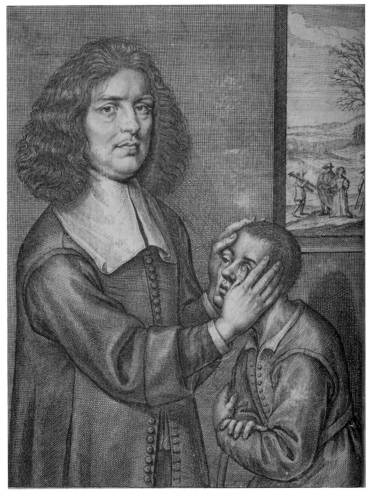

Valentine Greatraks, 1629–83, known as the 'Stroker', from Affane in Waterford, practised faith healing.
RCPI

The Londoners asked the Irish doctors to come to London instead, and to find out the facts for themselves. However they declared that they could not travel to London and stay there for a lengthy period because they could not afford to leave their private practice and business affairs in Ireland.

This could be interpreted as an 'own goal' by the Irish, or as an indication that they felt the King's offer to be less than sincere, or a little of both. The fact remained, however, that something had to be done, and one of the prime movers in finding a solution was Dr John Stearne.[5]

However, the way ahead was by no means simple, and the career of Stearne in itself demonstrated the importance of keeping in touch with the right people during those days of political upheaval and uncertainty.

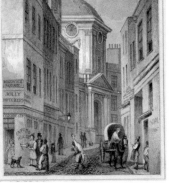

Royal College of Physicians, Warwick Lane, London
RCPI

Privileged background

Stearne was born in 1624 in Ardbraccan in Co. Meath, and he was the eldest of three sons of a Cambridgeshire man – also John Stearne – who had come to Ireland as an 'officer' of Bishop Theophilus of Dromore.

Stearne the younger entered Trinity College Dublin in 1639 at the age of 15, and became a Scholar in 1641. Due to the unrest in Ireland he fled to Cambridge, with a highly-influential recommendation from his grand-uncle, the famous Primate James Ussher, in whose house he had been born.

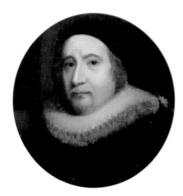

Primate James Ussher
TRINITY COLLEGE, DUBLIN

15

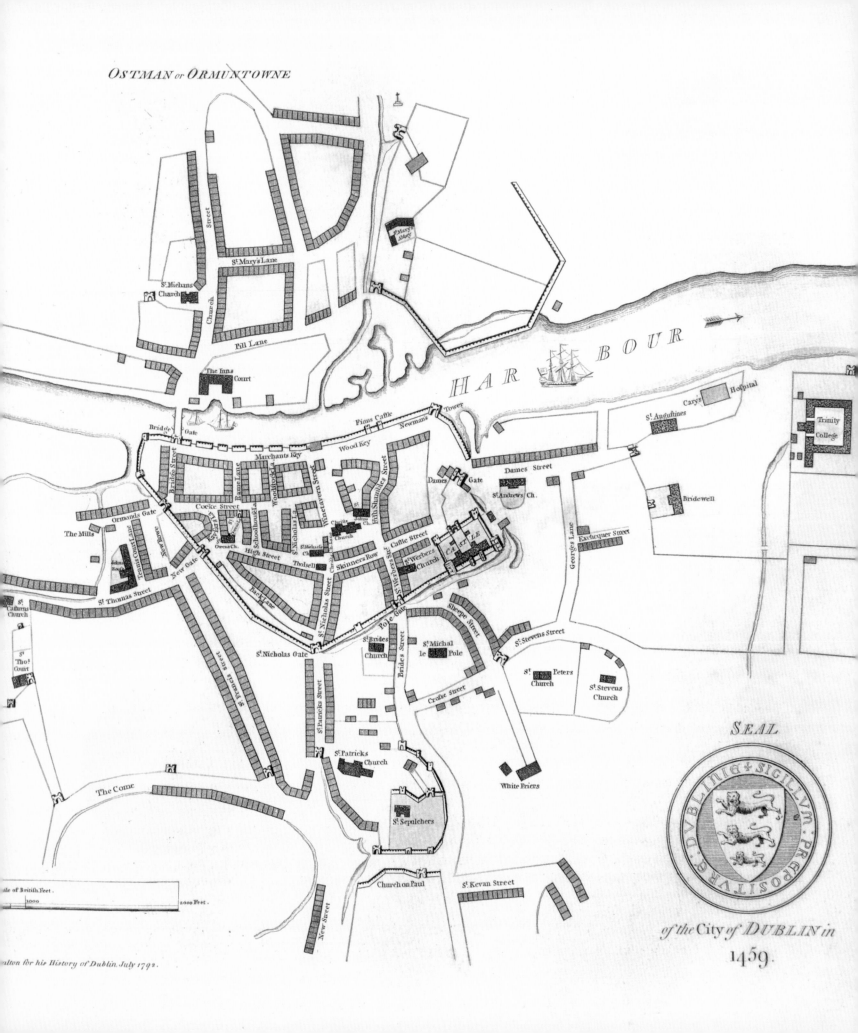

OSTMAN or ORMUNTOWNE

St Mary's Lane

St Michans Church

Street

Church

Pill Lane

The Inns Court

HAR BOUR

St Mary's Abby

Finns Castle

Tower

Carys Hospital

St Augustines

Trinity College

Bridge Gate

Newmans

Wood Key

Marchants Key

Dames Street

Dames Gate

St Andrews Ch.

Bridewell

Bridge Street

Pame Lane

Woodtool La

Winetavern Street

Fish Shambles Street

St

St Austins

Georges Lane

Exchequer Street

Cocke Street

St Nicholas La

St Johns Ch.

Ormonds Gate

Christs Church

Castle Street

CASTLE

St Michaels Ch.

The Mills

New Rawe

Schoolhouse La

St Nicholas

St Olines Ch.

Quens Ch.

High Street

Tholsell

Skinners Row

St Werbers Str

St Werbers Church

Johns Row

Tennis Court Lane

New Gate

Christs Ch. Lane

St Thomas Street

Back Lane

St Nicholas Street

Pole Gate

Shepe Street

St Catherns Church

St Thos Court

St Nicholas Gate

St Brides Church

Brides Gate

St Michal le Pole

St Stevens Street

St Peters Church

St Stevens Church

St Patricks Street

Crosse Street

St Francis Street

SEAL

St Patricks Church

White Friers

The Come

St Sepulchers

Church on Paul

St Kevan Street

New Street

SIGILLVM · PRÆPOSITVRÆ · DVBLINIG ·

of the City of DUBLIN in

1459.

Scale of British Feet.

1000   2000 Feet.

...alton for his History of Dublin. July 1792.

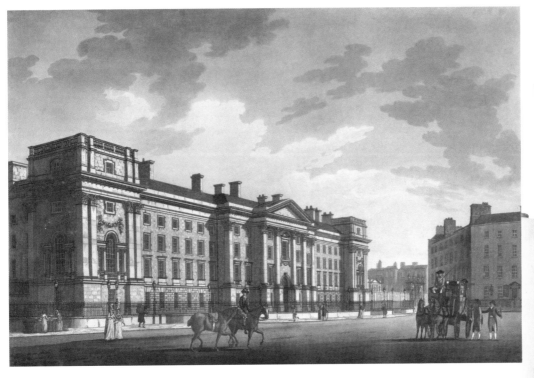

Engraving of Trinity College, Dublin from Malton's *View of Dublin*

RCPI

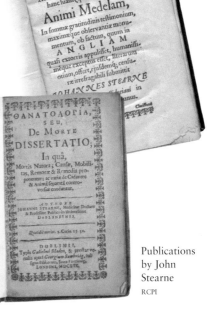

Publications by John Stearne

RCPI

It is thought that Stearne studied medicine at Cambridge, and graduated with a BA in 1642 and an MA in 1646, before the Civil War in England forced him to move again, this time to Royalist Oxford. Having survived thus far, he returned to Ireland in 1651 and was admitted to TCD as a Fellow for a probationary six months.[6]

Stearne not only survived but thrived in TCD, where he was confirmed in 1652 as Registrar and a Senior Fellow. In 1654, after some neat internal political footwork, he was able to establish a Fraternity of Physicians in Trinity Hall, a building that was situated just outside Trinity College. This was formerly a city prison, sited on what is now Dublin's Trinity Street.

Stearne had obtained the use of the premises from the Provost and Fellows of Trinity, and had indicated that if he were made President of the Hall, and allowed to live in part of it, he would have the building repaired at his own expense and would use it as a meeting place for physicians.

This began as a group who met to consider medical matters. It continued to meet, and in 1661, Trinity College approved a deed that Trinity Hall was, 'from henceforth forever converted to the sole and proper use and advantage of the study of medicine'. John Stearne became President of the Hall for life, and was allowed to have accommodation there. He was an influential polymath with his own large practice, and he developed the embryonic study of medicine in Trinity College.

He had also astutely survived the political turmoil of the times, and was clearly in the right place at the right time. In 1662 he was appointed the first Professor of Medicine at Trinity College, where he was also professor of Hebrew and Law. When King Charles II granted a Royal Charter on 28 June 1667 to establish a College of Physicians in Dublin, Stearne was confirmed as President for life.

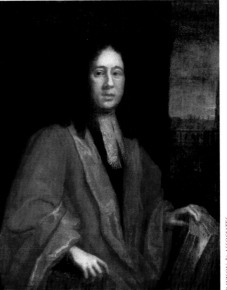

Portrait of John Stearne by Thomas Pooley

RCPI

OPPOSITE: The Fraternity of Physicians was based in Trinity Hall, a residence and teaching space for medical students situated just outside Trinity College. It was formerly a city prison, on what is now Dublin's Trinity Street, and is marked 'Bridewell' on this 1610 map.

RCPI

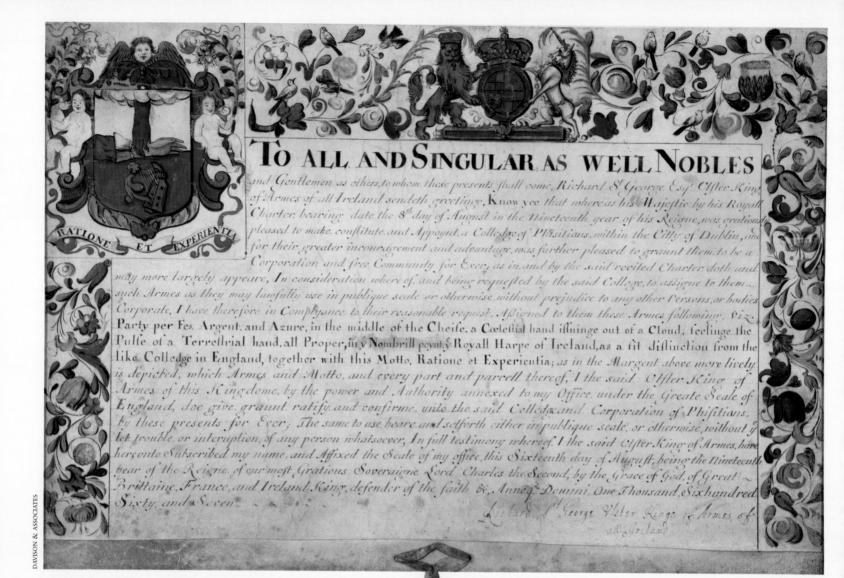

TO ALL AND SINGULAR, AS WELL NOBLES

and Gentlemen as others, to whom these presents shall come, Richard St George Esqr Ulster King of Armes of all Ireland sendeth greeting, Know yee that where as his Majestie by his Royall Charter, bearing date the 8th day of August in the Nineteenth year of his Reigne, was graciously pleased to make, constitute, and Appoynt, a Colledge of Phisitians within the City of Dublin, and for their greater incouragement and advantage, was farther pleased to graunt them to be a Corporation and free Community for Ever, as in and by the said recited Charter doth and may more largely appeare, In consideration where of, and being requested by the said College, to assigne to them such Armes as they may lawfully use in publique seale or otherwise, without prejudice to any other Persons, or bodies Corporate, I have therefore in Complyance to their reasonable request, Assigned to them these Armes following, Viz. Party per Fes. Argent, and Azure, in the middle of the Cheife, a Cœlestial hand issuinge out of a Cloud, feeling the Pulse of a Terrestrial hand, all Proper, in ye Nombrill poynt, ye Royall Harpe of Ireland, as a fit distinction from the like Colledge in England, together with this Motto, Ratione et Experientia; as in the Margent above more lively is depicted, which Armes and Motto, and every part and parcell thereof, I the said Ulster King of Armes of this Kingdome, by the power and Authority annexed to my Office, under the Greate Seale of England, doe give, graunt, ratify, and confirme, unto the said Colledge and Corporation of Phisitians, by these presents for Ever; The same to use, beare and setforth either in publique seale, or otherwise, without ye let, trouble, or interuption, of any person whatsoever, In full testimony whereof, I the said Ulster King of Armes, have hereunto subscribed my name, and Affixed the Seale of my office, this Sixteenth day of August, being the Nineteenth year of the Reigne, of our most Gratious Soveraigne Lord Charles the Second, by the Grace of God, of Great Brittaine, France, and Ireland King, defender of the faith &c, Annoq: Domini One Thousand, Sixhundred Sixty, and Seven

Richard St George Ulster Kinge of Armes of all Ireland

Grant of Arms to the Royal College by the Ulster King of Arms, 16 August 1667

RCPI

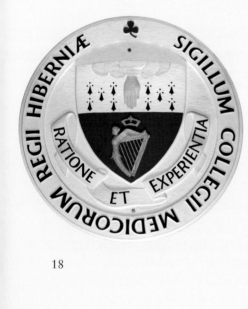

First Royal Charter

In an attempt to regulate medical practice, the 1667 Charter stipulated that no person might practise medicine within a seven-mile radius of Dublin, unless licensed by the College. It also named the first fourteen Fellows. Trinity College continued to allow the new College the use of Trinity Hall, and the Provosts and Fellows of Trinity had the power to elect succeeding Presidents of the new College of Physicians. Another important development took place in 1667, when the Ulster King of Arms made a Grant of Arms to the new College of Physicians. The Arms depict a celestial hand descending from a cloud to take the pulse of the temporal hand, over the Irish harp. The motto *Ratione et*

James Wolveridge was one of the early members of the Fraternity. Wolveridge's book was first published in 1670 in Ireland. The 1671 edition, published in London, is held by RCPI. It was one of the first books to be written in English on midwifery.

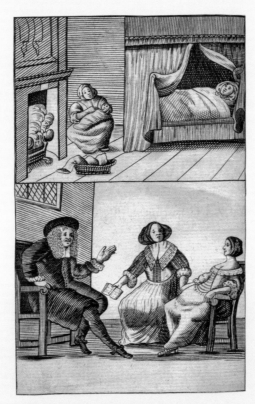

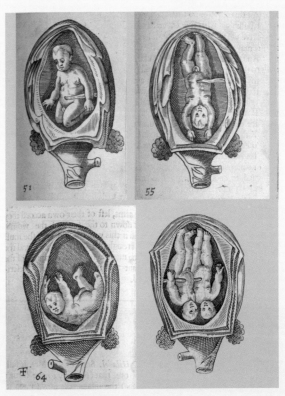

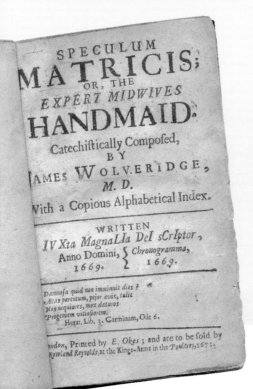

Illustrations from *The Expert Midwives Handmaid*, by James Wolveridge, 1671.
TOP: The nursemaid is shown with the baby and the mother is resting in bed.
BOTTOM: The physician is in discussion with the midwife and pregnant woman.
RCPI

Various positions of the baby in the womb from Wolveridge's book on midwifery
RCPI

Experientia (Reason and Experience) was also granted, and a version of the Arms remains in use today.

Unfortunately, there is no record of minutes for the Fraternity or for the early years of the College. However, there still exists a handsomely-bound book which was presented to 'The Fraternity of Trinity Hall on July 14, 1664 by a Thomas D'Olin, Gentleman'.

It was known in the College as 'D'Olins Book', and was meant for recording the Minutes. However, it remained empty for a decade, until 1674, and was then used to keep accounts. There are little or no other records of the early years of the College, apart from another account book dating from 1672, and which was also sparsely used.[7]

Unfortunately the story of the College's founder and first President, Dr John Stearne, came to an untimely end in November 1669, two years after he became President. He was only 45.

He had prior knowledge of his impending demise, and in his Will, which was written four days before his death, he requested that his body be interred in the Chapel of Trinity College. His wish was granted, and a memorial was erected on the north side of the Great Altar.

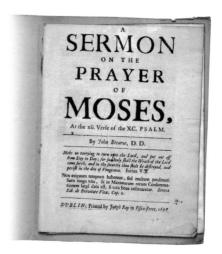

Title page of a publication, 1695 by John Stearne, Dean of St Patrick's Cathedral, Dublin and son of the College President.
RCPI

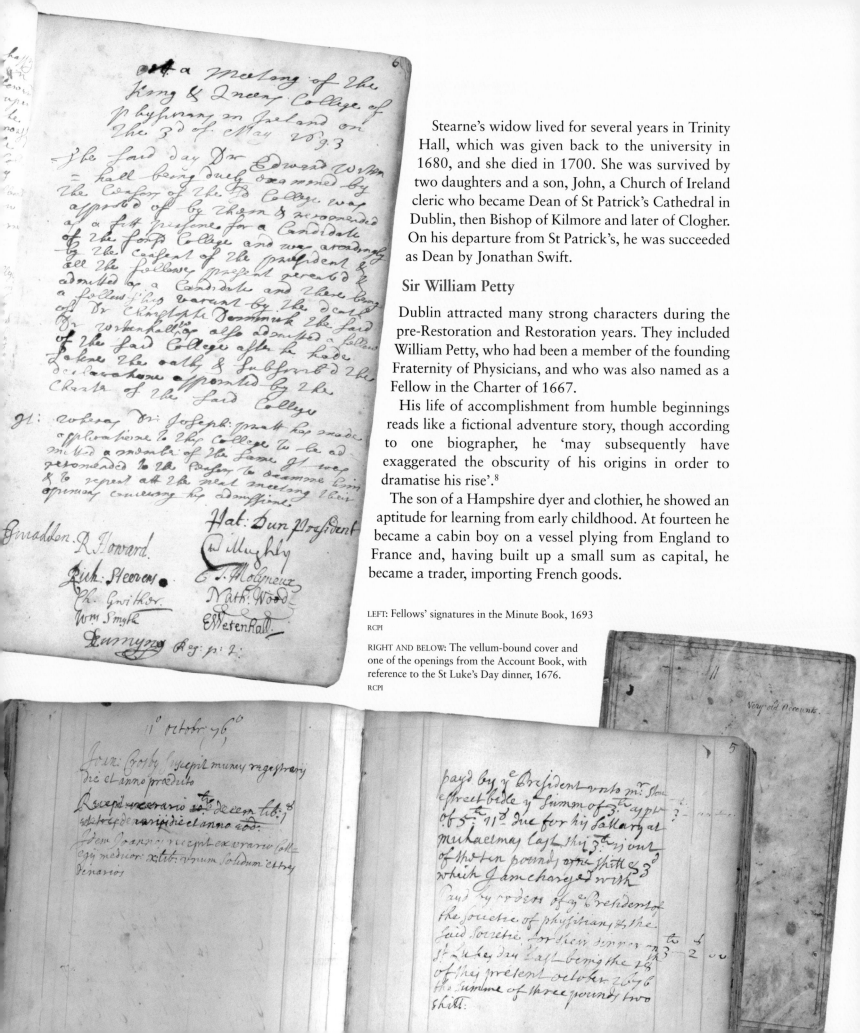

Stearne's widow lived for several years in Trinity Hall, which was given back to the university in 1680, and she died in 1700. She was survived by two daughters and a son, John, a Church of Ireland cleric who became Dean of St Patrick's Cathedral in Dublin, then Bishop of Kilmore and later of Clogher. On his departure from St Patrick's, he was succeeded as Dean by Jonathan Swift.

Sir William Petty

Dublin attracted many strong characters during the pre-Restoration and Restoration years. They included William Petty, who had been a member of the founding Fraternity of Physicians, and who was also named as a Fellow in the Charter of 1667.

His life of accomplishment from humble beginnings reads like a fictional adventure story, though according to one biographer, he 'may subsequently have exaggerated the obscurity of his origins in order to dramatise his rise'.[8]

The son of a Hampshire dyer and clothier, he showed an aptitude for learning from early childhood. At fourteen he became a cabin boy on a vessel plying from England to France and, having built up a small sum as capital, he became a trader, importing French goods.

LEFT: Fellows' signatures in the Minute Book, 1693
RCPI

RIGHT AND BELOW: The vellum-bound cover and one of the openings from the Account Book, with reference to the St Luke's Day dinner, 1676.
RCPI

After a broken leg curtailed his activities, Petty settled in Normandy where he developed his education. In an autobiography attached to his Will, he boasted that by the age of 15, he had a good knowledge of Latin, Greek, French, mathematics, geometry, astronomy and navigation.

From 1638–9 Petty was in the Royal Navy, and he retained a lifelong interest in shipping. He then furthered his education in Holland and France, and in 1646 he went to Brasenose College Oxford, where he received an MD four years later, and shortly afterwards became Vice Principal of the College. However, one biographer claims:

> As the university was purged of Royalists, Petty, pliant in both his political and religious principles, was elected into a Fellowship at Brasenose and in 1651 elected Professor of Anatomy.[9]

In 1650 he was admitted to the London College of Physicians, where he attracted widespread attention by reviving a young woman named Ann Green, who had been hanged for allegedly killing her illegitimate new born child.

She was described as 'being about twenty-two years of age, of middle stature, strong, fleshie and of an indifferent good feature'. She was declared dead by the local Sheriff, but when her body was brought to the dissecting rooms, William Petty, and a colleague named Willis, noticed signs of life.

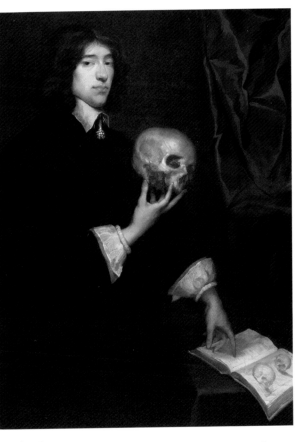

Sir William Petty, portrait by Isaac Fuller and, below, an account of his life.
NATIONAL PORTRAIT GALLERY LONDON

They speedily revived her with cordials and massage, warming her near-dead body by putting her in bed with another woman. In a story which would attract major headlines today from modern media, Ann Green was restored to health.

She lived for another fifteen years. There was also a happier footnote to her story. Petty and Willis not only obtained a pardon for her from the legal authorities, but also made a small collection to provide her with a dowry, and she married a man by whom she had several children.

In 1652 Petty came to Ireland as a physician with the Army. He was well-paid, and he had time to apply his many talents to help address the then ruinous state of the country. After extensive research he concluded that due to war, illness, famine and banishment, the population of Ireland had fallen from 1,466,000 in 1641 to 850,000 in 1652.

The remarkable Petty also showed an ability to balance the books in the provision of medicine for the Army, military hospitals, garrisons and other headquarters, and for a fee of £120 he saved the Government around £500 per annum. Such a person would be an invaluable Minister in the governments of the United Kingdom and Ireland today!

RCPI

In addition to his many other claims to fame, Petty mapped out and surveyed 22 counties in Ireland to help sort out the confusion over dividing land between former Cromwellian troops, as a means of paying arrears due to them. Hitherto this had been impossible because no accurate survey had existed. Petty carried out this huge task between December 1654 and March 1656. It was, and is, popularly known as 'the Down Survey', because it was the first to be set down in maps, and made Petty a personal net profit of £9,000 – a huge sum in those days.

Petty was politically astute and since 1655 he had built up a good relationship with Cromwell's son Henry, Major-General of the Forces in Ireland, who would employ him as his secretary. In 1659 he was elected to Westminster for the Kinsale and Bandon boroughs, and also West Looe in Cornwall. He chose the latter. Two years later however, he took his seat in the Irish House of Commons.

From 1659 he divided his time between Dublin and London, and was knighted in 1662. He had a huge range of interests, and was a founding member of the Royal Society of London and the Dublin Philosophical Society, of which he was the first President.

Following the Cromwellian land settlement, Petty became a rich landlord and owned some 18,000 acres in five Irish counties, which brought him an annual rental of £5,000–£6,000. Sir William also owned property in London and latterly lived in Piccadilly, where he died in 1687 from gangrene of the foot.

Even this brief outline of Petty's life and career provides an indication of the calibre of some of the men who helped to develop the Fraternity and later, the Royal College of Physicians of Ireland.

Trace map from the Down Survey of part of Sir Patrick Dun's Estate

'This trace (for so much) agreeth with the map of the Down Survey, taken in the parish of Fenogh, Barony of the Upperthird & County of Waterford, remaining on Record, in the office of His Majesty Surveyor General of Lands. Dublin Castle, 21st of Decem. 1751. Gab. Stokes Dep.y. Surv.r. Gen.l.'
RCPI

Scant Records

As noted earlier, there were scant records of the early days of the College, and after Stearne's death in November 1669 it seems that some three years elapsed before notice was given by Dr Margetson and Dr Howard that a new President might be elected. The Provost and Senior Fellows duly met and elected Abraham Yarner, who had come to Ireland in 1641 as an officer in the Lord Lieutenant's horse troop. He later became a Captain, and later Muster-Master General in Ireland. His career in Ireland was most successful, and in 1650 he became a Freeman of Dublin. Yarner, like Petty, had come to Ireland as a soldier-physician and

Narcissus Marsh, Provost of Trinity College, along with Petty, became one of the first members of the Dublin Philosophical Society. He contributed an early paper to that Society, called 'An Introductory Essay on the Doctrine of Sounds, Containing some Proposals for the Improvement of Accousticks', in which he apparently was the first to use the word 'microphone'.
Along with Marsh, William Molyneux, Patrick Dun, Allen Mullen and William Petty were founding members of the Dublin Philosophical Society.
MARSH'S LIBRARY, DUBLIN

stayed to make a significant contribution to the country, as well as greatly furthering his own career. In 1670 he received a knighthood.

The ubiquitous William Petty continued to attract attention, and he was asked by the Lord Lieutenant, the Duke of Ormonde to join with the new President in an inquiry into the alleged healing powers of a Dublin priest Father Finachty. Finachty had attracted a large following among Catholics and many Protestants over a wide area, with thousands of people following him

> ... even through bogs, woods, mountains and rocks, and desert places, whithersoever the people heard him, to have fled from the persecution of Cromwell's troops or governors.[10]

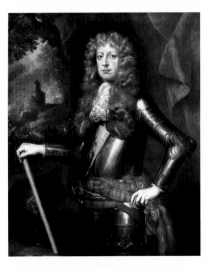

Portrait of James Butler, 1st Duke of Ormonde, by William Wissing. The Duke went into exile, with Charles II guaranteeing him favour with the monarchy after the Restoration.
NATIONAL PORTRAIT GALLERY, LONDON

However he was suspected of using exorcism, and he fell foul of the Catholic Church of the day. The Duke of Ormonde agreed to the request that Finachty should be asked to give a public demonstration of his healing powers, and Petty and Yarner were to select a wide range of people seeking help and willing to participate in the demonstration.

Yarner was not readily available, so Petty visited the priest to make his own assessment. Petty was shortsighted but not shortsighted enough to allow Finachty to continue his practices without some tangible evidence of his healing powers.

Accordingly Petty made a bargain with the priest, and told Finachty that if he cured him of his shortsightedness, he would attribute the healing to the work of God. The priest duly prayed for his distinguished patient, and it seems initially as if Petty's sight had improved, when he read the Bible which had thoughtfully been supplied by Fr Finachty.

However Petty soon discovered that his sight had not improved in any lasting way, even with a second attempt at a cure. The priest had failed to impress his eminent inquisitor, and rather than face the official trial ordered by the Lord Lieutenant, he wisely ceased his healing practices and discreetly disappeared into anonymity.

This intriguing episode must have been just one of many similar encounters throughout Ireland, as the physicians of the day tried to bring some discipline to an often chaotic spectrum of home cures, faith healings, the application of the wisdom of old wives' tales and other means of trying to help people in sickness and distress.

Unfortunately, one of the major problems for such legitimate physicians was the acute shortage of adequate medical facilities. William Petty, who was a philosopher and visionary in his own right, bemoaned the shortage of hospitals:

> ... for sick people, rich as well as poor, so instituted and fitted as to encourage all sick persons to resort unto them – every sort of such hospitals to differ only in splendour, but not at all in the sufficiency for the means and remedy of the patients' health.[11]

Petty argued that within such hospitals, medical students would learn more in one year, than in years in the outside world. Some of these thoughtful comments about hospital care from a distinguished commentator of centuries ago have a strikingly modern ring to them.[12]

Post-Restoration Development

The post-Restoration decades, during which the College was consolidating itself, brought with them a welcome period of relative political stability, and also prosperity. In 1663 and 1667 the Parliament at Westminster passed Cattle Acts which forbade the export of live animals from Ireland, in order to protect the English home market. However while this was economically damaging to Ireland, which had exported huge numbers to England, the loss was offset by a buoyant trade in Irish butter, which was particularly popular in France and which raised good prices in Holland.

On the social side, there were many fascinating comments from the new English settlers about the native Irish, including these remarks in one anonymous letter sent from the Curragh in 1683:

> The men are hardy, laborious and industrious, of healthful bodies and constitutions, able and enured to bear labour, and live to a great age, generally to seventy and eighty
>
> Their women [are] generally inclined to corpulency and thick-legged, which is occasioned by their loose garments, flat pumps and brogues, using little or no action or exercises, in or without their houses, having easy labour and being good nurses but bad housewives, not being used to any sort of manual labour except spinning, which, by reason of the suppleness of their fingers, they perform well.
>
> They are great admirers of music, yet their own songs are doleful lamentations as those of a conquered people, or as Jews in bondage or captivity. [12]

The post-Restoration stability and prosperity also helped the physical expansion of Dublin beyond its medieval limits. This era witnessed the development of

'The annexed view of the City of Dublin from an eminence in the Phoenix Park, by the draw-bridge of the Magazine. The park belongs to the Crown and contains one thousand and eighty Irish acres. On the north side of the river Liffey the dome of the Four Courts, the cupola of the Custom-house and the steeple of St Michan's Church can be seen. On the south side the Tower of Christ Church, the steeple of St Werburgh's Church and both St Catherine's and St Patrick's Cathedral are in view. At the bottom of the valley Steevens' Hospital for the relief and maintenance of curable poor persons.'

Notes to the plate and engraving from Malton's *View of Dublin*

RCPI

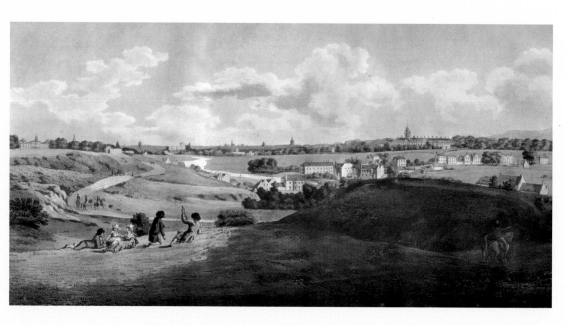

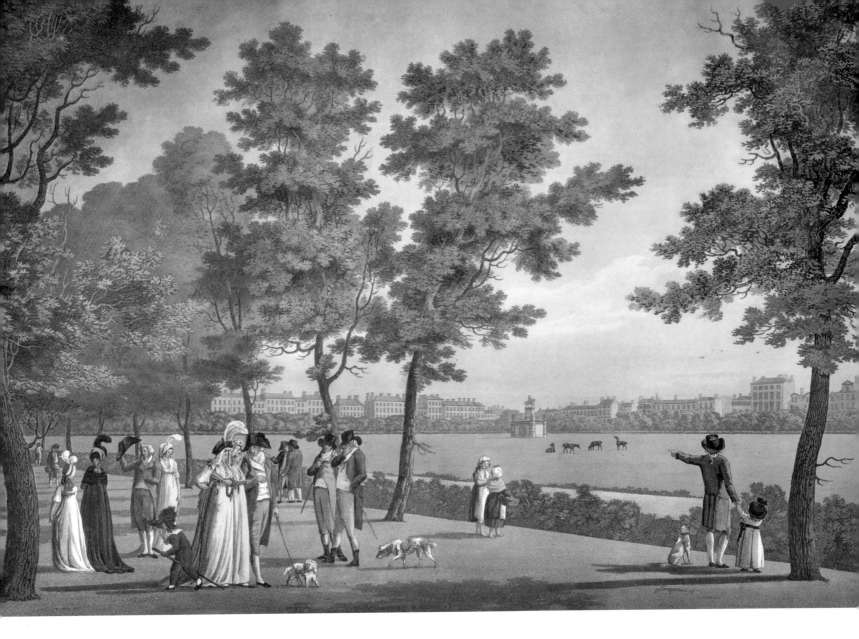

what later became the Phoenix Park, and in 1680 the laying of the cornerstone of the Royal Hospital of King Charles II at Kilmainham, which was initially intended for the treatment of injured soldiers who were no longer fit for service. It was completed in 1684, at a cost of £23,559 16s 11d.[13]

St Stephen's Green, which remains one of the jewels of central Dublin, was laid out, and plans were made for the development of Dublin port, and for the lease of land to the north of the Liffey, where citizens of means were encouraged to create quays 'for the advantage, ornament, and beauty of the city'.

These positive developments were well summarised by William Molyneux in a letter dated, 12 April 1684 to his brother Thomas, who was studying in Leiden and who later became a distinguished Fellow and President of the College:

> ... we are come to fine things here in Dublin, and you would wonder how our city increased sensibly in fair buildings. Great trade, and splendour in all things – in furniture, coaches, civility, housekeeping, etc.

St Stephen's Green was a popular place for Dublin society to meet. The notes to the plate remark that the Green was named after a church dedicated to St Stephen, which can be found on the map of 1610 but no longer exists.
From Malton's *View of Dublin*
RCPI

25

OPPOSITE: Text of the 1667 Charter copied into Dun's book and inset, portrait of Charles II.
RCPI

Despite this 'splendour', there was still widespread poverty and disease in the heart of the city and elsewhere, and the furtherance of a regulatory body for medicine, like the recently established Fraternity of Physicians, remained an urgent priority to help bring more discipline into a significantly unregulated situation.

The initial establishment of the College in 1654 and the grant of the Royal Charter over a decade later had been a long process. An influx of persons with medical expertise from England, some with European training, and from the European continent, also had important consequences for the improvement of medicine in Ireland. As one observer has noted:

> ... for the first time, in the early 1650s, Dublin possessed a critical mass of accomplished physicians, some with ties to the Royal College of Physicians in London, as well as to Oxford and Cambridge Universities.

A new sense of fraternity was now in evidence:

> ... bonds of professional affinity among professional physicians continued to transcend religious, political, and even cultural interests and identities ... Within just a few years, John Stearne advanced the process of giving that professional fraternalism formal, institutional expression in the foundation of the Royal College of Physicians in Dublin in 1654, and set the process of professionalism of Irish medicine onto a new plane.[14]

Another historian expertly summarises the vast changes in medicine and the Irish nation in those troublesome days as follows:

> ... between the Flight of the Earls in 1607 and the Battle of the Boyne in 1690, the form of Irish society was painfully broken and reset.
>
> By the end of the century the old Gaelic order had been definitively superseded by the new colonial power. As far as Irish medicine was concerned, this period certainly marked a fundamentally new start; the basis of the old order of carers – the old Gaelic medical families and the monastic hospitals – had been swept away by history, leaving a rump of variously qualified practitioners.
>
> The foundation of the Dublin Fraternity of Physicians, the precursors of today's Royal College of Physicians of Ireland, in 1654, can reasonably be seen as the very turning point of the tide.[15]

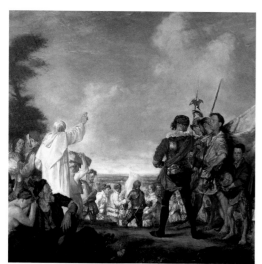

Detail from *The Flight of the Earls* by Thomas Ryan represented the exodus from Ireland of the cream of Gaelic society in 1607.
THOMAS RYAN

Dr John Stearne had made an important pioneering contribution to these historic developments, but the drive necessary to carry the work further was provided by another remarkable man, who was elected in 1677 as one of the College's fourteen Fellows. His name was Patrick Dun, and his life and legacy would prove to be of immense importance in the story of the College.

Carolus Secundus

Franciæ et Hiberniæ Rex, Fidei Defensor, et
nea pervenerint Salutem, Cum Regij Officij
hominum felicitatem omni ratione consulere,
indocti Artis Medicinæ Professores supplementur,
et instituentur, Ad Supremedic Collegium perpetuum, gravioris et doctorum
Medicinam publice exerceant in Civit: nra Dublin, in dicto Regn̄
et x Spatium Septem Miliarium, a dicta Civit undequaq3 versus.

Sciatis igitur quod nos de gratia nra speciali ac certa scientia
nris, Necnon de advisamento et consensu pdilecti et pquam dilec
Consiliarij nri Jacobi Ducis Ormondiæ Locum tenentis nri generalis
Gubernatoris, dicti Regni nri Hiberniæ ad juxta tenorem et effectum
Literarum, nostrarum manu nostra propria Signatarum, et sub Sig
apud Curiam nostram de Whitehall Vicessimo Octavo die Junij Anno
Septimo et nunc in Rotulis Curiæ nra Cancilariæ dicti Regni nri H

Dedimus, Confessimus, Constituimus et Ordinavimus quod
Medicinæ Doctor, Gulielmus Petty Miles, Edvardus Dynham,
Josephus Waterhouse, Gulielmus Currer, Robertus Waller, Thomas
Nathaniel Henshaw, Samuel Stillamore, Jeremiah Hall, Carolus
Johannes Unmusique, et Johannes Cusacke, omnes Medicinæ Docto
erunt vigore psentium, in re facto ad nomine unum Corpus corpora
et Communitas ppetua sive Collegium ppetuum per nomen Præsidentis et

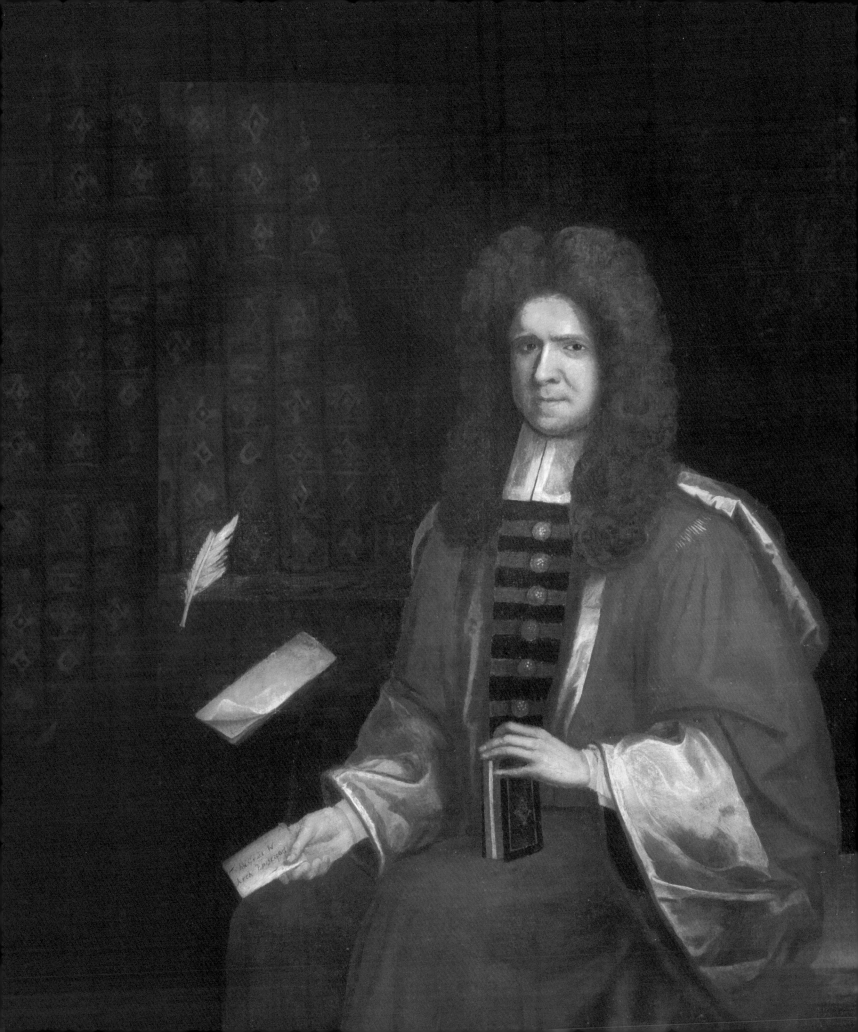

The Life and Times of Sir Patrick Dun

Patrick Dun, who was born in 1642 and died in 1713, was one of the most important figures in the history of the College. He was President for a record thirteen times and on his death, he left all his property in trust to the College.

The considerable income from Dun's estates was used to fund Professorships in Trinity College (despite his wishes that these should be established at the Royal College of Physicians), and also Sir Patrick Dun's Hospital in Dublin.

His life story was full of adventure and incident, and like Sir William Petty and several others, he demonstrated how a brilliant outsider could make his mark, and his fortune, in the troubled Ireland of the seventeenth and early eighteenth centuries, to the lasting benefit of the country.

Patrick was the third child of Charles Dun, a dyer and burgess of the city of Aberdeen. From the beginning he was well-placed to succeed in life, even though his great-grandmother had been burned as a witch.[1]

He was the grand-nephew and godson of Dr Patrick Dun, who was a benefactor of Aberdeen Grammar School, and the Principal and Medical Dean of the local Marischal College, where Dun studied Arts.

His further education was typical of the young high-flyers of his day. He studied in Valence and in Dauphine, France, and he later graduated in Medicine from Dublin University.

Patrick Dun had impeccable connections, and in 1677 he was awarded an MD *in absentia* from Oxford University, at the request of the then Chancellor, James Butler, Duke of Ormonde.[2]

A year or so earlier, he had been appointed Physician to the State and to the Lord Lieutenant of Ireland, by the same James Butler who had helped with the award of an Oxford degree. Dun settled in Ireland where he established an extensive and lucrative practice.

He quickly made his mark in medical circles, and became a Fellow of the College just a year after his arrival in Dublin. There is a record of an address given by Dun to the College on 4 April 1677, and afterwards he was treated to hospitality at the Castle Tavern, at a cost of 10s 6d, which would have funded a considerable spread in those days.[3]

Sir Patrick Dun
by Thomas Pooley
RCPI

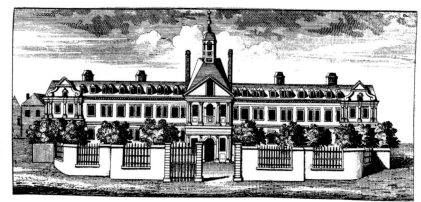

The west front of Trinity College, 1728 was later replaced by the present façade.
FROM BROOKING'S *THE CITY OF DUBLIN, 1728*

Prospering

While Dun prospered in his State duties and private practice, important developments were taking place at the College. In 1680, the physicians surrendered the use of Trinity Hall to Trinity College for a payment of £70, a very considerable sum in those days, amounting to the equivalent of £100,000 in today's terms.

It was also decided that the President of the College would be elected by the physicians themselves, who would then inform the TCD Provost and Senior Fellows of what had taken place. However there was one important clause which would create difficulties later on. They 'did oblige themselves to confirm the election of the President of the College of Physicians, provided the person elected were a Protestant of the Church of Ireland'.

In 1687 the College elected as President Dr John Crosby, a Catholic who not only had been a Fellow for some 13 years, but had acted as Treasurer from 1676–77.

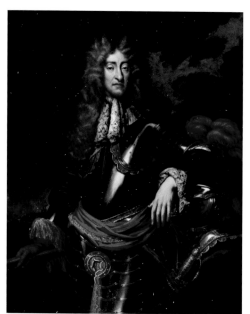

James II, whose daughter Mary married King William III
NATIONAL PORTRAIT GALLERY, LONDON

However this appointment was refused by TCD because he was a Catholic. This was strictly in accordance with the 1680 agreement. Trinity was clearly reluctant to accept a Catholic in the dangerous days when many feared a Catholic takeover by King James II .

Patrick Dun was elected President on June 24 1681, and he held the post continually until 1687. He was a leading figure at the College, and with his energy and drive, as well as his network of contacts, he was the ideal person to act as the public face of the Institution, while retaining great influence within the institution and within the profession as a whole.

Storm Clouds

However, with the succession to the throne of James II in 1685, following the death of Charles II, hugely important political and religious developments were casting a long shadow. The 25 years of Charles's reign had been relatively good for the Protestant population, but the elevation of the Catholic James boded ill for them, while Catholics, not surprisingly, looked toward better days in Ireland.

Some Catholic physicians persuaded the new King to consider the establishment of their own college in Kilkenny, but this proposal foundered in the stormy seas of contemporary politics and civil conflict.

Undoubtedly there was more trouble ahead, and in 1688 Dun decided to flee to England, with thousands of other influential Protestants who were fearful of their future in Ireland under James. Within a year, however, Dun returned to Ireland – this time as a physician to the invading army of the Protestant William III, who was literally carrying the battle to his Catholic father in-law, the hapless James II, on Irish soil. This was part of a pan-European war in which William, with other Protestant powers, as well the Pope, was ranged against the powerful Catholic Louis XIV of France. It was the last occasion in British history where two monarchs faced each other on the battlefield.

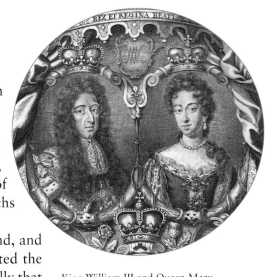

King William III and Queen Mary granted a new Royal Charter in 1692, by which the College was re-named 'The King and Queen's College of Physicians in Ireland'. The 1692 Charter, although heavily modified, is still the governing document of the RCPI today.

PHOTOGRAPH: DAVID SCOTT
GRAND ORANGE LODGE ARCHIVE

Much has been written elsewhere about the Williamite Wars in Ireland, and the victories at the Boyne, and decisively at Aughrim, which completed the Glorious Revolution. Indeed the memories of such victories, and especially that at the Boyne, remain alive today on the Unionist and Loyalist gable walls and the streets of the North, despite William's politically convenient alliance with the Pope.

Portrait of William III
RCPI

Patrick Dun, as one of William's leading physicians, served with him in the field, and on 27 July 1690 he was in the King's camp at Carrick-on-Suir. The previous night Waterford had surrendered, and the Army was marching to Clonmel, on the way to Limerick; subsequently the troops went into winter quarters.

By September Dun had arrived in Waterford, and wrote to his friend Dean William King that he was being relieved in the field by a

King William III

William III was no cardboard king, but in effect an astute monarch as well as a courageous soldier who led from the front – so much so that he was wounded in the shoulder by Jacobite artillery.

His wife Queen Mary was alarmed by news of his narrow escape. Prior to this she had written to him from London on 17 June 1690, shortly after he had landed with his troops in Carrickfergus.

She stated

> I cannot enough thank God for your being so well past the dangers of the sea. I beseech Him in His mercy still to preserve you so, and send us once more a happy meeting on earth. I long to hear from you how the air of Ireland agrees with you, for I must own, I am not without my fears for that, loving you so entirely as I do, and shall till death.

In her letter of 16 July, some days after the Battle of the Boyne, she was further alarmed at the news of her husband's injury:

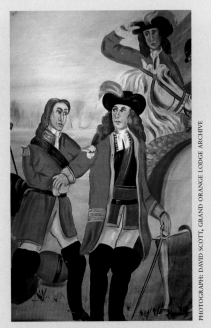

Detail from a banner illustrated with an image of William wounded at the Battle of the Boyne.

PHOTOGRAPH: DAVID SCOTT, GRAND ORANGE LODGE ARCHIVE

> I can never give God thanks enough as I live, for your preservation: I hope in His mercy that this is a sign he preserves you to finish the work he has begun by you: but I hope it may be a warning to you, to let you see you are exposed to as many accidents as others.[4]

William and Mary, who were cousins, had an arranged marriage as part of Charles II's European foreign policy. Mary was 12 years younger than William, and reportedly she had initially found him repulsive. However, as the above letters show, she grew to love him deeply, despite his long affair with one of her ladies-in-waiting, Elizabeth Villiers.

Notwithstanding Mary's obvious affection for William, he remained aloof from her, but he also depended on her for support, and after her death from smallpox in 1694, he grieved for her deeply. William, who was passionately fond of horses, died in 1702 following complications after a riding accident.

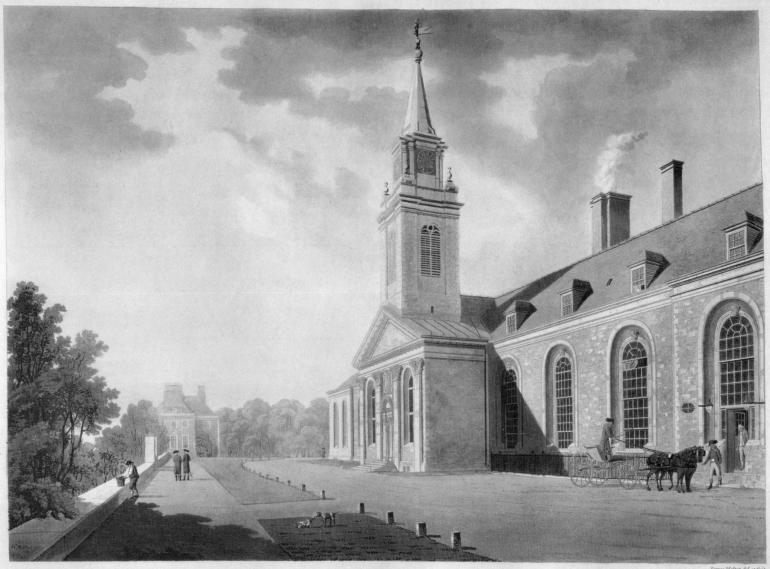

OLD SOLDIERS HOSPITAL, KILMAINHAM, DUBLIN.

London Pub.d by Ja.s Malton & G.Cowen Dublin. Feb.y 1794.

Engraving of the Old Soldiers'
Hospital, Kilmainham, from Malton's
View of Dublin
RCPI

Dr Le Can from the Royal Hospital in Kilmainham, where Dun was to take up duty as physician. Kilmainham, which had been completed only six years earlier, was also used as a base for treating war casualties, as an Irish version of the Chelsea Hospital in London.

Shortage of Supplies

Dun was also responsible for the reception of medical supplies for the army surgeons, and for despatching these to the various field camps in Ireland. His previous time in the field had given him experience of the rigours of combat, and when the War Secretary, George Clark was with General Ginkel near Athlone in 1691, Patrick Dun sent him:

> …a box containing two dozen bottles of the best claret I could get in Dublin, and two dozen bottles of Chester ale. At the same time I sent a lesser box, in which there is a dozen-and-a-half-potted chickens in an earthen pot; and

in another pot, four green geese. This is the best physic I advise you to take;
I hope it will not be as nauseous or disagreeable to your stomach – a little of
it upon a march.[5]

This may have been merely a ploy to impress the War Secretary, or perhaps an
example of the natural generosity of Patrick Dun, who knew how to keep in
with the right people. He certainly needed help at Kilmainham, where every
day he visited the sick and wounded, and saw their needs at first hand.
Sometimes the ferocity of ancient battles is overlooked by modern readers, but
Dun's correspondence underlines the suffering of human beings caught up in
the savagery, uncertainty and turbulence of war.

On 1 August, Patrick Dun wrote to the War Secretary, thanking him for his
financial contribution,

> … which came very seasonably to the relief of many in the Hospital who
> had spent all their money and lived upon credit. We all return to you our
> most humble and thankful acknowledgement for your favour and
> expedition.

However, Dun pulled no punches and described the
problems in Kilmainham. He stated:

> Last week the Hospital was so full of sick and
> wounded that we could not get beds for them. All the
> rooms, the great hall, most of the garrets, and second
> gallery were full … We have either spent in the
> Hospital, or sent to the marching hospital, all we had
> of some sorts of drugs, and have present use for some
> more. We are also daily wanting some utensils; about
> ten pounds sterling will suffice for our present
> necessity.

The number of casualties was overwhelming, and
Dun had to bring in extra temporary staff to cope.
They included, 'several supernumerary chirurgeons
and apothecary's mates, nurses, washers and porters …' The tale of woe
continued:

The Battle on the Bridge of Athlone,
by WC Mills
Williamite soldiers and Jacobites
fighting on the bridge, July 1691.
NATIONAL LIBRARY OF IRELAND

> Sir, we have at present in the Hospital 959 sick and wounded, most
> wounded. We have not a master chirurgeon with us.[6]

By the middle of the month there were over 1,000 wounded in the Hospital
and, 'about 116 lodged in Dublin for want of bedding'.[6]

Unfortunately, the War Secretary had sent insufficient money to cope with
the crisis, and the situation was so bad that Dun gallantly asked that his wages
be deferred in order to provide money for urgent hospital supplies. He was fully
confident that he would be reimbursed, but sadly after a lifetime of pursuit of
his just claim, and despite an agreement by Parliament to pay his arrears, he –
and his widow – ultimately received no recompense. This was not the first, or

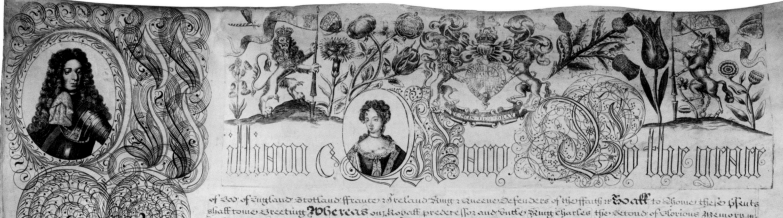

the last, example of a noble public servant receiving ignoble treatment by the State.

Following the decisive victory of the Williamite Army at Aughrim in 1691, peace was finally restored, and the business of everyday life in Ireland began to resume its normal pattern once again. This included the work of the College, of which Dun had been elected President on St Luke's Day in 1690.

New Royal Charter

Using his considerable influence, Dun set about seeking a new Royal Charter which would extend the remit of the College to all of Ireland. The College addressed a petition to the Lord Lieutenant Viscount Sidney, a personal friend of King William III, and the fact that Dun had served with the Monarch as one of his leading physicians in the field during July 1690 would have been a considerable advantage.

The doctors stated that the Charter of 1667 from King Charles II had been found:

… insufficient to compass that noble design, partly for want of power to correct and reform some abuses that have since crept in, or have been lately discovered, and partly because the power and jurisdiction granted by said Charter did not extend farther than 7 miles from the city of Dublin, so that your petitioners could not reform the inconveniences and abuses in the rest of the Kingdom, whereby the number of unskilful and illiterate practisers of physic had increased.[7]

Indubitably the situation had become worse rather than better since 1667, and a more effective Charter was needed. This was signed on 29 September 1692 by Queen Mary, who – as the eldest child of King James II – held the executive power, and not by King William himself.

The new Charter became effective on 15 December 1692, and despite significant modifications since then, it remains the governing document under which the College operates today. Its somewhat long-winded title 'The King and Queen's College of Physicians in Ireland', was changed in the nineteenth century.

Under the 1667 Royal Charter, there had been no religious discrimination, and several of the Fellows were Catholics. However the 1692 Charter imposed a religious bar, and the Fellows had to take an oath against Transubstantiation. Only seven men were named for the fourteen Fellowships available, these 'being the only Protestant surviving Fellows of the said late College'.

However the College was politely 'invited', to nominate more Fellows, and they produced seven more candidates, all Protestants. This discrimination against Catholics was partly due to a lingering fear of a Jacobite Restoration, and Archbishop King told an English friend, as late as 1712, that until the fear of the Pretender's return had been removed, or abated, the people would 'have no ears for nothing else'.

New President

Dun was named as the new President, and future Presidents were to be elected by the College, without approval from Trinity. Once again Dun's generosity was apparent. He had loaned over £31 to help pay for the £137 cost of obtaining the new Charter, and by the time all the expenses were covered, the College was left with just over £12.[8]

One of the most significant stipulations of the Charter was that any person wishing to practise medicine had to be examined by the College President and appointed Censors, except for graduates of Oxford, Cambridge or Trinity.

The College was also given jurisdiction over apothecaries and midwives, but one of the major challenges, as before, was in making this effective.

The 1692 Royal Charter imposed a religious bar on Catholics, as the Fellows of the College had to take an oath against Transubstantiation. The Roll of Fellows from 1692, showing the three oaths to be taken. RCPI

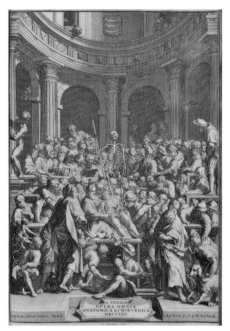

Illustration of the title page from Andreas Vesalius' *De humani corporis fabrica libri septem*, published in 1543. Note the dog and monkey, often used for the study of anatomy.
RCPI

'The Anatomy Lesson of Dr Nicolaes Tulp', 1632
Dr Tulp is pictured explaining the musculature of the arm to fellow medical professionals.
Rembrandt van Rijn
MAURITSHUIS MUSEUM IN THE HAGUE

The regulations needed the backing of the law, and attempts were made in 1693 and 1695 to pass the necessary legislation. However the apothecaries and surgeons had no regard for the new Charter or for this relatively 'upstart' College. Like physicians, they had been around for a long time, they had many influential contacts, and they proved to be formidable lobbyists. Their opposition was so strong that a Bill which came to the Irish House of Commons in 1695 was dropped.

Meanwhile an agreement was reached between the College and Trinity for the examination of candidates for a degree in medicine, but it was not until early in the next century that the University opened its own Medical School.

Regardless, the first meeting of the new College was held on 7 January 1693, less than a month after the Charter was granted, and for more than 100 years the meetings were held in the various Presidents' houses, until a special room was set aside in Sir Patrick Dun's Hospital, which was finally opened in the early part of the nineteenth century.

Dissections and other grisly tales

One of the important clauses of the 1692 Charter was the provision for the College to annually obtain for dissection the bodies of six criminals who had been executed, provided that subsequently their remains were decently buried at the expense of the President and the Fellows.

One pressing concern for the seventeenth-century Irish physicians was the advancement of the study of anatomy, and an important figure in promoting this was Sir William Petty. He had retained his lifelong interest in anatomy, and

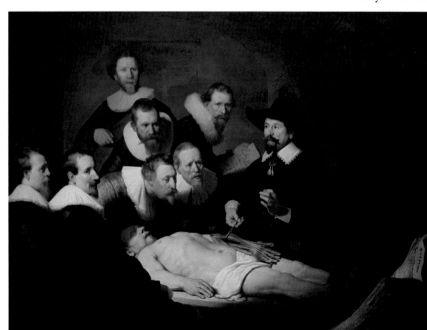

had given a talk to the College on this subject as early as 1672. The surviving records provide fascinating details of an anatomical dissection of a recently executed criminal in 1676. A warrant for the body was obtained at a cost of £1 3s, and soldiers were employed to protect the body from any attempt at a retrieval by friends or relatives. The soldiers were paid 13s 6d, plus 3s 10d to buy drink. Then, to pay for the burial after dissection – which the law required – a coffin was purchased for 4s 6d.

Prior to this, however, the College had to provide a dissecting table costing 6 shillings, and a cutler was paid 5s 5d for cleaning the dissecting instruments. Meanwhile the sexton of the nearby St Andrew's Church was paid 6d for keeping a dog which was

An engraving of the mature Sir William Petty.
He considered anatomy, just like his contemporaries, to be the basis of genuine progress in medical knowledge; 'The real art of medicine cannot be older than anatomy'.[9]
RCPI

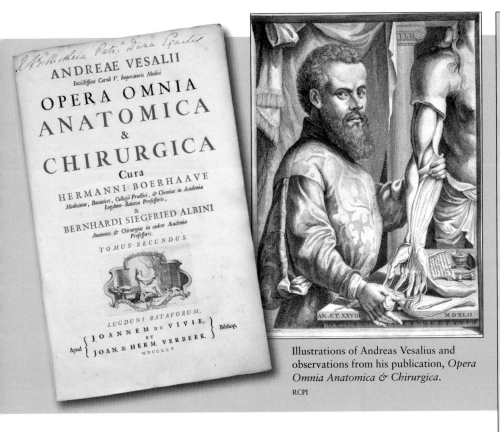

Illustrations of Andreas Vesalius and observations from his publication, *Opera Omnia Anatomica & Chirurgica*.
RCPI

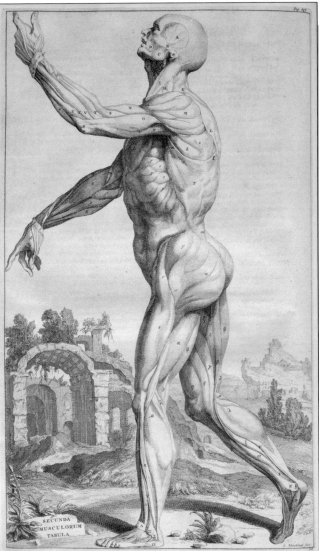

Vesalius established a new approach to anatomy in the sixteenth century, basing his methodology on first hand observation at dissections.
RCPI

also used as part of the research, in the days when animals – usually a monkey or a dog – were used for the study of comparative anatomy.[10]

Until the nineteenth century the term 'dissection' also covered what is now known as a post–mortem, and the earliest reference to this in Ireland was an account of 'extraordinary charges' to the Lord-Deputy Sir William Fitzwilliam in the last decade of the sixteenth century. These included a fee of 10 shillings paid to a surgeon, William Kellye, 'for opening the corpse of Anthony Grenehan, deceased'.

As well as this passing reference, the earliest known surviving report of a post-mortem in Ireland was that performed on the remains of a Lady Dorcas Lane, who died in July 1671 from a case, most likely, of 'uterine carcinoma'. Her husband, Sir George Lane, who was well-placed in the corridors of power, had been a private secretary to Charles II prior to the Restoration and to the Lord-Lieutenant, the Duke of Ormonde after the Restoration.

In the 1684 minutes of the Dublin Philosophical Society which was established in 1683 with Petty its first President, there was an account published of a dissection made by a surgeon named Patterson on an executed criminal. His body had been procured by Patrick Dun, who publicly and somewhat controversially advocated the practice of anatomy.[11] Dun was also a leading member of the Dublin Philosophical Society. It had connections with the Royal Society in London and the Philosophical Society of Oxford University, as well as close links with Trinity and with the Royal College of Physicians of Ireland.

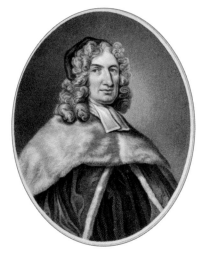
Archbishop William King
ST COLUMB'S CATHEDRAL, DERRY

Its members included Archbishop King, Dean Jonathan Swift, and other leading figures of the day. In all, there were ten doctors, which amounted to a quarter of the membership, and a significant number of the papers presented and discussed had to do with medical matters.

The Society's objective was to encourage research, and it published papers which helped to promote Dublin in international scientific circles. However, it had a relatively short existence partly due to the tumultuous political developments of the period, and ceased to meet early in the eighteenth century. However, it ultimately helped to inspire the foundation of the Dublin Society in 1731 (which became the Royal Dublin Society in 1820), and the Royal Irish Academy.

The Elephant Man

Allen Mullen, elected in 1684 as a Fellow of the Royal College of Physicians, was an outstanding scientist and physician in seventeenth-century Ireland. The son of a Patrick Mullen of Ballyculter, Co Down, he graduated from Trinity College with an MB in 1679 and an MD in 1684. Mullen was a leading member of the Dublin Philosophical Society, and he contributed over half of the papers read at its meetings.

These included accounts of a wide range of topics, including dissections, vivisections and injections, as well as experiments on animals, including the respiration in a dog.[12]

Mullen had a lucrative medical practice among the gentry, and he was famed for curing gout 'for which he used a vegetable which may have been colchicum infused in brandy'.[13]

An expert anatomist, he also made his name by the dissection of an elephant which had accidentally died in a fire while on exhibition in Dublin. His colourful account of this episode was given to the Royal Society of London through William Petty, and is one of the earliest surviving accounts of the anatomy of an elephant. Another noted contribution to the Royal Society was on the eye of animals, and details of both papers were published in a book in 1682.

Mullen was also well-known for an experiment in trying to determine, through animal trials, the likely weight of blood in a

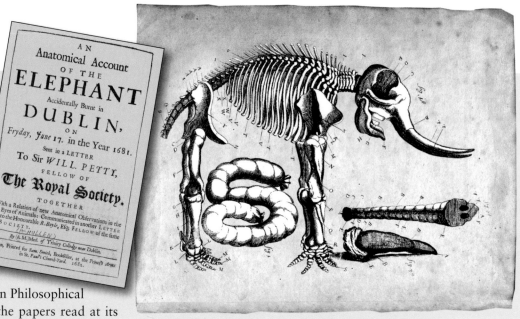
The title page of Allen Mullen's 'Anatomical Account of the Elephant' ..., with an illustration of the elephant's skeleton.
ROYAL COLLEGE OF SURGEONS IN IRELAND

human being, but his estimate was too low because he was unaware that some blood remains in a corpse after an alleged 'complete' drainage.

His personal life was dramatic, and he left Ireland in 1686 after a 'scandalous' love affair. He was keenly interested in the early work of Hans Sloane, another north of Ireland man, whose bequeathed collections would form the British Museum, London, in 1759. Mullen fitted in easily to the social and scientific life of contemporary London.

In 1690 he set off for the West Indies in the hope of making his fortune through the exploitation of valuable minerals. Sadly, however, he fell into over-zealous company in Barbados, drank too much, and developed a fever, from which he died. His early death at 37 was a major loss to the development of medicine in Ireland.

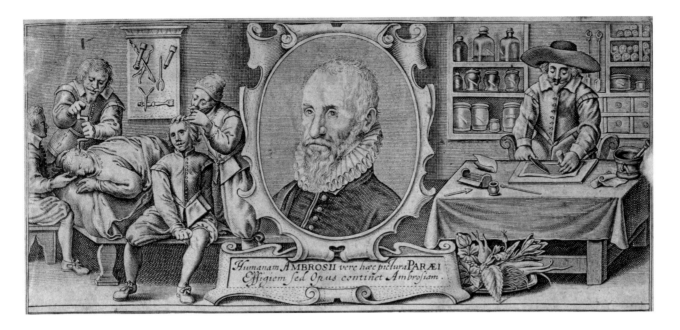

Detail from the title page of Ambroise Paré's *The Works of that famous Chirurgion Ambrose Parey. Translated out of Latin and compared with the French, 1649.*
Paré was a barber surgeon and a pioneer in surgical techniques and battlefield medicine especially in the treatment of wounds.
RCPI

The elephant in the room

The most striking account of a dissection was that of an elephant which had been accidentally burnt to death while on exhibition in Dublin. Dr Allen Mullen dissected it, working day and night in the warmth of a hot June, while soldiers kept a curious public at bay. Subsequently the canny owner of the elephant obtained the skeleton and did a roaring trade by exhibiting it, instead of the former animal.

In 1693, only a few months after the second Royal Charter was granted, the College obtained the body of an executed criminal, which was duly dissected, but not properly buried. A London bookseller, John Dunton, who visited Ireland in 1698, later wrote about a skeleton which was thought to have been that of the executed malefactor and which ended up in the library of Trinity.

Not all procedures went according to plan, and in 1699 the body of an executed criminal was rescued from the College by family and friends before a dissection could begin. There are continued references to anatomical dissections in 1707 and 1708. However, once the School of Physic was open at Trinity shortly afterwards, it was allowed obtain its own bodies for dissection and further warrants from the College were no longer necessary.

Reckless behaviour

By 1692 Patrick Dun's reputation was secure as President of the College. However, banana-skin slips by prominent figures were as common in the seventeenth century as they are today, and within a year Dun was being rightly criticised for his reckless public behaviour.

Early in 1693 he had an altercation with a College Censor and former College President, Dr Ralph Howard in York Street, Dublin, where both had just shared in a consultation with a patient. Suddenly Dun drew his sword and made for Howard who retreated with his back to a wall and called out for a policeman to come to his aid. Fortunately, a number of passers-by who had noticed what was happening, had pulled the senior doctors apart before any real damage was done. However, both men were left to face the wrath of the College and, even worse, the ridicule of the public.

It appears that Dun had suspected Howard of trying to usurp him as State Physician, an influential post he had held for the previous 17 years. The College authorities were furious, and censured both men. According to a record of March 1693:

> There having happened an unhappy difference betwixt Dr Dun, our present President and Dr Howard, one of our present Censors, upon the College interposing, they have both unanimously and without reserve submitted to the decision and determination of the College, and the censure of the College being read to them, they accordingly allowed of and complied with it, and are now, in presence of the College, returned to their former friendship.[14]

Behind the flowery language there was the stark message to both men: 'Make it up to one another-or else!'. Dun by then was aged 51, and he should have had more sense, even if his early experience as a soldier-physician with King William on the battlefield had got the better of him.

Not surprisingly, the satirists, had a field day. *An Epigram on the Late York Street Duel* stated:

> O valiant doctors! Will you now give o're?
> Have you so many killed, you'll kill no more?
> Yet (by long practice being cruel grown)
> As other lives, will you destroy your own
> A favour this is, for by doing this,
> You damn yourselves, lest you should murder us.

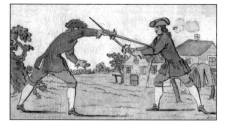

Illustration of a typical seventeenth century duel

This is a record of the Royal College of Physicians' pained reference to the famous 'duel' in March, 1693, between two of its most distinguished figures, Sir Patrick Dun and Dr Ralph Howard.

RCPI

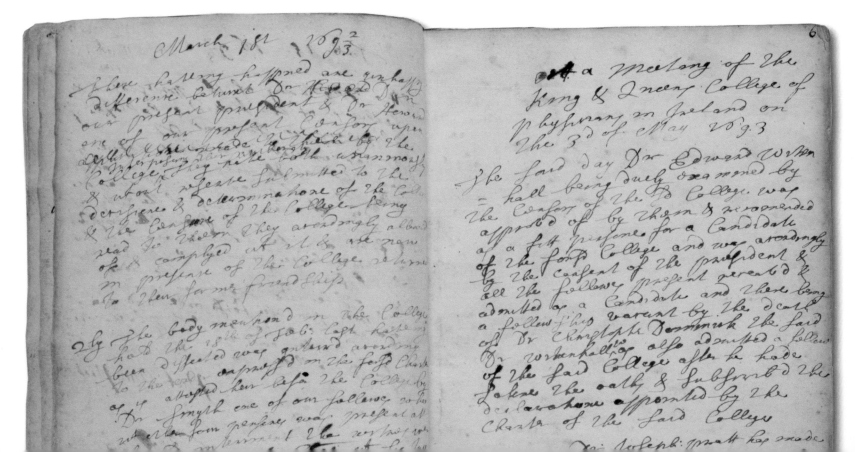

A poem titled *The Duel between two old Physicians* and attributed to Jonathan Swift, added to the amusement:

> As for the motives most men doubt,
> Why these two doctors did fall out,
> Some say it was Ambition;
> And thus one did undermine
> The other's credit, with design
> To be the State's Physician.

This is certainly not the best writing that Swift ever produced, but he had made his point. Then, as now, the news agenda moved on, and Dun gradually regained his mantle of prestige and authority.

Business as Usual

The daily business of the College continued, and on 3 May 1693 Dr Edward Wetenhall was admitted as a Fellow in their first formal examination procedure under the new Charter. A few weeks later a Gilbert Hamilton was approved as the first Licentiate allowed 'to practice physick'.

By the end of the tumultuous seventeenth century, the College had been firmly established, and while it was still relatively small, it was on the way to fulfilling, as best it could, its objective of bringing some order and structure to the proper practice of medicine. Sir Patrick Dun, who had done so much to consolidate the reputation of the College, was still looking firmly to the future. In a deed of 1704 he outlined his vision:

> … to make provision for one or two professors of physic to read public lectures and make public anatomical dissections of the several parts of human bodies, or bodies of other animals; to read lectures of osteology, bandage, and operations of surgery; to read botanic lectures, demonstrate plants publicly; to read public lectures on materia medica, for the instruction of students of physic, surgery, and pharmacy.[15]

The outworking of this enormous agenda, which Dun reiterated in his Will of 1711, would take many years to fulfil, but when he died of a fever during a Dublin epidemic in 1713, he had already outlined a blueprint which would prove to be of enormous benefit to the College, and also to the practice of medicine throughout Ireland in the remaining decades of the new century: a century which would provide its own challenges, setbacks and achievements.

Dun had been a member of the College for over 30 years, and during this long period he had missed only 28 meetings. As President 13 times and a Censor on five occasions, his record has not been surpassed, and his reputation remains secure as one of the most important figures in the history of the College.

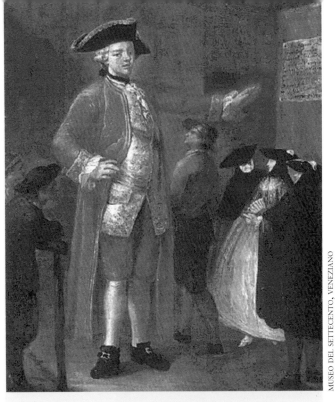

A portrait of the Irish Giant, Cornelius Magrath. *Ritratto del Gigante Magrat* by Pietro Longhi (1702–85). Magrath was visiting Venice as part of his exhibition tour of Europe.

The Irish Giant

The *London Daily Advertiser*, 1752, Cork, July 24 – 'There is now in this city one Cornelius Magrath, a boy 15 years 11 months old, of a most gigantic stature, being exactly 7 feet 9 inches three Quarters high, he is clumsy made, talks boyish and simple, he came hither from Youghal where he has been a year into Salt Water for Rheumatic Pains which almost crippled him, which the Physicians now say are growing pains, for he is grown to the monstrous Size he is of within Twelve months.'[16]

Cornelius Magrath was born in 1736. He suffered from a disorder of the pituitary gland which led to the production of an excess of growth hormone. Due to his extreme height, he was exhibited in Cork, Dublin, London and many cities throughout Europe. On his return to Dublin in 1760 he was invited to play the part of the giant in a pantomime, *Jack the Giant Killer*, in the Theatre Royal, Dublin. However he was suffering from a fever and died shortly afterwards of an ague.[17]

His dissection caused great interest among the medical fraternity. The professor of anatomy at Trinity, Robert Robinson, is reputed to have advised his students that to steal the body was no hanging matter so long as 'not a rag or a stocking is taken with it'.[18]

The students duly went to Magrath's wake and managed to secure the body, which was dissected before Magrath's friends awoke to find him gone. The skeleton remains in Trinity.

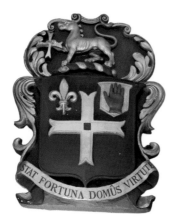

The Molyneux Arms hang in the entrance hall of the College.
DERMOTT DUNBAR

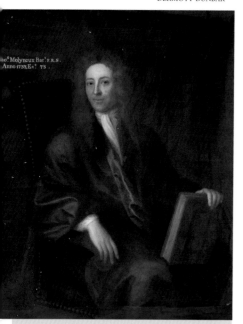

Sir Thomas Molyneux
1661–1733

Sir Thomas Molyneux was one of the outstanding Irish physicians of his era. He was elected President of the Royal College of Physicians of Ireland on four occasions and like, Sir William Petty, he was a polymath.
Sir Thomas held every major medical post in the country, including Professor of Physic at Trinity College, Physician-General to the Irish Army and the first State Physician in Ireland. He became Ireland's first medical Baronet, and died at the age of 72.

PAINTER UNKNOWN, 17TH CENTURY
© NATIONAL MUSEUMS NORTHERN IRELAND COLLECTION, ARMAGH COUNTY MUSEUM

The Age of Reason and Unreason

When Sir Patrick Dun died on 24 May 1713 his all-important Will could not be found. Five days earlier he had attended a College meeting for what proved to be the last time.

In the spring of 1713 there was an epidemic sweeping through Dublin, and Dun 'fell into a fever'. He was treated by 'blistering', but on 23 May, Bishop John Stearne – son of the founder of the College – who was visiting Sir Patrick daily, wrote to Archbishop King, Dun's long-term friend, expressing his worst fears.

King, who had Dun's Will locked up in a bedroom in the Archbishop's Palace, had left Dublin for Bath, where he was being treated for a severe attack of gout, and he had taken the key of the house with him.

On hearing this, Dun's nephew Patrick Mitchell, the then President of the College, immediately had his uncle's house sealed off, and all his trunks locked up.

Not surprisingly, this raised the ire of the formidable Lady Dun, who had already taken an intense dislike to her husband's nephew, and this began a gargantuan tussle over the details of the Will, which lasted until Lady Dun's death in 1748, and indeed beyond that date.

Fortunate

In fact the College, which was to become the major beneficiary, was fortunate that there was a Will at all. Patrick Dun had only finally decided to draw it up on 16 November, 1711, about 18 months before he died, and after three or four years of constant persuasion from Archbishop King.

Most leading physicians of the day had lucrative practices, and few were richer than Thomas Molyneux who built a mansion to accommodate his large family. Molyneux was elected President of the College on four occasions. Like Sir William Petty, he was a polymath, and he held every major medical office, including Professor of Physic at Trinity, Physician General to the Irish Army and the first State Physician in Ireland. In 1730 he became Ireland's first medical baronet, and died in 1733 at the age of 72.

Dun had no children alive at the time of his death, and few beneficiaries, so the College was able to benefit from his estate particularly generously, at least in the longer term.

Sir Patrick had married at 52, which was relatively late in life in the seventeenth century. The wedding took place some 18 months after his infamous duel with his fellow physician Dr Ralph Howard – so he might have felt in need of a woman's touch as a steadying influence in his life!

His wife Mary Jephson came from a well-known family, and her grandfather had been a Privy Councillor. The marriage took place in St Michan's Church in Dublin on 11 December 1694, and almost three years later, they had a son called Boyle, who died at an early age. Consequently Sir Patrick left the bulk of his real and personal estate to the control of two trustees – his cousin Patrick Dun, who lived in Scotland, and the previously-mentioned Patrick Mitchell. The income was to be paid to Lady Dun while she remained a widow.

The details were complex, and as the medical historian, Eoin O'Brien, has noted:

> Few estates can have been as badly managed as that of Sir Patrick Dun. His wishes were ignored or, at best, misinterpreted; his estate at Waterford was mismanaged; his library was poorly cared for, and many books that would today be priceless heirlooms were lost or stolen; his Will was the subject of a number of law suits, and Parliament had to intervene on no less than two occasions.[1]

Talk of the Town

Certainly the Dun legacy would have been the talk of the town in the drawing-room society of eighteenth-century Dublin which was still small enough for

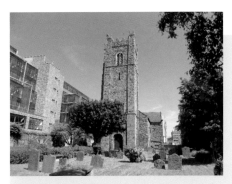

St Michan's Church, Dublin

The great and the good of Dublin society, including a number of leading physicians, were buried in the vaults of St Michan's until there was a natural move away from the city as it became more populous. When some of these vaults eventually gave way, five mummies were exposed. They survive due to the perfect atmospheric conditions.

BELOW: View from Capel Street looking over Essex Bridge, Dublin from Malton's *View of Dublin*.
The scene shows 'the confluence and ceremonious intercourse … of the town made by the river. … Parliament Street is a broad, handsome thoroughfare, composed of well-constructed houses, entirely inhabited by traders, with very splendid shops'.[2]
This illustration from 1790 shows the daily military parade from upper Ormond Quay to the guard of the Castle.
RCPI

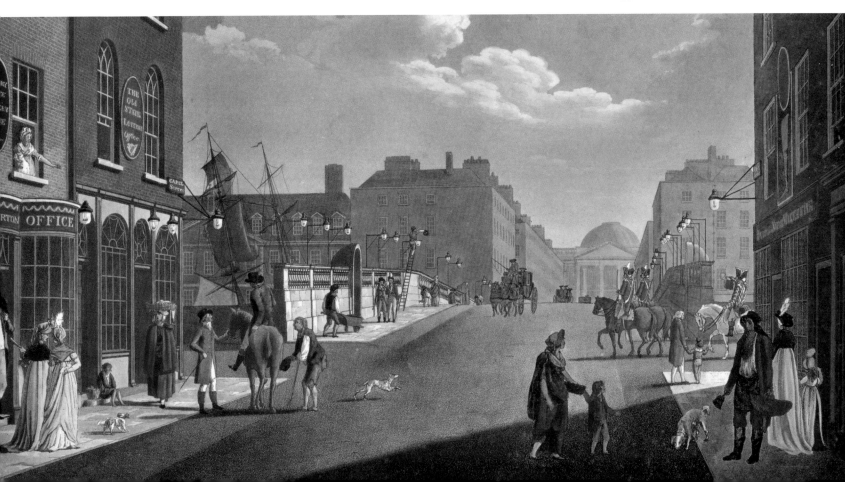

The Dun Estate

Perhaps the most interesting collection of papers are the Estate papers of the trust lands. The estates comprised the lands of Templeverick, Bonmahon, Shanakill, Ballinard, Kilmoylan, Portnaboa, Curraghnagarraha, Ballyduane, Lisnagerah, Killameeleane and Curraghbolinlea, all in County Waterford. Dun had purchased the lands at the beginning of the eighteenth century from the Duke of Ormonde. Some of the original title deeds survive, as well as a large collection of eighteenth and nineteenth century leases, estate correspondence, rentals and agents' accounts, giving insight into the estates' tenants.

Papers relating to the Bonmahon Estate
RCPI

Management of the estates seems to have been a continuing source of trouble to the College.

In 1824, when Edward Hill, a Fellow of the College, visited the estates, he lamented that the suggestions in his previous report had been ignored and suggested that, 'the College rests in absolute ignorance of their affairs; no one of them having ever seen the estates'. He suggested that someone from the College needed to visit the estates to gain a full understanding of them, and to work to reduce the ongoing hostility between the College and their tenants. The most profitable part of the estates was the copper mines, but there was some confusion as to whether the College owned these, resulting in a number of legal cases.

Relations between the College and their tenants clearly did not improve, as the number of papers relating to legal cases taken by the College against their tenants for non-payment of rents shows. At the end of the nineteenth century the lands were sold to the tenants under the Land Commission. The trust itself continued until 1961 when it was finally wound up.[3]

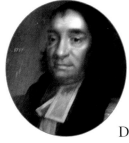

Bishop John Stearne
CLOGHER CATHEDRAL

gossip to flourish and for information to leak out gradually, unlike the instantaneous revelations of today's social media.

Lady Dun herself was a forceful character, who did not easily take advice, and who constantly took offence. She was particularly annoyed that Dr Mitchell was a co-executor of her husband's Will, and she accused Dr Mitchell and his wife of undermining 'her husband's affection for and confidence in her'.[4]

Lady Dun was so difficult at times that she provoked the anger of even the thoughtful Bishop Stearne who was trying to comfort her. She was so tiresome on occasions that Stearne decided to visit her only on condition that she behaved herself 'more moderately'.

However, Archbishop King, ever the diplomat, advised him:

> She is naturally of a quick and vivid sense, and her passions very eager and keen, and if the sense of religion and a very good understanding did not restrain her, they would be extravagant enough; but in such cases as her Ladyship's, the most religious think they may indulge themselves, nay many think it a duty, and therefore she has to be dealt with another way.[5]

While this legal and medical soap-opera was playing itself out, the nature of Irish society itself was changing. This was the century of the Penal Laws and the drive towards Catholic Emancipation, and even, in the latter period, of rebellion against the Crown.

As Professor RF Foster has noted:

> To be a Protestant or a Catholic in eighteenth-century Ireland indicated more than mere religious allegiance: it represented opposing political cultures, and conflicting views of history.[6]

To some extent this view could still be applied to parts of the island of Ireland today.

Ascendancy

Sir Patrick Dun, as a leading Protestant, was buried at St Michan's Church, where his son had been baptised and buried. His close connection with this fashionable church in itself symbolised how the College was the preserve of the Protestant Ascendancy, and would remain so for quite some time.

By 1716, just three years after Dun's death, around two-thirds of Dubliners were Protestants, but by 1800 or so, the numbers of Protestants had dwindled by a third. However it was not until the early twentieth century, as the 1911 Census demonstrated, that even half of the physicians in Dublin were Catholics.[7]

Changing Times

The first half of the eighteenth century also witnessed significant changes in the attitudes to medicine, and within medicine itself. In the Age of Enlightenment,

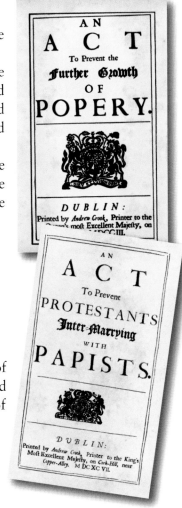

The Irish Parliament passed the Penal Laws against Catholics and Dissenters in the early eighteenth century, to maintain the power of the Anglican Ascendancy. Their prohibitions encouraged many Dissenters, particularly in Ulster, to emigrate to America. Catholic Emancipation was not achieved until 1829 through the leadership of Daniel O'Connell, 'the Liberator'.
LINEN HALL LIBRARY

The Westmoreland Lock Hospital

During the eighteenth and nineteenth centuries many hospitals would not admit patients suffering from venereal diseases, leading to a need for a dedicated hospital. George Doyle established the Westmoreland Lock Hospital in 1755 for their treatment.

The name 'Lock Hospital' dates back to earlier leprosy hospitals, which were known as 'lock' hospitals, from the French *loques* – rags that were used to cover the leper's lesions. Lock Hospitals were developed specifically for the treatment of syphilis.

The Westmoreland Lock Hospital was relocated to Townsend Street in 1792, as this was considered an ideal location, given the larger size of the hospital and its proximity to the city centre. It was named in honour of John Fane, 10th Earl of Westmoreland, who was Lord Lieutenant of Ireland at the time and sponsored the move to Townsend Street. This move was also significant as it signaled a shift in the importance of acknowledging and treating venereal disease.

From 1819 men were no longer admitted to the hospital. There were fewer men seeking treatment, partly because of the reduced military presence in daily life after the Battle of Waterloo in 1815. Men instead were treated for sexually transmitted diseases at Sir Patrick Dun's Hospital or Dr Steevens' Hospital. The Lock Hospital continued to treat women, many of whom were prostitutes. High levels of prostitution in Dublin were partly the result of the presence of large British garrisons in the city in the nineteenth century. At the time it was believed that the female body was not only 'the principle vector of the disease, but also its source'.

John Fane, 10th Earl of Westmoreland, from an engraving colourised by Robin S Taylor

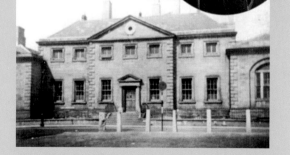

with its emphasis on reason, illness was much less regarded as a punishment from God for wrongdoing, and there was a growing realisation that people could take some measures of their own to help stave off, or to combat, ill-health.

There was also an awareness that the spread of some of the epidemics which occurred all too regularly might have much to do with poor sanitation and other threats to health. By the mid-century, there were still high death tolls due to fevers, smallpox, old age and other causes, as well as high infant mortality. Generally people of all classes suffered greatly, and many died from what would be regarded today as routine and treatable illnesses and disorders.

Despite the elegance of parts of Georgian Dublin and other urban areas in Ireland, many thousands of people lived in poor, cramped and foul-smelling conditions, and the importance of fresh air, exercise and proper diet was only gradually being recognised.

In a somewhat amusing observation, the author, Tony Farmar, notes that some people regarded regular sex as beneficial to good health, but not so the sister-in-law of the Duke of Leinster. He had been trying cunningly, and evidently vainly, to spread this novel idea, which had been concocted, no doubt, by the eighteenth-century 'brotherhood'. She concluded:

> I should quarrel with the Duke of Leinster, as I do with all men that fancy that they are so mighty necessary to a woman's health and happiness; it's abominably indelicate and I don't believe a word of it. I'm sure one sees many an old virgin mighty well and mighty comfortable.[8]

However, there were serious observations at the time as well, including the potential importance of a calm mind and steady demeanour in the bearing and control of illness, which would certainly strike a note with modern society. Sterne, the author of *The Life and Opinions of Tristram Shandy*, noted that:

> A man's body and his mind are exactly like a jerkin, and a jerkin's lining; rumple the one, you rumple the other.

Sterne, incidentally, was an Anglo-Irish novelist and Anglican clergyman, who was born in Clonmel in 1713, and died of consumption in London in 1768. He was distantly related to John Stearne.[9]

Important Developments

The story of the Royal College of Physicians of Ireland is closely entwined with that of Trinity College, and also with the significant contribution of a small group of physicians and other medical men who helped to change the face of medicine in that important period of Irish history.

For the greater part of the century, the key to the relationship between the Royal College and Trinity was contained in the Will of Sir Patrick Dun, who nearly a decade before his death had outlined clearly the requirement for a more ordered approach to the education of future doctors. This encompassed the need for a medical establishment in Ireland, so that students could be educated at home without having to leave the country, as so many before them had been obliged to do. The Trinity School of Physic (Medicine) was established in 1711, and in 1715 a Charter was set up to establish a professorship funded by Dun's bequest. The holder was to be known as the King's Professor of Physic in the City of Dublin, because the incumbent would be appointed by Royal Charter.

However it took almost two years to make an appointment. After a series of formal examinations, a Dr Robert Griffith was appointed the first King's Professor of Physic. He had been appointed a Lecturer in Chemistry at Trinity in 1711, when he was also President of the College for the second time in six years.

The Professorship had been established as quickly as possible because it was the first step to making Sir Patrick Dun's will legally operative, but the appointment was literally academic. Dr Griffith could not be paid until the death of Lady Dun, who was entitled to the income from her husband's estates; therefore he was not obliged to give lectures. In fact Lady Dun long outlived Dr Griffith, who was King's Professor for only three years. He died in the latter half of 1720, at the age of 58.

Slow Progress

Progress on implementing Dun's Will was slow, and it was not until 1725 that a Deed was signed to transfer Sir Patrick's land in County Waterford to the Royal College of Physicians for a nominal ten shillings, although Lady Dun retained the rents and profits accruing from the estate. The settlement of his personal estate was another matter, and it took years of legal wrangling with Lady Dun, until she finally agreed in 1740 that the legacy estimated at £1,200 would be handed over to the College.

However she lived to the age of 95 – a noteworthy longevity for the eighteenth century – and the final estate was valued at £1,217. This was a less than a quarter of the £6,000 valuation at the time of Dun's death some 36 years earlier, and doubtless much of the money had melted away in long and costly legal battles.

Shortly after settling the lawsuit with Dun's widow, the College decided to create three King's Professorships, as foreseen by the visionary Sir Patrick, and this was ratified by an Act of Parliament in 1742.

However it was not until the death of Lady Dun several years later that two more Dun's Professorships were created, to add to the Chair of Physic which had been held for 27 years by Professor Robert Griffith's successor, Dr James Grattan, who died in 1747. In 1749 Dr Henry Quin was elected as the new Professor of Physic, Dr Nathaniel Barry became Professor of Chirurgery and Midwifery, and Dr Constantine Barbor was appointed Professor of *Materia Medica* and Pharmacy.

An indenture between Patrick Dun and the Duke of Ormonde concerning the Dun Estates
RCPI

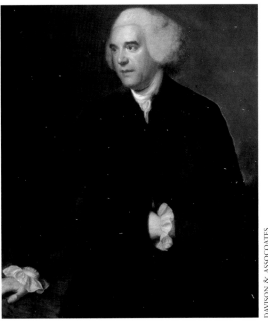

Dr Nathaniel Barry, who became the Dun's Professor of Chirurgery and Midwifery in 1749.
Portrait attributed to Thomas Hickey or Robert Hunter
RCPI

47

By mid-century therefore, Dun's vision was being fulfilled, but only by piecemeal methods and painfully slowly. Each Professor was to be paid around £90 per annum, and their lectures were to be delivered without charge at Trinity, and in Latin. In 1752 there were further regulations concerning these appointments, and as time progressed, the Professors' salaries increased because of the rising income from Dun's estate.

Sinecures

The three Professors stayed in office for a total of 112 years, but it is doubtful if they actually did enough to justify their salaries, which in any case were not always paid properly. The posts seemed to be little more than sinecures. By 1783 the situation was so unsatisfactory that the College launched an inquiry to determine how the Professorships could be made more effective.

After lengthy discussions, and disagreements, between the College of Physicians and Trinity, a further Act was passed in 1785, which made legal provision for four Professorships, though it would take more than 40 years for the fourth Chair to be filled. Another major problem was the lack of a teaching hospital. It was all such a long way from Sir Patrick Dun's visionary Deed of 1704 and his Will of seven years later. Unfortunately, the disputes over the allocation of money from Dun's estates dragged on tiresomely as the century progressed. By 1793 the income totalled more than £1,300 annually, and even though some rents were in arrears, this was a huge sum by today's standards.

However as the century drew to a close and just as it seemed as if progress was being made, a major disagreement threatened to split the College. On the one side was Professor Robert Perceval, who was the President of the Royal College of Physicians for a short period in 1799, but resigned when he was appointed to the Chair of Chemistry at Trinity. On the other side was the Professor of Botany, Dr Edward Hill, who was also President of the College of Physicians on six occasions between 1782 and 1813.

Determined

Both men were greatly determined, but did not agree on how to use part of the income from Dun's estate. Perceval, who like many of his contemporaries had been educated at Leiden, saw the urgent need for a proper teaching hospital in Dublin in order to prevent many aspiring Irish students from going abroad for training, and also to ensure the survival of the Dublin School of Medicine.

Eighteenth-century statistics underlined the need for such an establishment. No medical degrees were conferred in Dublin betweeen

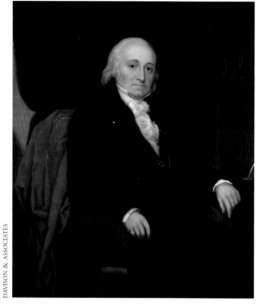

Professor Robert Perceval recommended the setting up of a teaching hospital in Ireland, so that medical students would no longer need to travel abroad to attend teaching universities such as Leiden in Holland. Portrait by William Gillard

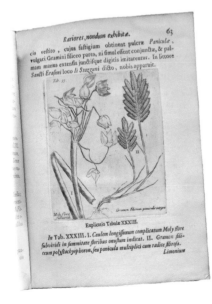

An illustration in Bocconi's *Plantae*

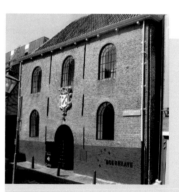

Originally the nunnery of St Caecilia in Leiden, the building became municipal property after the Reformation and shortly before 1600, was converted into a 'plague hospital and madhouse'. In 1635 it became a University hospital. It was here, around 1720, that Herman Boerhaave gave his famous sickbed lessons that drew medical students to Leiden from around the world. The building became Museum Boerhaave in 1991.

1724–40. In Edinburgh, which had a good reputation for clinical teaching, some 800 students graduated in medicine in the last quarter of the eighteenth century, including 237 who were Irish.[11]

In his timely pursuit to offer a viable alternative in Ireland, Professor Perceval urged the College to set aside funds from Dun's estate to build a clinical teaching hospital, but Hill resolutely opposed this, and argued that the money should be spent on a 'Garden of Physic' i.e., a botanical garden. From the

A brief history of the Botanic Garden

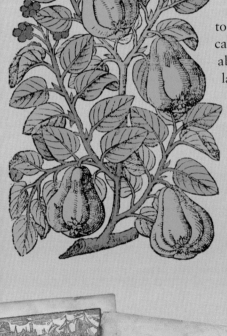

Trinity College initiated a physic garden on the main College campus in 1687 to provide plant material to support the teaching of medicine. By 1773 this garden had become derelict, and was partly used to dump offal from the Anatomy Department. There was a short-lived attempt to establish a garden in Harolds Cross to the south-west of the campus, but by 1806 the College Physic garden was finally abandoned, and a Botanic Garden established in an area of land leased in Ballsbridge. Over the next one hundred years this garden developed considerably, and held an important and varied collection of plants. Notable curators of this Garden include JT Mackay, credited with producing the first Flora of Ireland, and FW Burbidge, who was well-known for his exploration of the Kinabalu region of what is now Sabah, and for his work on the collection and hybridisation of narcissus.

The Garden celebrated the tercentenary of the College in 1892, with the presentation of a massive specimen of the tree fern *Todea barbara*, originally a gift from the Royal Botanic Garden, Melbourne. A cutting of this plant still thrives in the present Garden. The position of Curator was abandoned after the death of Burbidge, and as a result the Gardens ceased to develop. This was partly redressed with the appointment of an assistant curator in 1950. In 1965 a plan was put before the College Board to relocate the Gardens to Trinity Hall, an accommodation complex in Dartry. This move was approved, giving the Gardens better long-term security, as the Trinity Hall site is freehold. The move was completed over 1966 and 1967; two modern hotel complexes now stand on the site of the former Ballsbridge Garden. Many important plant specimens were transferred to Dartry, including a 25 foot tall Ginkgo and various cycads.[11]

Hibernicarum by Thomas Molyneux
RCPI

The Chelsea Physic Garden, founded in London in 1673 as the 'Garden of the Society of Apothecaries' was originally situated at Westminster. The plants were moved to Chelsea in 1676.

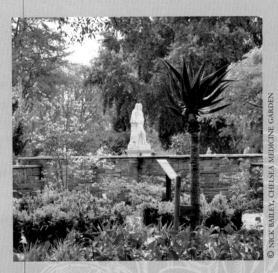

© NICK BAILEY, CHELSEA MEDICINE GARDEN

A new garden of medicinal plants was opened in 2014 with a new statue to the Ulsterman Sir Hans Sloane. The statue was donated and unveiled by the Earl Cadogan (a descendant of Sir Hans Sloane) and sculpted by Simon Smith after the original from 1737 by John Michael Rysbrack (1694–1771). The original statue was erected in the Garden by the Apothecaries in 1737, as a token of their gratitude after Sir Hans Sloane covenanted the Garden to the Worshipful Society of Apothecaries. Sir Hans Sloane was responsible for introducing the use of *Cinchona* (Peruvian bark) as a cure for malaria, and the active ingredient, quinine, is still used to save millions of lives.[12]

Hans Sloane, 1660–1753

Born in Killyleagh, Co Down, Sloane was a distinguished physician and a Fellow and President of the Royal Society, London. His vast collection of books, plant and other specimens formed the basis of the British Museum. He was created a baronet by King George I in 1716.

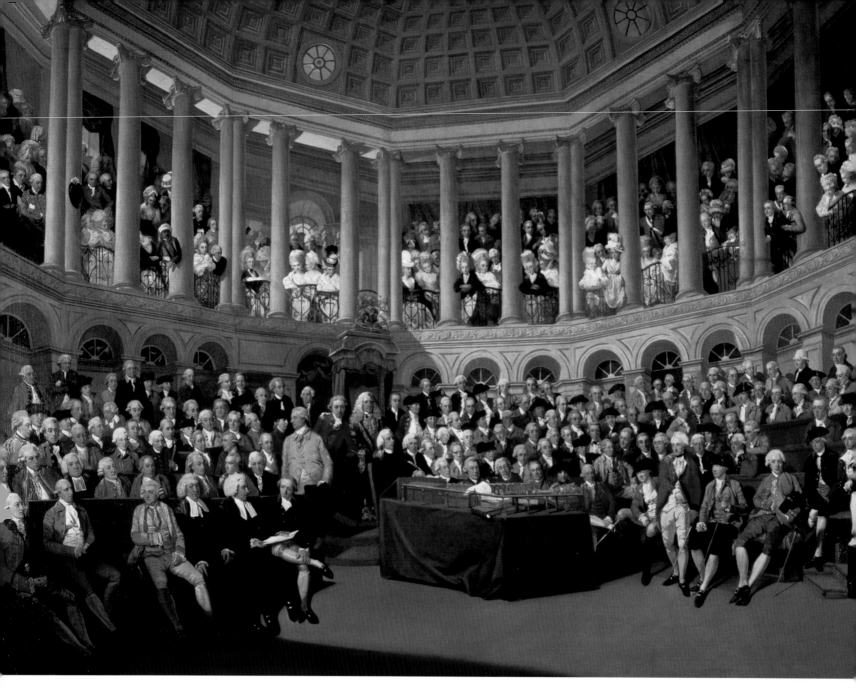

The Irish House of Commons, 1780.
Henry Grattan, the 'patriot' politician,
stands to the right of the table.
Painting by Francis Wheatley
LEEDS CITY ART GALLERY
BRIDGEMANIMAGES

earliest times botanical gardens had been an indispensible part of most of the great European teaching centres because they grew many of the plants then used in the practice of *materia medica*.

There had been a botanical garden at the Dublin Botany School which was established in 1711, but it had been encroached upon by buildings, and disappeared totally by 1773. Hill's dream of a physic garden was not well-received, particularly by Perceval who believed that it would be a waste of scarce money.

He was roundly criticised in turn by Hill, who, with the classical bitterness of academics on the war-path, described Perceval as:

> ... a self-sufficient, vindictive gentleman, singularly obstinate in his own opinions, and unwearied in the pursuits of such objects as a mind intent on higher thoughts would abandon to the ordinary course of common events.[13]

By modern standards Hill's objections seem ill-placed, but in the context of his time, the subject of botany was as important as the study of medicine. Despite Hill's coruscating rhetoric, however, the views of Perceval prevailed, and he was instrumental in the passing of the 1800 School of Physic Act.

This was one of the the last Acts passed by the Irish Parliament before its dissolution under the Act of Union, and it determined that a hospital to facilitate clinical teaching would be established with the money from Sir Patrick Dun's estate, and that this building would be named after him.

Significantly, the Act also removed the College's discretionary powers in the further management of Dun's estate. This followed an Inquiry by a Committee of the Irish House of Lords in 1799, which examined how the College had applied the funds from Dun's estate to build 'a Hospital for clinical lectures', although that had not been Dun's intention.

The Lords' Committee were scathing about the way in which the Royal College of Physicians had used, or misused, the funds, although in a lengthy history of the College Professor John Widdess concluded that:

> ... while the Lords' Committee might well have formed an unfavourable opinion of the College as administrators, it was either grossly misinformed or deliberately unjust in certain particulars.[14]

Despite Widdess' attempt at mitigation, the administration of the College in the eighteenth century had not been impressive.

The Physic Act of 1800 was immensely important, though the grudging Professor Hill suspected that Perceval had used his influence with the Attorney General Lord Clare in getting his way, and he scathingly denounced 'the unnecessary private conversations of this restless busybody'.[15]

Indeed Lord Clare was less than popular, particularly because of his judgement in a lawsuit between the Professors and the College over remuneration. The appeal to the House of Lords was heard on 8 February, 1796. The Lord Chancellor, none other than Lord Clare himself, declared that the appeal by the Professors must be considered

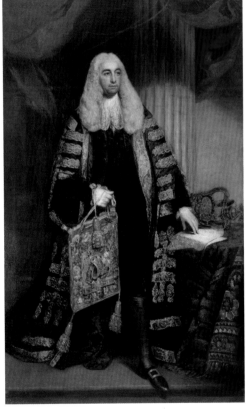

> as a gross and shameless fraud ... it seems to me to be most perfectly clear that they should be scouted from a Court of Equity with shame and disgrace.

Not surprisingly the Professors' Appeal was dismissed. When Lord Clare died several years later, it was said that, 'curses and a shower of dead cats' rained upon his grave. The history of eighteenth century law and medicine in Ireland was nothing if not colourful.[15]

Portrait of John Fitzgibbon, Earl of Clare (1749–1802), c. 1799–1800 Painting by Hugh Douglas Hamilton. Fitzgibbon was an outspoken Irish Attorney-General who made enemies. It is said that following his burial 'curses and a shower of dead cats rained upon his grave'
NATIONAL GALLERY OF IRELAND

Milestone

In reality, the Physic Act of 1800, so disliked by Professor Hill, was another important milestone in the long history of the College. It finally settled the long-running disputes over the Dun's estates, and also the unsatisfactory situation regarding professorships, which also had long been an area of dispute.

Three King's Professors of the Institutes of Medicine, the Practice of Medicine, and Materia Medica and Pharmacy were to be appointed at a fixed salary, and a Professorship of Midwifery was to follow, when it was thought fit and when funds were available. This Chair was not filled until 1827.

The new Physic Act also stipulated that the King's Professorship, originally reserved for Protestants, could be open to anyone, 'who professed his faith in Christ'. Significantly, the Fellowships of the Royal College of Physicians were now also opened to Catholics, if they took an Oath of Loyalty to the King. The Act also stipulated that medical graduates of Trinity could no longer be admitted to the College of Physicians without examination – a privilege previously granted in the 1692 Royal Charter. They would now have to sit the same examination as anyone else.

By the end of the eighteenth century the College of Physicians, because of its individual strengths and despite some of its collective weaknesses, had made its mark in the training of medical students, and promised much for the future. It had survived as an Institution throughout another century of political and social change in Ireland, and a number of its colourful and able Presidents and others had made important advances in the development of healthcare in Ireland.

These developments and the rich texture of political and social life in Ireland, which formed an important backdrop to the story of the Royal College of Physicians, will be further considered in the following chapter.

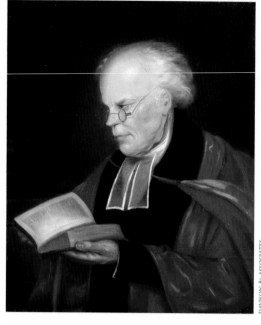

Professor Edward Hill opposed the use of Dun's inheritance to fund a teaching hospital, as proposed by Professor Robert Perceval. Hill supported the idea of a 'Physic Garden'.
RCPI

DAVISON & ASSOCIATES

The Irish Parliament,'is situated on College Green, and is placed nearly at right angles with the west front of the College (Trinity) ... The contiguity of two such structures give a grandeur of scene that would do honour to the first city in Europe'.[16]

From Malton's *View of Dublin*
RCPI

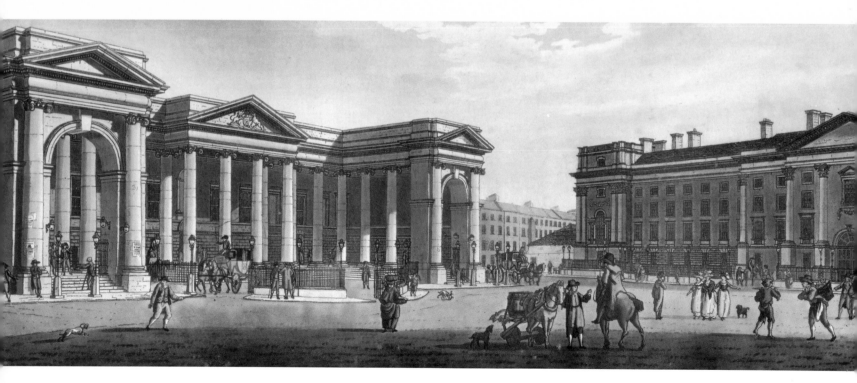

Hospitals, Healing and Hope

Much of the story of the Royal College of Physicians of Ireland in the eighteenth century has a strong focus on the long and tortuous outworking of the Will of Sir Patrick Dun. During the same period, however, there were significant advances in Irish medicine.

A number of hospitals were established in a country which had none since King Henry VIII's dissolution of the monasteries in the mid-sixteenth century. The success of these new institutions was due to the vision and hard work of several outstanding individuals. Some of these people were Fellows or Licentiates of the College of Physicians, supported by wealthy and philantrophically-minded members of the public.

During this period the physicians, surgeons and apothecaries continued their long-running tussle over their respective roles and status, though this would be settled by the end of the nineteenth century, when the often abrasive divisions between these groups were breaking down. Meanwhile in the eighteenth century, surgeons had finally freed themselves from direct association with the Barber-Surgeons' Guild, and established their own Royal College of Surgeons in Ireland in 1784.

By the end of the century there was a discernible order in the map of Irish medicine, compared to the relative chaos of the previous years, and although much remained to be done, there was at least a framework in place which became part of the basis that had its part to play in the great leap forward in the next century.

All of this happened against a changing background of political uncertainty, culminating in the 1798 Rebellion and the subsequent Act of Union of 1801 when a whole new order was established. There were also natural disasters such as the 1740 Great Frost and the resultant devastating famine, as well as important developments in the architectural, social and cultural life of the island.

The impetus for creating hospitals arose partly from the medical profession's need to create teaching establishments, as well as helping to ameliorate the wretched conditions of the poor, in a country where there was such a huge gap in living conditions.

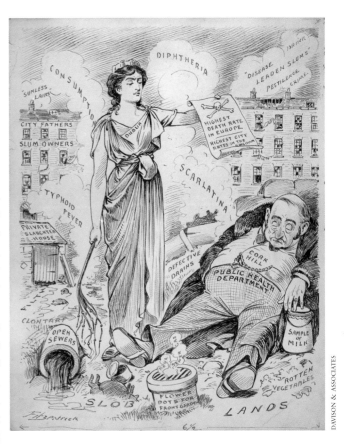

A cartoon by the Irish artist Thomas Fitzpatrick (1860–1912), produced for his publication *The Leprechaun*. The cartoon relates to public health issues in Dublin in the 1910s. It gives important insight into the social and environmental problems of this period of history and touches, none too subtly, on their effects on the health of the general populace. We see the terrible conditions of life in Dublin's slums at this time, including disease, defective drains and open sewers. The vested interests of the Dublin Corporation Members, many of whom were also slum owners, are also being attacked. Living conditions had barely improved during the previous century.
RCPI

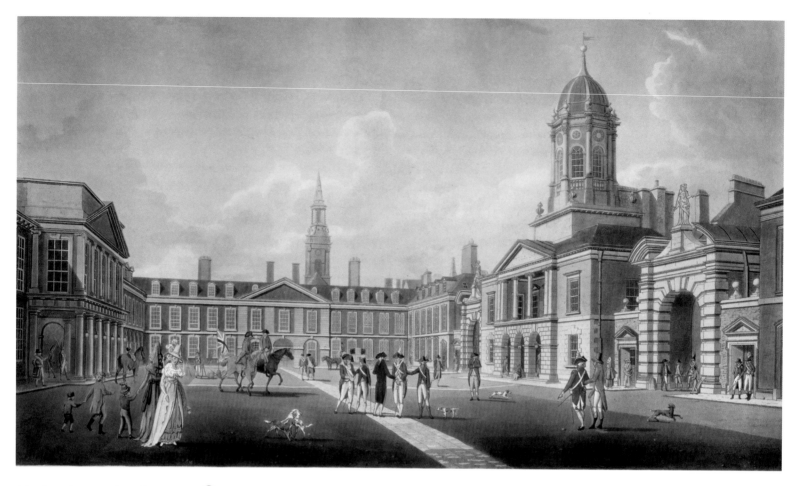

The Great Court Yard, Dublin Castle.
Until 1922, Dublin Castle, off Dame
Street, was the seat of British rule in
Ireland, and is now a major Irish
government complex.
From Malton's *View of Dublin*

RCPI

Contrasts

The Irish writer Brendan Behan once satirised the Ascendancy as 'a Protestant on a horse'. Without doubt the members of the Ascendancy – landlords, aristocrats, Anglican clerics, and members of the professional classes – saw themselves as a cut above the rest, and although they were never totally secure about their political status in an Ireland where the Westminster Parliament still made key decisions, many of them took advantage of their considerable wealth and privileges as members of a ruling, yet minority Establishment.

By contrast, the Catholic sense of dispossession was acute, as noted by one historian:

> It took different forms as social and political circumstances changed, but its essential proposition was constant: the land of Ireland had been stolen from its rightful owners and given to strangers whose title to it might be good in English law, but was morally illegitimate.[1]

The historian Dr Jonathan Bardon underlined the almost obscene self-indulgence of some of the Protestant gentry, surrounded by a sea of poverty and hordes of people lacking most of the basics of life. He quoted the fifth Earl of Orrery, who in 1736 wrote of the gentry thus;

> Drunkenness is the touchstone by which they try every man ... It is a Yahoo that toasts the glorious and immortal memory of King William in a bumper without any other joy in the Revolution than that it gives him a pretence to

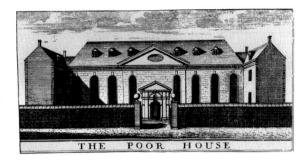

THE POOR HOUSE

drink so many more daily quarts of wine. The person who refuses a goblet to this prevailing toast is deemed a Jacobite, a papist and a knave.[2]

Such distasteful self-indulgence contrasted sharply with the dire poverty in so much of the rest of the country. The medical historian, Dr John Fleetwood highlighted in particular the unhappy fate of illegitimate and unwanted children, which was one of the touchstones of an unbalanced and socially dysfunctional society. He described the Dublin of 1728, where malnutrition and close personal contacts between people in the crowded poorer areas led to the 'devastatingly rapid' spread of diseases.[3]

In 1703 the Irish Parliament had passed an Act to establish a workhouse, which eventually also tried to make provision for the physically and mentally ill. A further motive for founding the workhouse was, 'to preserve the lives of illegitimate children and the educating and instructing of them in the Protestant religion'.[4]

Following a House of Lords' Commission in 1730, a part of the Dublin workhouse was made into a foundling hospital:

> At one of these gates (in the hospital) there was a basket fixed to a revolving door. Those who wished to abandon a child placed it in a basket, rang a bell

The Dublin Workhouse was opened in 1703 and continued as such until 1730, when it became a foundling hospital. It survived as the South Dublin Union, now St James's Hospital.

'The interior, a vast hall occupying the whole of the centre block, 120 feet by 40 and lofty in proportion, was one of the noblest architectural spaces in Dublin ... Unhappily it was seen by hardly anybody except those whose misery prevented them from getting any good of it.'[5]

BROOKING'S CITY OF DUBLIN

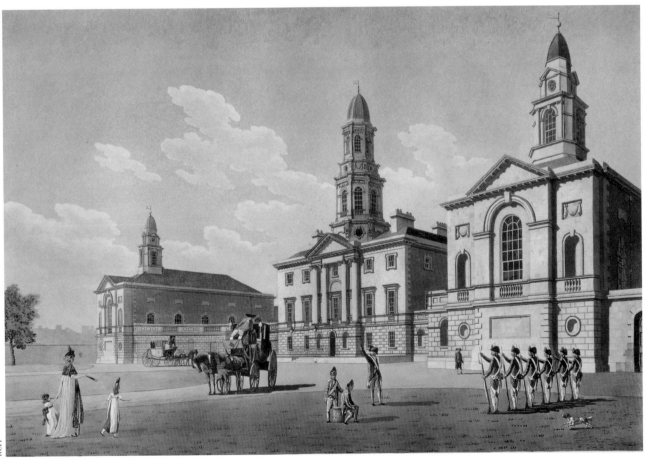

'The Blue-Coat Hospital, originally in Queen Street, Oxmantown, was founded in 1670 by Charles II, with a Charter and a Grant, of the ground whereon it stood. It was at first intended as an asylum for the aged and infirm poor of the city, as well as their children, but the funds proved unequal to such extensive charity. After 1680, boys only were received, and the number increased from about 40 to 170, the present number (1794) supported by voluntary contributions.
The children admitted to the Hospital must be the sons of reduced freemen. The Corporation of Merchants supported a mathematical school here, for the instruction of ten boys in navigation, for the sea service. The children are dicted and cloathed, carefully instructed in reading, writing and arithmetick; and when properly qualified, apprenticed, with a fee of £5 each, to Protestant masters.'[6]

From Malton's *View of Dublin*

The building in the centre is the Hospital, with the school to the left and the chapel to the right.

and left. Within a few minutes the door was turned from inside, and the baby was received by a porter who could not see the depositor.[7]

Meeting the need

The need was obvious, and the steady establishment of a number of voluntary hospitals helped to meet that demand. During the eighteenth century, 37 hospitals were opened, comprising eight in Dublin and 29 in the rest of Ireland. Some 23 of these were established as County Infirmaries by an Act of the Irish Parliament in 1765, but many of the latter did not have the services of a physician.

The vast majority of the physicians were attached to the Dublin hospitals, though they were not necessarily Fellows or Licentiates of the College of Physicians. A considerable number of them maintained their own practice independently. A 1774 poem, written by John Gilborne, mentions 61 outstanding physicians, but only 24 had a Fellowship or Licentiate in Medicine from the College. However, physicians at the top of their profession were usually well-connected to the College.[8]

Dublin Hospitals

In 1718 six Dublin surgeons opened modest premises in Cook Street at their own expense. This became known later as the Charitable Infirmary, and it was the earliest of its kind in Ireland. When it moved into No 14 Jervis Street, it became the Jervis Street Hospital.

One of the most important medical institutions of the early eighteenth century was Dr Steevens' Hospital, which opened in 1733.

Richard Steevens had become a Fellow of the College following the granting of the second Royal Charter in 1692. He was President of the College twice – the second time in 1710, although he died on 15 December, shortly after his election.

He had made a fortune in medicine, and the very day before his death, he made a Will, leaving his property in trust to his twin sister, Grizel. He intended that after her death the residue of the estate would be used to establish a hospital, but his strong-minded sister was unwilling to countenance any delay in providing help for the poor and needy.

She remained a spinster and therefore retained the properties, and she was always a staunch supporter of her brother's initiative to establish a hospital. However she had a struggle to make his vision a reality. His Will was not legally established until 1713; meanwhile she

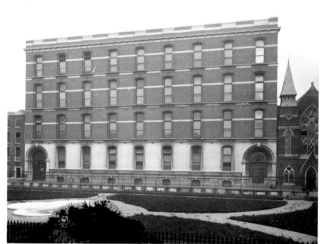

Dublin Evening News, 10–14 July, 1733
An invitation to the public, (bar a few exclusions noted at the bottom), suffering from ill-health to present themselves, with their certificates of poverty, on Mondays and Fridays at the Dr Steevens' Hospital.
NATIONAL ARCHIVES

The Charitable Infirmary

Jervis Street Hospital
NATIONAL LIBRARY OF IRELAND

Archbishop King
RCB LIBRARY

petitioned Queen Anne with plans for a hospital in Phoenix Park. This was thwarted by the death of the monarch in 1714, but Grizel Steevens pressed on with her efforts, with the backing of Archbishop King.

She lived frugally, and when she appointed trustees in July 1717 to build a hospital, she vested in them £2,000 of her own money. By the time the hospital was opened in 1733, she had personally contributed some £14,000 to the project, and very wisely she decided to take up residence in the building when it was finished.[9] Indeed it was understandable that, having poured so much time, energy and her soul into such a grand and worthy undertaking, she wanted to make sure that it would work out properly.

Grizel Steevens nominated Edward Worth to be a Governor and a physician at the new hospital. He was a Fellow of the College, and he was twice nominated as President, an honour which he mysteriously declined on both occasions. It has been suggested that this may have been due to an obscure dispute with the College.[10]

Worth was a chronic invalid, and he died in 1733 at the age of 55, shortly before the Steevens' Hospital opened. However, he donated the then large sum of £1,000 for its upkeep, and also his magnificently-bound collection of some 4,500 books. Professor John Widdess, the one-time Honorary Librarian at the Worth Library, stated glowingly:

> … [this] rich collection – not confined to medicine – contained no less than twenty-one books printed before 1500, and a number of fine Dublin bindings, is the monument of a scholarly physician.[11]

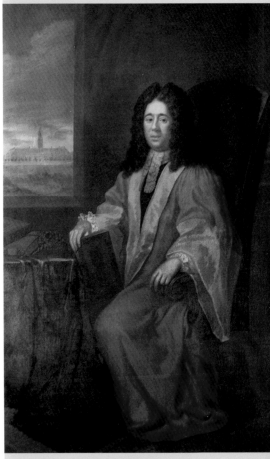

Portrait of Edward Worth, 1676–1733
COURTESY THE TRUSTEES OF THE EDWARD WORTH LIBRARY

Dr Edward Worth

The book collection assembled by Edward Worth, a notable Dublin physician, is one of the lesser-known treasures of the city's cultural inheritance. It is housed in Dr Steevens' Hospital, an institution of which Worth was a Governor and major benefactor.[12]

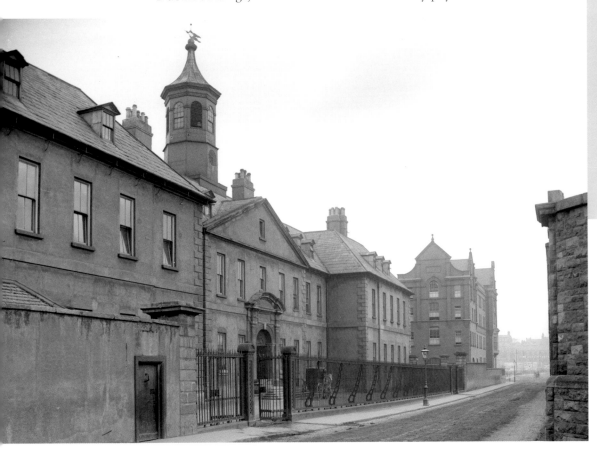

Dr Steevens' Hospital
NATIONAL LIBRARY OF IRELAND

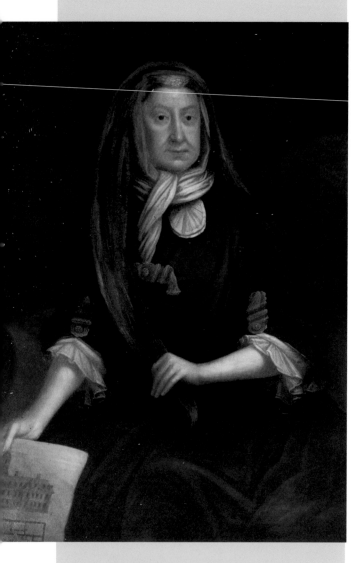

Grizel Steevens

Grizel Steevens, 1654–1747, was the twin sister of Dr Richard Steevens. After his untimely death in 1710, his Estate was inherited by his sister who worked tenaciously and tirelessly to establish Dr Steevens' Hospital, which opened in 1733.

She lived frugally, and donated £14,000 of her own money to the project. Grizel Steevens had accommodation in the hospital from the time it opened, and lived there until her death in 1747.

It is said that she often wore a heavy veil, in an attempt to retain her anonymity when carrying out her considerable work for charity, and when walking in the grounds of the Hospital. Her portrait by Michael Mitchell still hangs in the former Dr Steevens' Hospital, which is now a centre for the Health Service Executive.

By the time Grizel Steevens died in 1747, aged 93, the routines and reputation of the Hospital had been well-established, and this was partly due to the leadership of the Governors, who were also physicians. From the start, they set out clear instructions about how it would operate.

They stipulated that the physicians were to be accompanied by the first surgeons, and their chief duties on the days of attendance, were to examine the new admissions:

> This was not done in the wards, but in a committee room. When the patient had been prescribed for, his or her subsequent care fell to the second surgeon, who also acted as apothecary. He kept the drugs, mixed them, and handed the medicines to the nurses for administration'.

A contemporary report on the procedure at St Bartholomew's in London provided an insight to what may also have been happening in Dublin. 'The physician came in, accompanied by the apothecary, and sat down at an armchair at the head of the table. The apothecary stood to one side, and on the other side, the sister of the ward.'

The patients, if possible, sat on benches on each side of the table, and moved to the physician's right so that he could see them in turn. The apothecary took down the prescription, the matron held a towel:

> … and after seeing each patient, the physician washed out his mouth with water into a bucket, and rubbed his hands with the towel.[13]

Despite the medical theatricality of such encounters, the physicians only occasionally visited the wards. As a profession they were well-paid, with a physician receiving a guinea for a consultation at his own rooms, and two guineas for a home visit. The consultations were very different from those of today, and there was no detailed physical examination of the patient. The physician would attach great importance to the pulse, as well as an examination of the urine or stools, and most significantly, the patient's account of the symptoms of his or her own illness.

Physicians were busy men, and obviously they could not see every patient. However, there were always ingenious ways of combining duty with financial rewards, and some physicians were not above meeting surgeons and apothecaries at coffee houses to prescribe medication, for a half a guinea, on strength of a verbal outline of the symptoms. This must have been one of the earlier examples in Ireland of cut-price medicine, but a prescription from a physician at secondhand was better than no prescription at all.[14]

More Hospitals

A year after the opening of Dr Steevens' Hospital, Mercer's Hospital was established, with a capacity of ten beds. It was the vision of Mary Mercer, who a decade earlier set out to build a refuge for 'twenty poor girls'. By 1734 it had become an institution for people suffering from

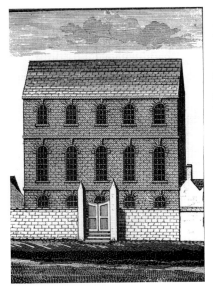

Mercer's Hospital

> ... diseases of tedious and hazardous cure, such as falling sickness, lunacy, leprosy, and the like, or of such other diseases ... as the trustees think proper.[15]

In 1738, to help raise funds, a concert took place at St Andrew's Church, at which music by Handel was performed:

> ... with the greatest decency and exactness possible ... at which their excellencies the Lord Justices and 800 persons of the first quality attended.[16]

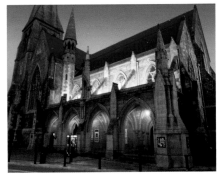

St Andrew's Church
DUBLIN TOURISM

This was just four years before the first performance of Handel's *Messiah* in Dublin, and the composer's music, and that of others, featured regularly in other concerts to raise funds for voluntary hospitals and other good causes, which literally tuned in to the wealthy Dublin audiences' appreciation of eighteenth-century music.

Charles Lucas 1713–71

Charles Lucas was born in 1713 and became penniless following the death of his father in 1727, when the boy was 14. However, he rose to become a leading apothecary, doctor and politician.

Lucas was initially apprenticed to a Dublin apothecary and this provided him with a means of bettering himself, though the trade 'was notorious at the time for fraud, malpractice, adulteration of medicines and the use of poison'.[17]

One of his earlier achievements was to campaign successfully for legislation to control apothecaries, and he was partly responsible for the important 1733 Act, which granted the Royal College of Physicians the power to regulate the trade.

Lucas was an outspoken politician on behalf of citizens' rights, and, as a member of Dublin Corporation, he fell foul of the authorities when he claimed that, 'there was no general rebellion in Ireland since the first British invasion that was not raised or formented by the oppression,

instigation, evil influence or connivance of the English'.[18]

Not surprisingly he had to flee for safety to the Isle of Man and from thence to London and continental Europe, where he studied medicine in Leiden and Paris.

He was later pardoned by King George III, and he returned to Ireland where he successfully contested a Dublin seat in the Irish Parliament. He played an important role in medical reform, and his most important legacy was the Lucas Act of 1761.

This greatly extended the powers of the Royal College of Physicians to inspect all apothecaries, and also to give them the right to complete a Pharmacopoeia to catalogue and deal with the mixing of medicines.

Lucas suffered severely from gout, and he died, aged 58, on 4 November 1771. He was honoured with an imposing funeral, and interred in the family burial ground at St Michan's.[19]

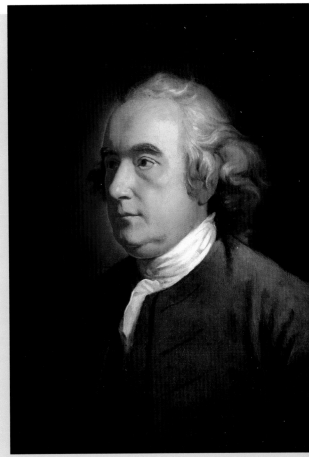

Portrait of Charles Lucas by Thomas Hickey
RCPI

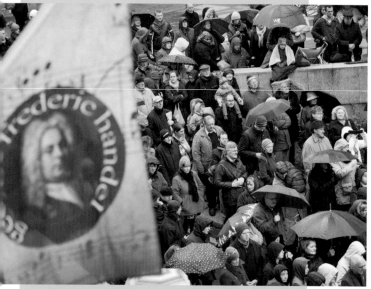

Handel's Day, 2013
Our Lady's Choral Society performed 'Messiah on the Street' on Dublin's Fishamble Street, on the 271st anniversary of its first performance in 1742 .

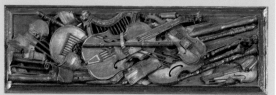

George Frideric Handel

The music of Handel was popular with eighteenth-century Dublin audiences of the great and good, and his works featured frequently in fund-raising concerts for voluntary hospitals and other good causes.

The disastrous famine of 1741 resulted in many thousands of hungry and sick people flocking to Dublin, where the hospitals were overwhelmed with patients. A large sum of money was needed to help, and Handel was invited to Dublin, where he gave his first performance of *The Messiah* in the new Musick Hall in Fishamble Street, Dublin in April 1742, to great, and obviously lasting, public and worldwide acclaim.

This first performance, for which the composer, the musicians and the singers had given their services free, raised the then large sum of £400, which was divided between local charities, including the Charitable Infirmary, the Charitable Music Society and Mercers' Hospital.

RIGHT: The organ (dated 1724) in St Michan's Church on which Handel is said to have practised *The Messiah* in advance of the first performance.
ABOVE: In front of the gallery is the Organ Trophy, a carved wooden piece which depicts 17 musical instruments and was installed in 1724.

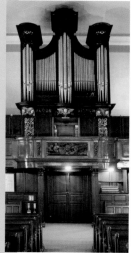

In 1743 a Hospital For Incurables, later the Royal Hospital, Donnybrook, was established to help patients with food, shelter and relief from their distressing illnesses. Some 13 years later, the Meath Hospital was established and it enjoyed particular prominence in the nineteenth century, due to the outstanding work of its physicians, who will be mentioned in more detail later.

First Maternity Hospital

The Dublin 'Lying-In' Hospital which was opened by Dr Bartholomew Mosse in 1745, was the first maternity hospital in the British Isles, and received widespread recognition.

Mosse was a remarkable eighteenth-century Irish obstetrician who specialised as a male midwife and was granted one of the very few Licentiates in Midwifery from the College of Physicians.

During his practice in Dublin he encountered widespread poverty and despair, which was greatly increased by the influx of many thousands of desperate and impoverished rural people seeking employment in the cities, after the ravages of 1740 Great Frost and the subsequent famine.

The highly-motivated Mosse was determined to found a Lying-In hospital for destitute mothers, and also to provide more widespread training in midwifery. He had a number of influential patrons, including the Rt Reverend Robert Clayton, the Bishop of Clogher, who also had a Dublin residence in St Stephen's Green, at the site of the future Department of Foreign Affairs. Clearly many of the eighteenth-century Anglican prelates in Ireland were men of affluence as well as influence.

Rt Rev Robert Clayton Bishop of Clogher, one of the influential patrons of the hospital
CLOGHER CATHEDRAL

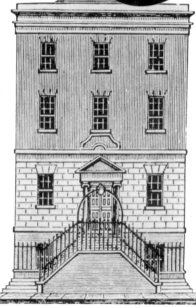

The new Lying-Inn Hospital opened in March, 1745, and during the first twelve-and-a-half years of its existence it catered for 3,975 mothers, who were delivered of 4,049 children.

The innovative hospital was so successful that the eminent nineteenth-century surgeon, Sir William Wilde, writing about it over a hundred years later century later, claimed that it had:

... an unrivalled superiority, not only in the British Isles, but (and we speak advisedly, having visited all the others of note upon the Continent) in Europe also.[20]

Meath Hospital, 1744

Mosse was not only a remarkable humanitarian, but also an entrepreneur who raised large amounts of money through lotteries, concerts and other performances to fund a more suitable premises for the Hospital because the original building – a former theatre in George's Lane – was proving too small for its purpose. These fundraising concerts included performances of Handel's Oratorios in 1746–48.

The Rotunda

Eventually Mosse acquired the site on which the Rotunda now stands. He also commissioned at his own expense a landscape gardener to lay out a Pleasure Garden, which was to become another fundraising venture for a larger Lying-In Hospital.

Mosse employed a distinguished architect, the German-born Richard Cassells, who had designed several well-known Dublin buildings, including Leinster House. The new Lying-in Hospital was opened on 15 March 1757 by the Lord Lieutenant, having received a Royal Charter in the previous year. It later became popularly known as 'The Rotunda', with its distinct tower and cupola.

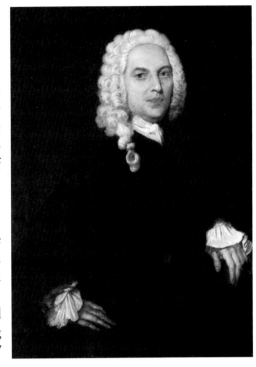

Bartholomew Mosse
ROTUNDA HOSPITAL

The Lying-in Hospital from Malton's *View of Dublin*
RCPI

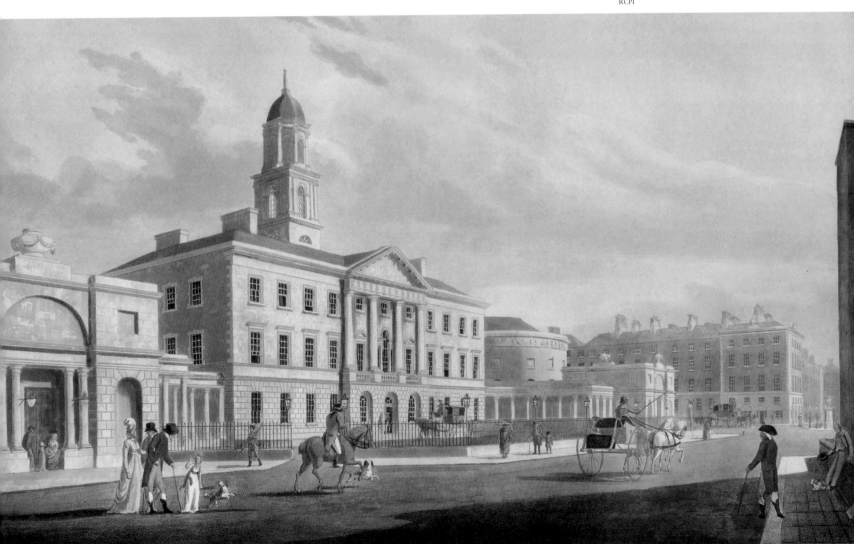

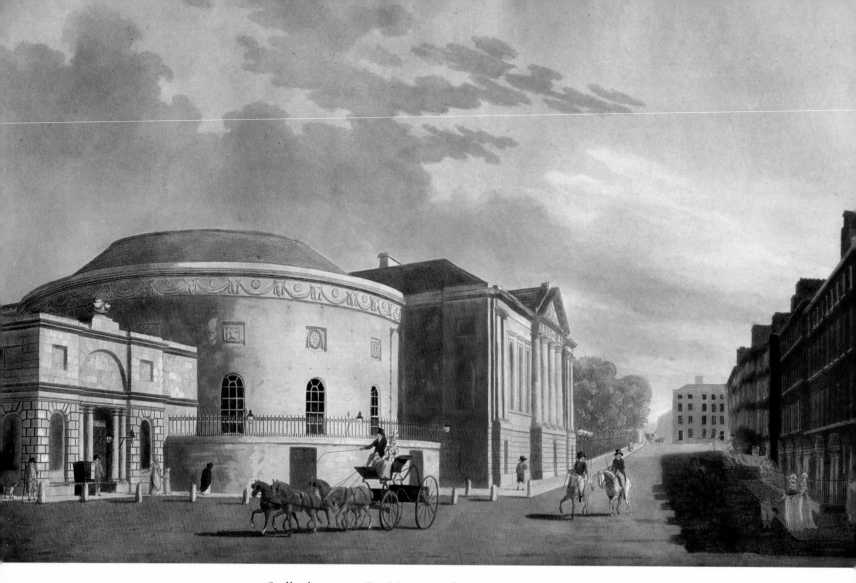

The Rotunda Rooms from Malton's *View of Dublin*.

'The New Rooms are superb; they consist of two principal apartments ... the lower is the Ball; the upper is the Supper and Tea Room. There is a smaller ball-room on the ground floor ... Besides weekly concerts in the winter season, there are here held subscription balls, supported by the first nobility and gentry ...[21]

RCPI

Sadly, however, Dr Mosse – who was the first Master of the Hospital – did not live to see the fulfillment of his vision for the construction of a large auditorium on the site, called the 'Rotundo', which was used for fundraising concerts and other activities.

He died, literally worn out, on 16 February 1759, at the age of only 46, and he was succeeded as Master by Sir Fielding Ould. Mosse was buried in an unmarked grave at Donnybrook, which lay undiscovered for over 200 years, after the graveyard had been taken over by Dublin Corporation to make a small public park.

A proper memorial stone to this inspiring man was erected and officially unveiled in 1995, on the 250th anniversary of the establishment of the first Lying-In Hospital in 1745.

An article published in the *Dublin Quarterly Journal of Medical Science* to mark the centenary of the Hospital paid a fulsome and much deserved tribute to its founder:

Men will labour diligently for their own advancement, either directly or indirectly; but how seldom do we see an individual give his time, his talents, bodily and mental labour, and his wealth, to the sole purpose of raising up an asylum for the relief of suffering, and at the same time, for the improvement of his own profession without the prospect – nay, we may say without the possibility – of an adequate reward?[22]

Sir Fielding Ould, the hospital's second Master from 1759–66 faithfully carried out Mosse's wishes for the construction of the new auditorium, which survives today as the Ambassador Theatre, and also the magnificent chapel in the hospital building, which lay at the heart of Mosse's religiously-inspired vision. This continues to be used as an ecumenical place of worship. It is especially notable for the Baroque stucco work by Cramillion, and for its ornate Venetian window.

Sunday promenades

The unique atmosphere of those eighteenth-century 'Sunday Promenades' was well captured by a contemporary visitor from London, who noted that:

> … except (for) some beds given, and endowed by private donors, the funds for the support of this charity, are raised from musical entertainments and from subscriptions to a right of walking in the garden at all times.
>
> They have built a large circular room called the Rotunda. Here they have an organ and orchestra for concerts, in the wet evenings of summer, and for balls in winter.
>
> Nay, it is something more than all these, it is a polite place of public resort on Sunday evenings. On these nights, the Rotunda and gardens are prodigiously crowded, and with the price of admission, being only sixpence, everybody goes.
>
> Whether this entertainment be strictly defensible, in a religious point of view, I shall not determine; but if the goodness of the end may in any instance be pleaded in jubilation of the means, I think it may in this.

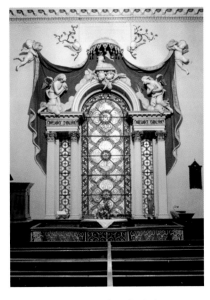

The ornate Venetian chapel window at the Rotunda
ROTUNDA HOSPITAL ARCHIVE

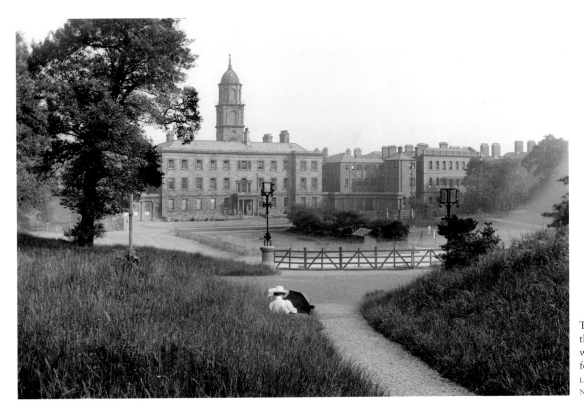

The gardens at the rear of the Rotunda Hospital were open to the public for a subscription.
LAWRENCE COLLECTION
NATIONAL LIBRARY OF IRELAND

63

However it seems rather a matter of wonder, that London, so fond of amusement, and so ready to accept new fashions of dissipation, has not struck out something similar for passing those hours, which on some people sit so heavy; and which may, after all, be spent in a much worse manner.

On these nights, the Rotunda and gardens are prodigiously crowded. It would perhaps benefit the charity, if the price were doubled, for though it might exclude a great many, it would, I think, bring more money.

On the other hand, it must be confessed that the motley appearance gives an air of freedom; for the best company attends, as well as those to whom another sixpence might be an object.[23]

Serious Dispute

Sir Fielding Ould was a distinguished obstetrician with a large Dublin practice, and he was present at the birth of a number of historic figures, including the Duke of Wellington. Ould was knighted in 1760, and this gave rise to the often-quoted poem by a Dublin wit:

> Sir Fielding Ould is made a Knight,
> He should have been a Lord by right;
> For then each lady's prayer would be,
> O Lord, good Lord, deliver me!

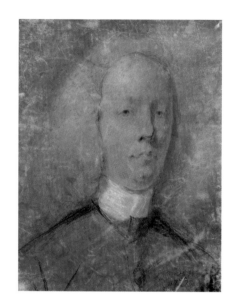

Sir Fielding Ould, 1710–1789,
Male Midwife, 1759
Charcoal with white highlights on card
by Thomas Hickey

Ould made a significant contribution to Irish medicine, and his book titled *A Treatise on Midwifry* was regarded as one of the truly original major obstetric works published in English, and included a number of important observations as well as practical advice on the subject. As noted previously, one of the earliest books on midwifery written in English was by a Trinity graduate James Wolveridge. It was published in 1671, and included material from other earlier works.

Sir Fielding Ould's book was dedicated to the College of Physicians, but his hitherto cordial personal and professional relationship with the institution deteriorated badly in 1756, when he applied to the College, and also to Trinity College, for permission to be examined in Medicine.

Field had been at Trinity earlier in his career, chiefly as a dissector, but he had left without a degree in Medicine. His application to both Colleges led to a major rift between the two institutions, which had worked together closely for over six decades.

The College of Physicians looked down on midwifery, and had determined back in 1736 that no-one who practised midwifery should become a physician. They decided that no-one could hold both their Licentiate in Medicine and their Licentiate in Midwifery. Despite the fact that they did not have the power to prevent people from practising both, they steadfastly refused to examine Fielding, by now a highly-distinguished figure, for a medical degree.

To some this might appear as snobbery, but it was more than that – it was also about the nature of the medical profession and how it should develop, as well as partly because the Rotunda were issuing their own Licentiates in Midwifery, which they had no right to do.

However Trinity College went ahead and awarded Fielding a medical degree in 1761. By doing this they were breaking their existing agreement with the Royal College of Physicians. Those at the College were greatly offended, and made changes to their links with Trinity. This coolness persisted for over 20 years, but wiser counsel eventually prevailed, and in 1785 Sir Fielding Ould and several other obstetricians were admitted as Licentiates of Medicine.

One medical historian claimed however that 'the relationship between the College of Physicians and Trinity College would never again be as close as it had been before this dispute'.[24]

Swift's Hospital

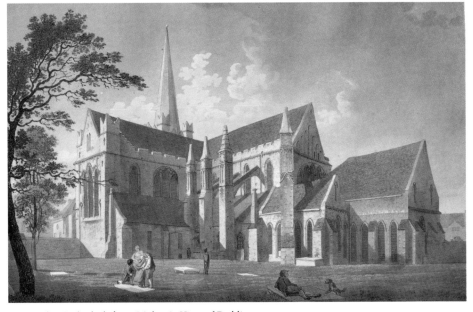

One of the pre-eminent figures in Irish society was Jonathan Swift, the Dean of St Patrick's Cathedral; he was also a writer and satirist of international stature.

With commendable Christian generosity and pragmatism, he left in his Will the huge sum of over £10,000 for the establishment of a haven of refuge and treatment for the incurable and insane. It opened in 1756, some eleven years after his death.

According to his bequest, it became known as St Patrick's Hospital, and Swift, as always, had the last word. He described his donation thus, in his final *Verses on the Death of Dr Swift*:

Bust of Jonathan Swift in
St Patrick's Cathedral, Dublin

He gave the little wealth he had
To build a house for fools and mad;

St Patrick's Cathedral, from Malton's *View of Dublin*.
RCPI

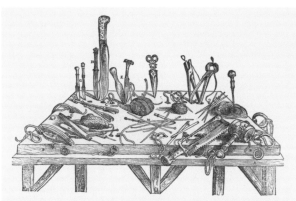

A series of eighteenth-century surgical instruments

Dr Samuel Clossy

Dr Samuel Clossy, who was elected as a Fellow of the College in 1761, was a pioneer in the study of morbid anatomy. A medical graduate of Trinity College, he worked briefly at Dr Steevens' Hospital, at St George's Hospital, London, and also at Mercer's Hospital, where he was appointed as a physician in 1761.

One of his seminal works, published in 1763, was *Observations on some of the diseases of the parts of the human body. Chiefly taken from the dissection of morbid bodies*. However, his zeal for dissection was not without its dark humour.

Clossy himself described the case of an Elinor Proudfoot, aged 20, who was admitted to Mercer's in 1762. She was complaining of a pain in her hips, which had spread to her thigh and leg, and down to her ankle. Within a month she had developed a large abdominal tumour, which Clossy thought to be 'most likely ovarian'.

However in a neat twist of dry humour, Clossy himself noted that in November his patient had left the hospital 'for fear of being dissected'!

Somewhat surprisingly, Clossy left for New York, hardly a year after his prestigious appointment to Mercer's. He did well in America and eventually became Professor of Anatomy and Natural Philosophy at King's College, later the University of Columbia.

Clossy fared less well during the American War of Independence, and he left New York in 1780. On his return to London he somewhat optimistically sought compensation from the authorities for the loss of his salary and property in New York.

However shortly before his death, he received another kind of compensation, literally without price, when, on St Luke's Day 1784, he was 'unanimously elected as an Honorary Fellow of the College of Physicians'.[25]

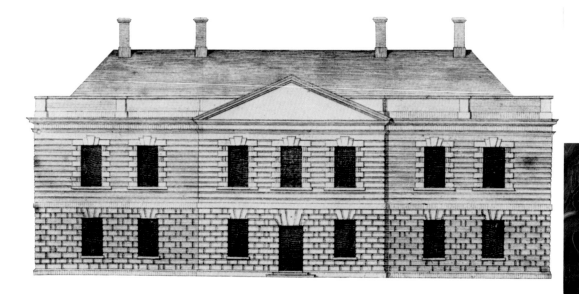

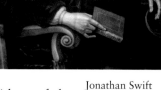

Jonathan Swift
BELFAST CATHEDRAL

And showed by one satyric touch
No nation wanted it so much.

Among Swift's wide range of associates was his doctor, a Dr Richard Helsham, Professor of Natural and Experimental Philosophy, and later of Medicine, at Trinity. Helsham was President of the College of Physicians in 1716 and 1725. Swift was close to Helsham, whom he described in1729 as:

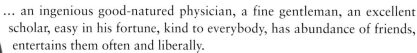

> ... an ingenious good-natured physician, a fine gentleman, an excellent scholar, easy in his fortune, kind to everybody, has abundance of friends, entertains them often and liberally.
>
> They pass the evening with him at cards, with plenty of good meat, and wine, eight or a dozen together. He loves them all, and they him.
>
> He has twenty of these at command. If one of them dies, it is no more than 'poor Tom'. He gets another, or takes up with the rest, and is no more moved than at the loss of a cat. He offends nobody, is easy with everybody. Is not this the true happy man? [26]

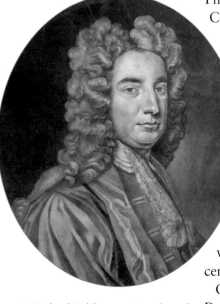

Dr Richard Helsham was President of the Royal College of Physicians in 1716 and 1725, and also also a friend of Dean Jonathan Swift. Helsham died in 1738 and gave instructions that: 'before my coffin be nailed up, my head be severed from my body and that my corps be carried to the place of burial by the light of one taper only at the dead of night without Herse or Pomp attended by my Domesticks'. [27]

RCPI

Swift's slightly barbed compliments to Helsham also provide a fascinating vignette of the rich social life of a successful Irish physician in the eighteenth century.

One of the richest and most fashionable physicians of the period was Dr Henry Quin, who as mentioned earlier was also a King's Professor of the Practice in Medicine, a Fellow and seven times President of the College of Physicians. He was known for his good 'bedside manner', and he had a large and lucrative practice. He was described by the well-connected socialite, Mrs Delaney, a member of Swift's circle, as, 'a very sensible, good physician, and an ingenious and agreeable man'. [28]

One historian has noted that:

> Although Quin did not contribute to any medical advancements, he promoted the development of modern medical teaching, and was a generous patron of the arts. [29]

He held much-appreciated soirées in his home at St Stephen's Green in Dublin, and he developed some particularly interesting hobbies. He became interested in collecting old gems, and set up a laboratory in Dublin to study the reproduction of gems, with the assistance of a stone-cutter and modeler, James Tassie. Quin soon recognised Tassie's creative skills, and encouraged him to go to London where he became considerably successful in the development of gem imitations.

Quin also became the patron of the medallist William Mossop, and also the seal-cutter, John Logan, at a time when young craftsmen greatly needed benefactors.

Henry Quin also had an eye for business and property, and was an original subscriber to the Bank of Ireland, to which he gave the considerable sum of £5,000. On his wife's death he acquired a large fortune. He died at his home in St Stephen's Green in 1791, at the age of 74, and left a large portfolio of property worth around £70,000.[30]

Quin was not a polymath like William Petty or Thomas Molyneaux, but he was a physician who did very well for himself indeed in eighteenth-century Ireland.

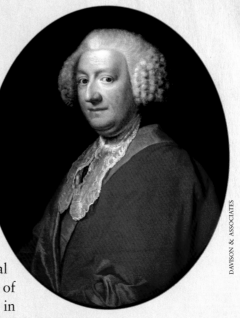

Dr Henry Quin, 1718–91 by an unknown artist

Dr Quin was President of the Royal College of Physicians seven times. He was described by a member of Dean Jonathan Swift's circle as, 'a very sensible, good physician, and an ingenious and agreeable man'.
RCPI

Hard Times

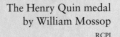

The Henry Quin medal by William Mossop
RCPI

However, not every physician enjoyed such affluence. Dr John Rutty, who became a Licentiate of the College of Physicians in 1729, was a Quaker, and lived austerely in rented rooms in Little Mary Street. He was a good man and a good physician, but unfortunately many of the patients he treated were unable to pay him, though some may have been unwilling to do so. He noted in his diary:

… the medical profession exhibits strongly the vanity and wickedness of the world, where the more work, the less pay-a pretty handsome supply of paupers, but few of the rich-much medical work and little wages. Lord give patience! Eight patients and not a penny.[31]

Rutty was a considerable scientist in his own right, and the Royal College of Physicians gave him a subsidy to publish his wide-ranging *Essay Towards a Natural History of the County of Dublin*, which was published in two volumes in 1772.

One of the College of Physicians' most noteworthy Licentiates in Medicine was Dr Robert Emmet, who was Physician and *ex-officio* Governor of St Patrick's Hospital for more than 30 years. His record was unequalled in the Hospital, where the first Physician had been Dr Robert Robinson, a Fellow of the College of Physicians, and the son of a College President, Dr Bryan Robinson.

It was said of Dr Robert Emmet that he personally examined and treated every patient he admitted in the first five years of his appointment, without a salary.

Turkish Delight

In sixteenth and seventeenth century Dublin there were many exotic characters. One truly outstanding figure was a Dr Achmet Borumbodad, a Turkish physician who arrived in Dublin in 1771.

He persuaded the local physicians and doctors to back his scheme for erecting public healing baths on the Dublin Quays. They supported him with a petition to the Irish House of Commons for financial help, and he received some £400 of public money for his project. The College of Physicians also gave him £50.

Some 800 people were treated in the Baths in 1774–5, and a very large sum of well over £5,000 was spent on their enlargement. Around 10,000 people were treated between 1775–81, but Dr Borumbodad found himself in serious financial difficulties, as he still owed nearly £2,300 to the builders.

He appealed to Parliament for further help, and promised that if this was forthcoming, he would make the Baths public property, suggesting that they be placed under the governance of the College of Physicians.

No more was heard of the petititon to Parliament, or of 'Dr Borumbodad', who allegedly had fallen in love with a Miss Hartigan and declared his true Christian identity as a Patrick Joyce from Kilkenny.

However, the duplicity of the 'Turkish' physician had a positive ending, in more ways than one. In 1784 'Dr Borumbodad's' premises were sold to the Commissioners for 'Making Wide and Convenient Streets', and their work from 1785 onwards created a network of Georgian roads and squares which became the architectural glory of Dublin.

Their initiatives were complemented by the extraordinary creativity of the architect, James Gandon, whose designs included those of the Custom House and the Four Courts.

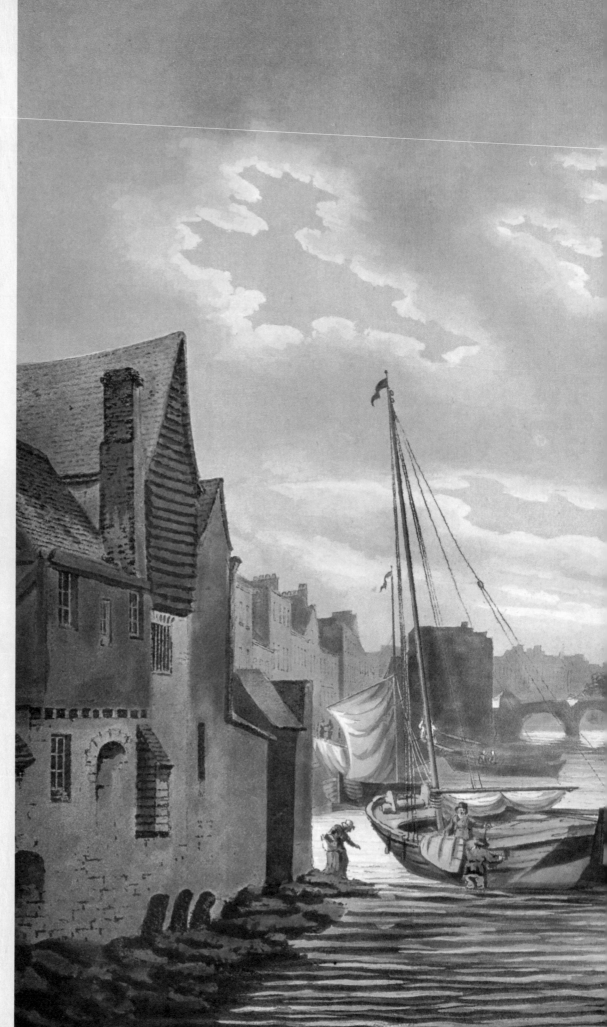

The Law Courts, and the river Liffey beside which the 'Turkish' physician, Dr Achmet Borumbodad allegedly set up his Healing Baths.
From Malton's *View of Dublin*
RCPI

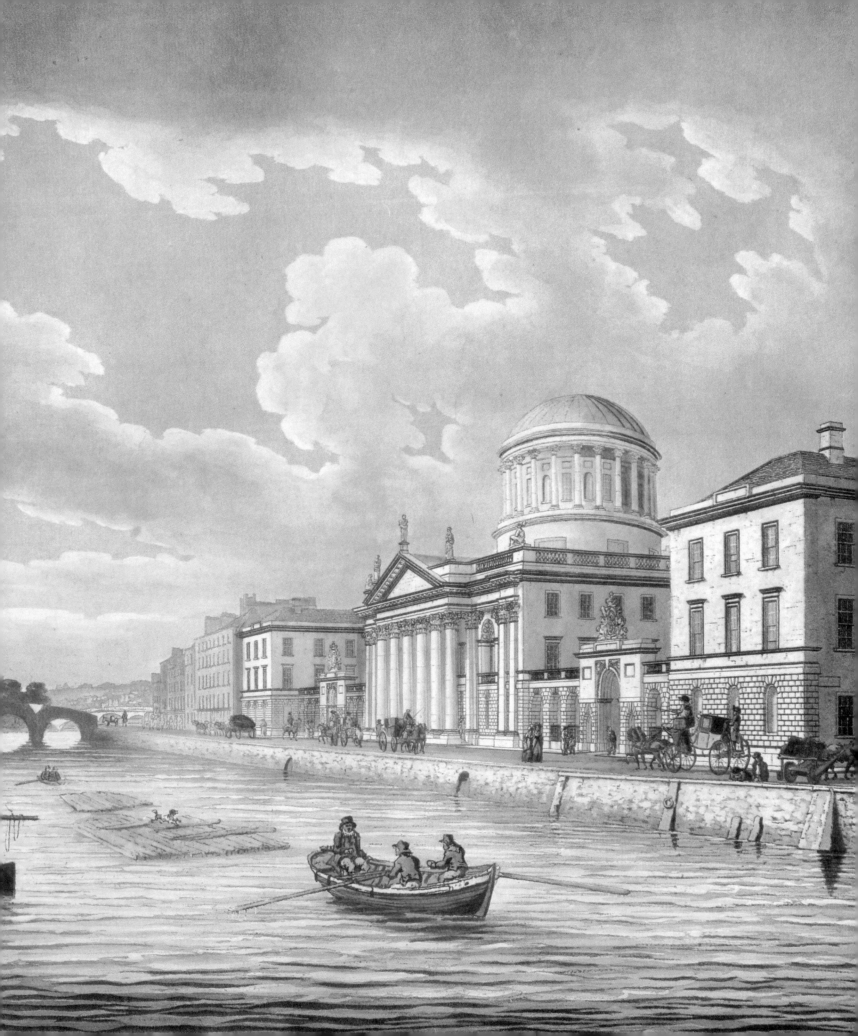

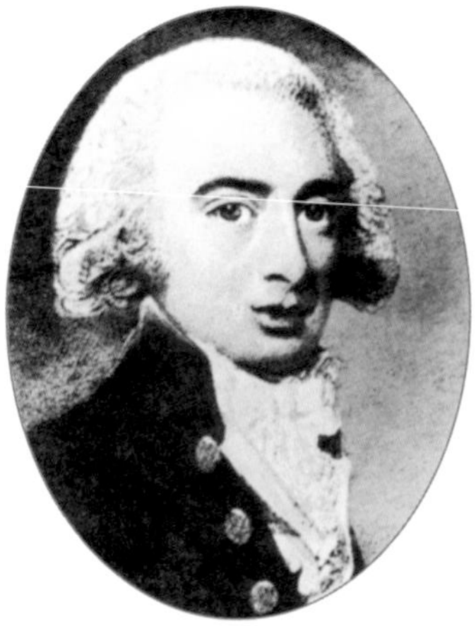

Dr Robert Emmet

Powerscourt House which underlines the elegance and prosperity of parts of eighteenth-century Dublin
From Malton's *View of Dublin*
RCPI

His fellow Governors were so impressed that they subsequently granted him an annual fee for his services, and he played a leading role in the Hospital's management. He was appointed Treasurer in 1777, and six years later the Governors presented him with a silver plate 'as a Memorial, not compensation'.[32]

Dr Emmet's professional life was exemplary, and he attended his last Board meeting on 3 May 1802. He died the following December, but he was spared the personal tragedy of witnessing the execution of his son, Robert Emmet, the Republican who made a memorable speech from the dock before he was hanged in Dublin in 1803, following an attempted uprising. His brother Thomas had been imprisoned for his part in the 1798 rising, but he had later emigrated to New York where he pursued a successful legal career.[33]

The dramatic story of the Emmet family over two generations graphically encapsulates the history of the growing importance of medicine in the country

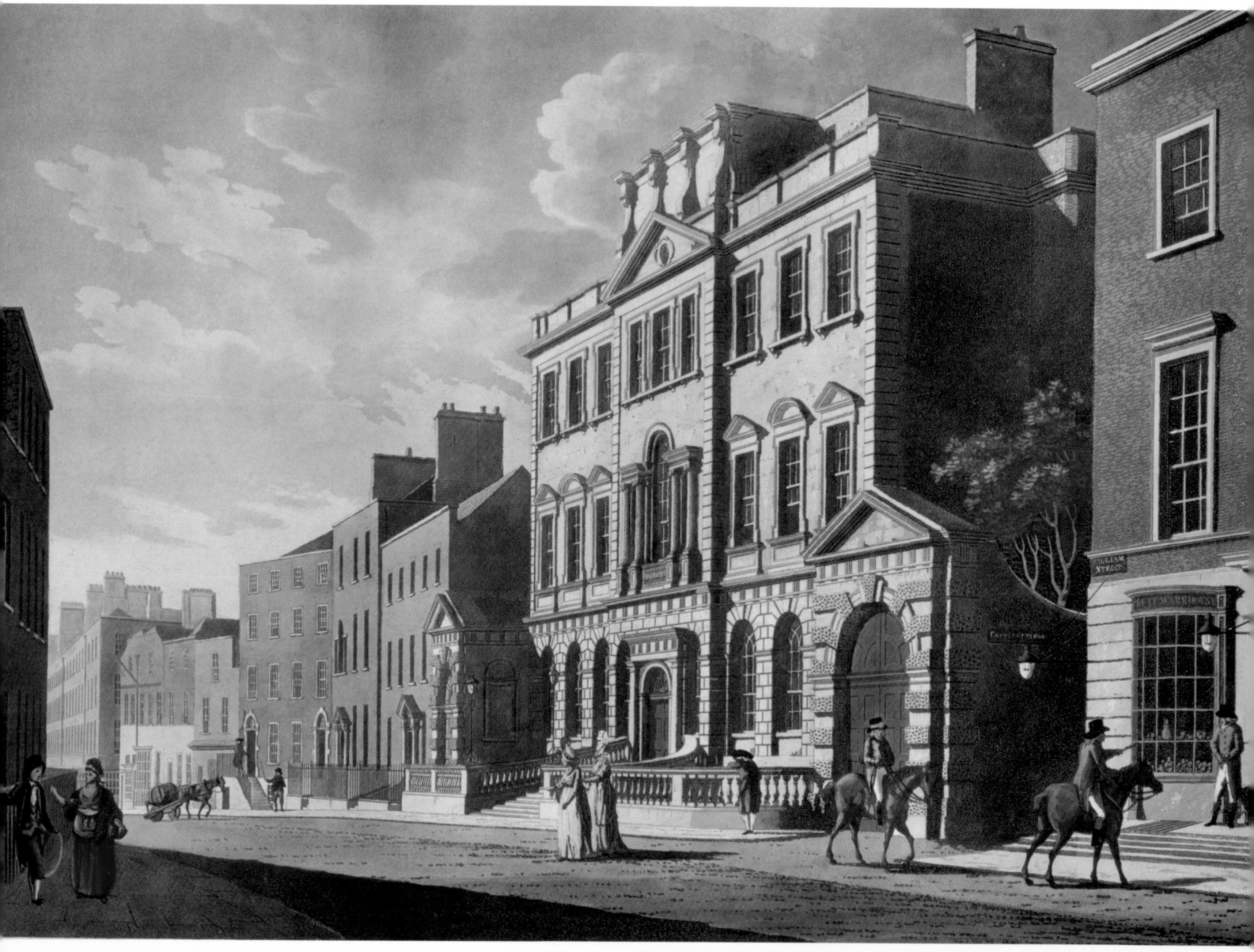

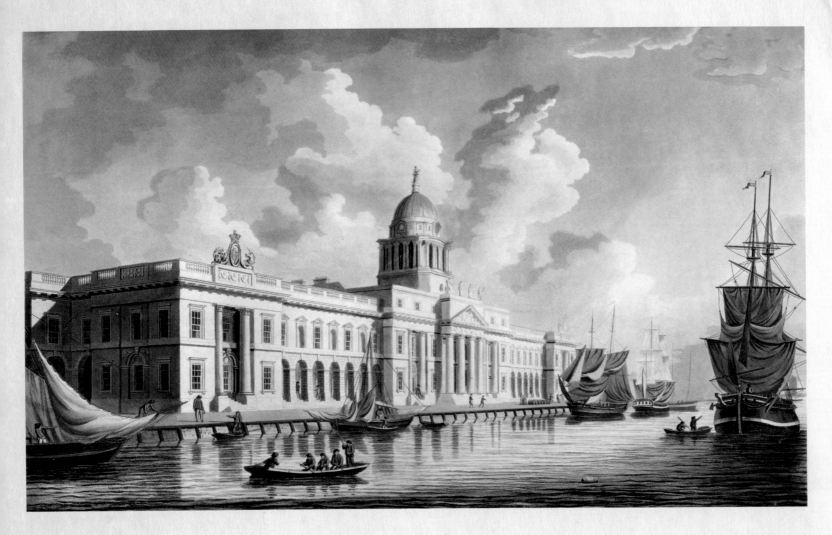

against the background of political and social turbulence of the eighteenth-century.

The Act of Union of 1801 produced an entirely new political relationship between England and Ireland. Only time would tell whether or not this would be an improvement on what had gone before.

The new century, however, would also see what came to be known as the Golden Age of Irish Medicine. However, without the assiduous eighteenth-century groundwork carried out by the Royal College of Physicians of Ireland and the other institutions and individuals who brought discipline and organisation to medical practice, this new 'Golden Age' would scarcely have been possible.

The Four Courts from Malton's *View of Dublin*
RCPI

The engraver and watercolourist James Malton (1761–1803) was employed as a draughtsman in the office of the famous architect, James Gandon, known for building the Four Courts (1786–95), the Custom House (1781–91) and King's Inns (1795–1815).

'Malton's prints are, arguably, the most important series of engravings of eighteenth century Dublin.'[34]

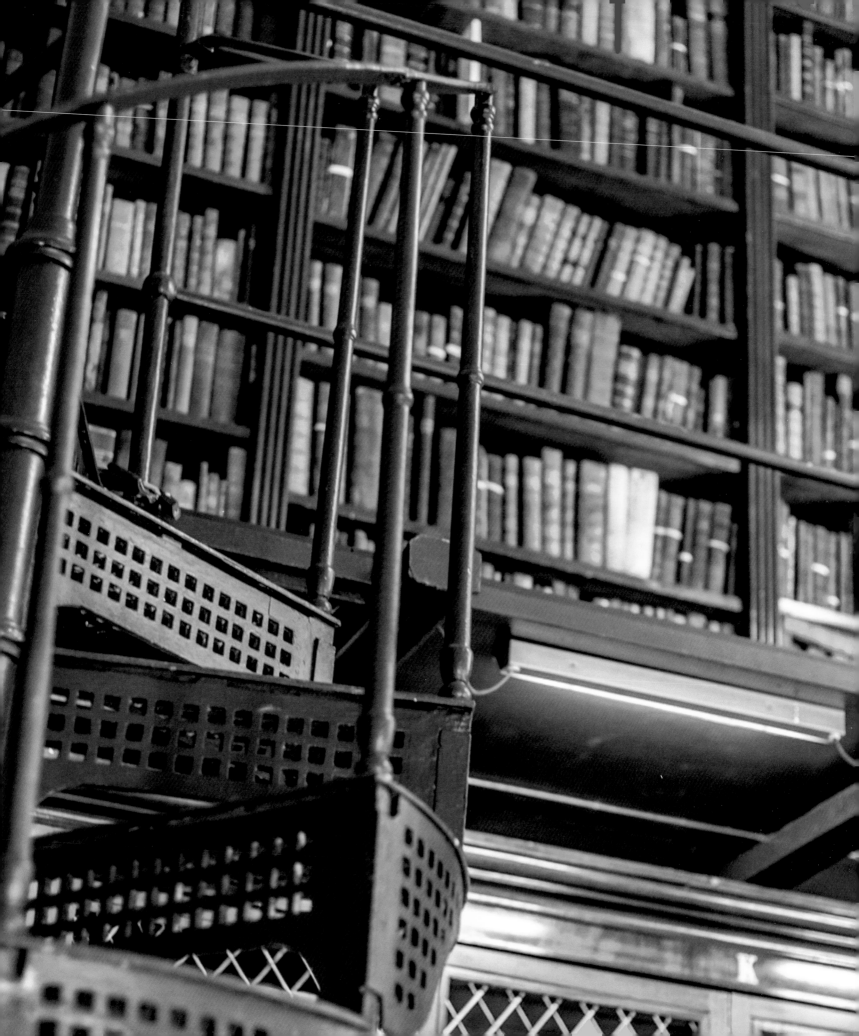

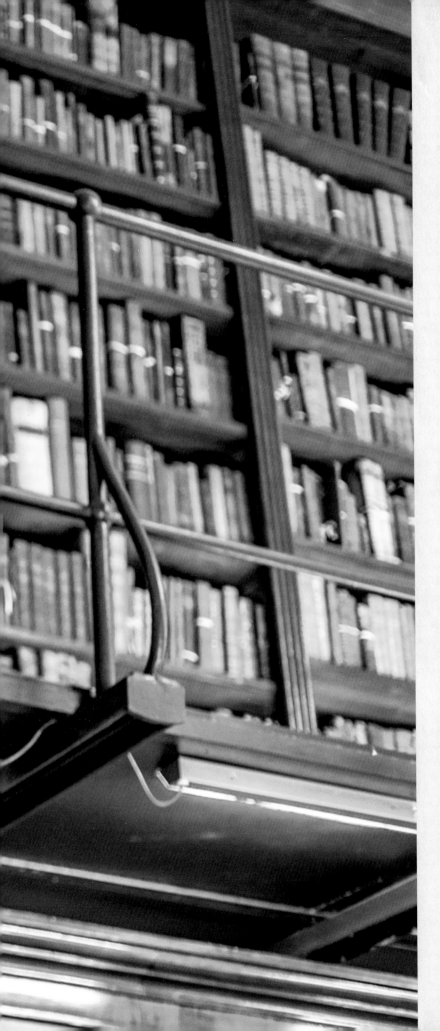

Dun's Library
Vision and Reality

The twists and turns in the history of Dun's Library match the complex story and fluctuating fortunes of the College of Physicians over the past four centuries. Its establishment was part of the vision of Sir Patrick Dun, and while its evolution was difficult and sometimes painful, it is today an outstanding historical medical library.

In his Will of 1711, Sir Patrick outlined his ideas for a library with typical clarity. He stated:

> I would give my books for the lawful use of the sd Professors and College of Physicians … [they must] give Bond and security to keep and preserve the sd Library and all and every Book and Books in it, and if any should be lost or wanting, to pay for or purchase another of the same kind, the same paper and edition or better, in the room thereof.[1]

Dun also stipulated that the Professors should be given access to his library which was kept in his house on Inns Quay, and that this room should also be used as a meeting place for the College, which at that stage did not have its own premises.

This arrangement worked well for several years, and for each of the years from 1714–16 the College Treasurer stipulated that a guinea be paid to Lady Dun's servant for his trouble in attending the College, and half a guinea to Lady Dun's maidservant. Unfortunately, however, the relationship with the difficult Lady Dun deteriorated and, when she left for a long stay in Bath in 1717, and kept her Dublin house locked up, the College had neither meeting place nor access to their library.

However there was an important development in 1725. Dun's real estate was conveyed to the College, and on 16 January the following year the Minutes recorded that Dr Helsham should deliver the contents of Dun's Library and catalogue to Dr Cope, one of the College Censors.

The College finally had possession of the books. And in one of those peculiar twists of fortune which make history so fascinating, the successful transfer of the Dun Library was in fact a rare stroke of luck. Just a few years later, on 1 September 1728, Dun's house was very badly damaged by a fire which would most probably have destroyed his entire library of books, had they still been on the premises.

A report in the Dublin Intelligence newspaper underlined the extent of the damage:

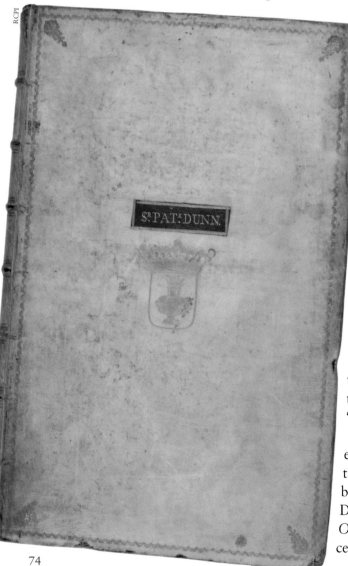

So great a loss as was here was not sustained by any fire in the city these many years, the house being exceeding full of exceeding valuable goods, as well as clothes, plate and linen, little of which were saved for the owner, that part of them which was unconsumed being mostly taken away, several of the mob barbarously expressing there was no pity due for the loss.

Unknown Quantity

One of the problems about Dun's Library is that no-one knows the exact content of the original collection which was bequeathed to the College .

Harriet Wheelock, RCPI's Keeper of Collections, has underlined that the catalogue of the Library transferred to the keeping of Dr Cope in 1726 has not survived, nor have any of the manuscript catalogues or reports on the Library which were compiled during the eighteenth century.

She said: 'We do know from a statement made to an Irish House of Lords Enquiry in 1742 that there were some 300 volumes in the Library at that time, which were held by the then Registrar Dr Henry Quin and that the catalogue was "in a chest of lumber with the old books"'.[2]

This is hardly encouraging. However in 1794 the earliest existing catalogue of Dun's Library was published showing that, of the 1,179 titles listed, only 112 were published before 1713, and therefore could possibly have belonged to Dun. Yet only one of these, Marcello Malpighi's *Opera Omnia*, which was published in 1687, can be identified with certainty as having belonged to Dun, whose name is on the title page. It is clearly the same signature which is on the relevant Minute books of his time with the College.

Harriet Wheelock has suggested that the reason why so little is known about Dun's Library and why many of the original contents have been lost, lies in the nomadic existence of the College: 'It had no permanent home during the eighteenth century. Meetings were held in the houses of the different Presidents and moved the library from house to house on several occasions.'

Ownership

The administration of Dun's estate proved difficult, as has been noted earlier. Although the College had full ownership of the property, following the death of Lady Dun in 1748, disputes continued about the use of the money, and it took Acts of the Irish Parliament in 1741, 1785 and finally in 1800 to settle the matter. The most important of these Acts, for the Library, was that of 1785 which virtually guaranteed its survival.

It stipulated that:

> … [the] surplus of the clear rents and profits of the said Sir Patrick Dun's estate after the payment of the yearly salaries shall be applied to the support of clinical lectures, for purchasing medical books for the use of the students in physic.[3]

It was decided that the books would be kept in the medical lecture room at Trinity, and that one of the King's Professors would be appointed as Librarian, and would give a Bond of Security for the books, as had been directed in Dun's Will.

Furthermore, the Librarian was to be in attendance twice a week to give out books to Fellows and students as requested, and to make sure that a full catalogue was kept; Dun's name was to be stamped on the covers of all the books.

Irregularities

So far, so good, but much depended on the ability and commitment of the Librarian. On 19 September 1787, Dr Stephen Dickson, the King's Professor of the Institutes of Medicine, became the first Librarian, and received large amounts of money from the estates to buy new books.

Thus within seven years there was a record of over 1,100 books in Dun's Library, but by 1797, Professor Dickson had lost his position as Librarian and

Marcello Malpighi's *Opera Omnia*, published in 1687, can be identified with certainty as having belonged to Dun.
RCPI

was reprimanded by the College. Worse was to come, and two years later he was deprived of his Fellowship for having been absent from the meetings of the College for two years without leave.

Not surprisingly Professor Dickson disappeared from view, and it seems likely that he left Ireland. His reasons for lying low, and leaving the country entirely, became clear in a subsequent inquiry which discovered irregularities in the Library accounts. A catalogue of 1800 revealed that many books which should have been in the Library had been 'lost by Dr Dickson'. In other words, the first Dun's Librarian had been 'brought to book' three years earlier, but the precious volumes themselves remained lost.

Happily, a turning-point for the Library came with the 1800 Physic Act, which determined that funds would be used to build a Sir Patrick Dun's Hospital, and the Library was to be safely kept in the new building.

Harriet Wheelock notes that:

> Properly housed and cared for by diligent librarians, the Library was finally
> what Dun had intended – namely, a library for the students and Fellows.
> Funds were also made available to ensure that the collection was developed,
> and kept as up-to-date as possible with the advances in medicine.[4]

From the early nineteenth century onwards, the Dun's Library was steadily improved. One of its great benefactors was the peppery Regius Professor of Physic in Trinity, Dr Edward Hill, whom we met in a previous chapter.

He was appointed the Dun's Librarian in 1819, when he was 78 and in his eightieth year, he produced a manuscript catalogue of the Library. Like subsequent Dun's Librarians, he donated many of his own important books, and helped greatly to strengthen the collection.

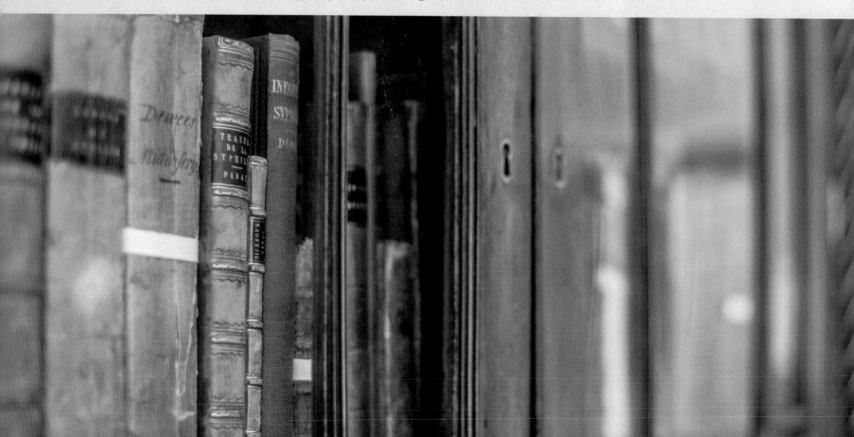

His successor, Dr TH Orpen produced a second printed catalogue in 1827, which showed 1,419 entries. That was an increase of just 300 books in more than three decades, but the collection was growing steadily. When Orpen published a catalogue supplement in 1832, there were another 325 entries – a five-year increase which matched the input of the previous 30 years.

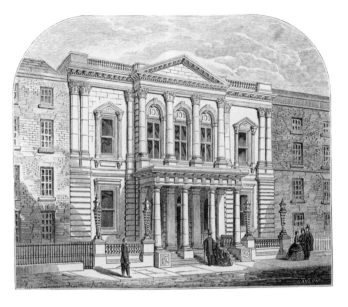

Breakthrough

A major breakthrough in the history of the Dun's Library was its relocation to the new College headquarters at 6 Kildare Street from 1864. At last the Library had a purpose-built location, and it was not just a lending library but also offered a reading room for Fellows and Licentiates.

Engraving of the façade of the Royal College of Physicians, No 6 Kildare Street, Dublin, based on Murray's plans published in the *Irish Builder*, 1862
RCPI

For the first time, a non-medical person was appointed to run the Library, while a Fellow of the College was elected as Librarian. The first appointee was Dr Thomas Belcher, who was also one of the first historians of the College.

Harriet Wheelock summarises the advances thus:

> The move to Kildare Street provided space for the development of the collections. The nineteenth century is the best-represented period in the Library's Collections, with an extensive and important range of books, pamphlets and journals, which have a special focus on Irish medicine.[5]

There are collections from several particularly notable Fellows, including the obstetricians Fleetwood Churchill, Sir Arthur Macan and Thomas Wrigley Grimshaw, a physician and Registrar General for Ireland, as well as books on eye diseases from Arthur Benson, and on mental illness from Dr Connolly Norman.

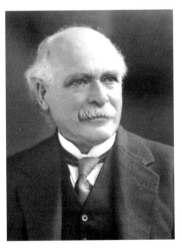

Dr TPC Kirkpatrick
RCPI

Difficulties

Towards the end of the nineteenth century, funds for the Library had decreased because of the reduction in income from Dun's estate, and this serious problem remained during the early 1900s. However the College was fortunate in its appointment of Dr TPC Kirkpatrick as Registrar in 1910. During his term of office, which lasted until his death in 1954, he also became the *de facto* Honorary Librarian.

A keen bibliophile and a medical historian, he did much to promote and protect the Library, partly by donating many items to the collection, and encouraging others to do so. Some of the unique and most important items in Dun's Library were gifts from Dr Kirkpatrick.

Sadly, however, the Library began to decline after his death, and the Librarian Gladys Gardiner had so many responsibilities related to the administration of the College that she had little time to devote to Dun's Library.

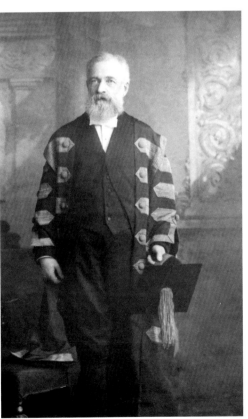

Thomas Wrigley Grimshaw
RCPI

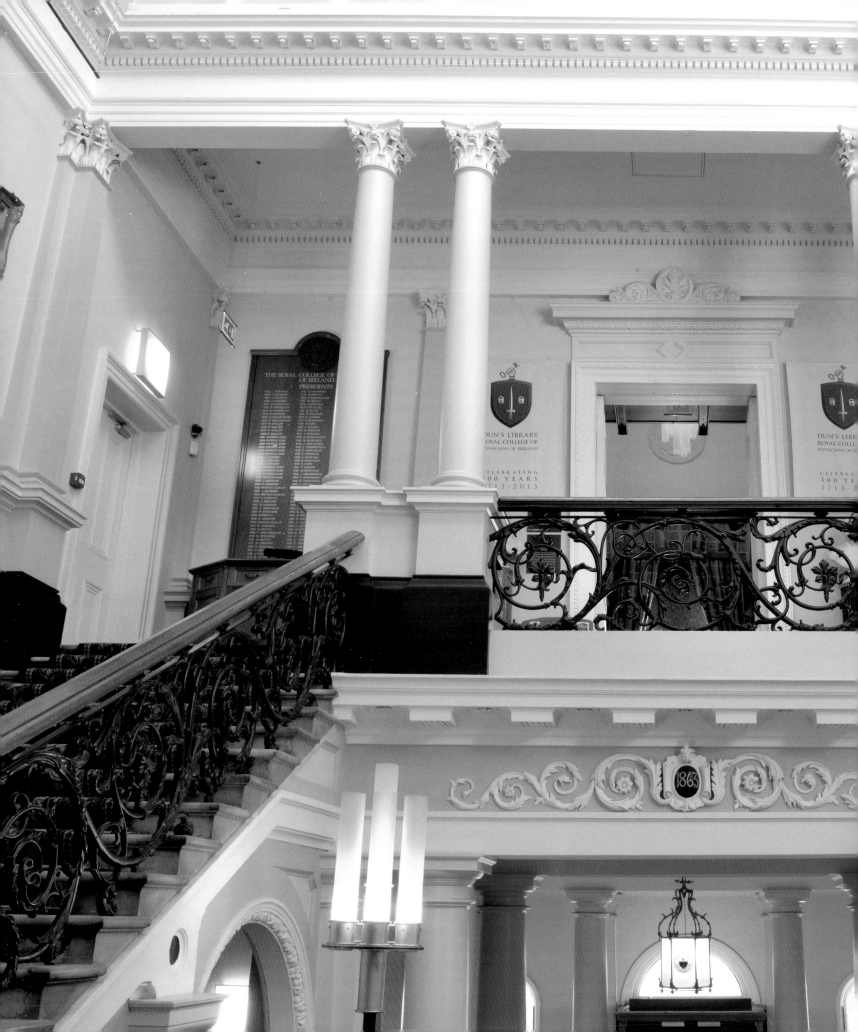

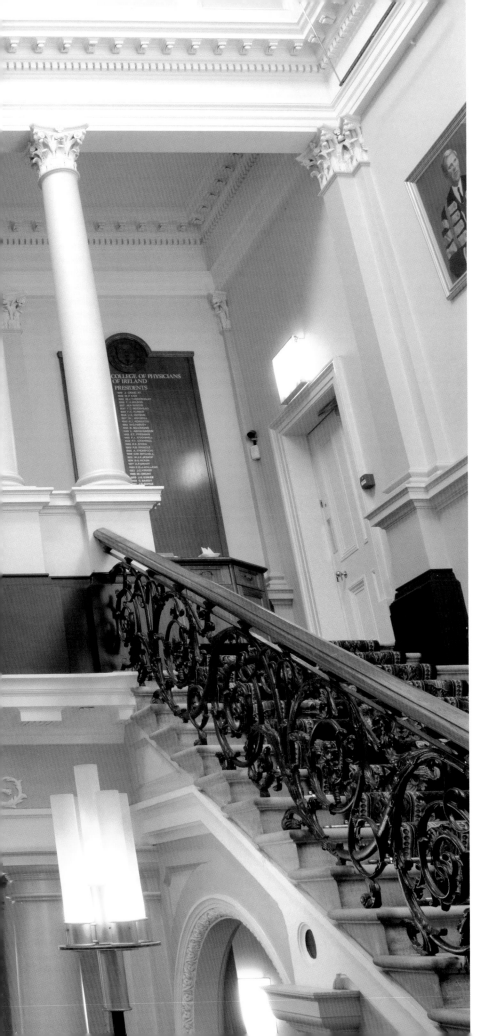

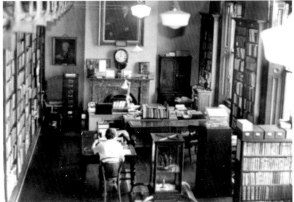

Dun's Library, 1960s
RCPI

In 1971, a Wellcome Trust Report outlined the serious decline in the following blunt terms:

> Sir Patrick Dun's Library is well on the way to being chocked as a useful entity by the failure to adapt to modern conditions. The sad thing is that one of the most valuable medical libraries in the British Isles should have remained virtually static for the past fifty to one hundred years; a historical library, which, to speak frankly, masquerades as a current one, occupying as it does an area which is visited for the most part by readers who have no desire to consult old books.

Scathing

Such scathing criticism challenged the College fundamentally, and recent decades have witnessed a renewed interest in Dun's Library. As Harriet Wheelock observes:

> Essential conservation on the books has been carried out, and is continuing. A current e-cataloguing project is opening the contents to a worldwide audience, and with the archive and other collections held by the Heritage Centre, Dun's Library has become one of the most valuable resources for the study of the history of medicine in Ireland.
>
> As Dun intended over 300 years ago, his Library is still in the home of the College in Kildare Street, and it is available for the use of all Members and Fellows. It is also available to anyone with an interest in the history of medicine in Ireland.

The staircase leading to Dun's Library, 2014
DERMOTT DUNBAR

No doubt, Patrick Dun himself would heartily approve of the translation of his eighteenth-century vision into its subsequent and up-to-date reality.

The Importance of Not Being Discreet …
Sir William Wilde and the RCPI

Oscar Wilde, the famous Irish author, playwright and wit, noted in his 1890 novel, *The Picture of Dorian Gray*, that: 'There is only thing worse in the world than being talked about, and that is not being talked about.'

However a man who was greatly talked about in his lifetime was Oscar's father, Sir William Wilde, a distinguished eye-and-ear surgeon, and the author of important works on archaeology and folklore. He was also an accomplished medical historian, and is still regarded as one of the great figures of the 'Golden Age' of Irish medicine.

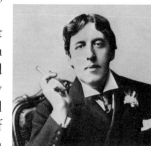

Oscar Wilde
FROM *OSCAR WILDE VOL 1,*
BY FRANK HARRIS, 1916

Prowess and Scandal

Sir William attracted widespread attention for his medical prowess and his achievements as a world-renowned doctor, but also for his colourful personal life which would have kept today's tabloid press busy with stories about his amorous adventures.

As a surgeon, Wilde was not a member of the College of Physicians but he had a strange, and indeed unique, link which proved to be of long-term benefit for the College.

Sir William had had three illegitimate children before his marriage to Jane Francesca Agnes Elgee, a poet who published her work under the pen name 'Speranza'. In later life he had a liaison with a Mary Josephine Travers. However Wilde's affection for Miss Travers waned, apparently because she had become very demanding. Then as now, however, hell hath no fury like a woman scorned, and Mary Josephine refused to allow the matter to fade away quietly.

She accused Wilde of various indiscretions, and of assaulting her sexually during a consultation: an accusation which naturally displeased his long-suffering wife. Somewhat inadvisedly, Lady Wilde expressed, in writing, her strong objections about her husband's alleged lover, and Miss Travers sued her.

This became a cause célèbre in the Dublin of the day, and although Miss Travers won her case, it was a somewhat Pyrrhic victory. She was awarded damages of only one farthing, although Lady Wilde was left to pay hefty legal costs.

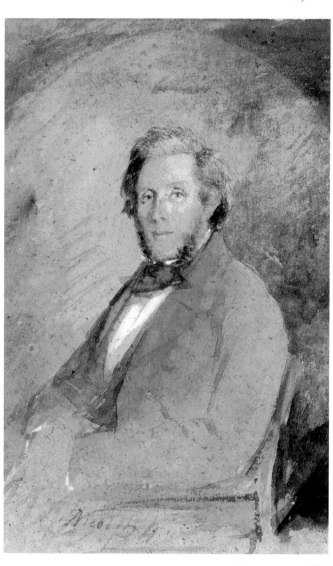

Sir William Wilde, 1815–76, father of Oscar Wilde, was a distinguished eye-and-ear surgeon and also an important author and medical historian. His work on the 1851 Census has been described by Sir Peter Froggatt as, 'one of the greatest demographic studies ever conducted'. It became a standard reference work on the Great Famine.[6]

Portrait by Erskine Nicol
NATIONAL GALLERY OF IRELAND

Innocent

An innocent victim however of this social debacle was Mary Josephine's father, Dr Robert Travers, a Fellow of the College of Physicians, and also Professor of Medical Jurisprudence at Trinity College.

Significantly, Dr Travers was also for some thirty years the Assistant Librarian at Marsh's Library. This was a Church of Ireland library, and the oldest 'chained' library in Dublin.

Dr Travers had also amassed a considerable personal library which contained important medical books, as well as others dealing with history, natural sciences, theology and other topics. He intended to leave his collection to the Marsh Library, and after such long service as an Assistant, he had well-founded expectations that he would be appointed as the Librarian.

This did not happen, and people surmised that this may have been because he was not a member of the Church of Ireland, which required that the Marsh Librarian had to be an Anglican. This sounds plausible, but another even more important factor may have been the public scandal surrounding his daughter and Sir William Wilde.

Snubbed

Whatever the reason for Dr Travers' non-appointment, he felt snubbed by Marsh's Library, and he left his important collection of books to various other institutions, including Dun's Library.

So, ironically, Sir William Wilde and Miss Mary Josephine Travers were instrumental in helping to bring an important collection to the College!

Sadly, however, the whole episode damaged Wilde's reputation, and after his wife's libel trial he spent more and more time at his country home in the Corrib region. However he is best, and deservedly, remembered today as one of the most significant figures Irish medical history.

Dr Paul Darragh
Dun's Librarian

Dr Paul Darragh, the current Dun's Librarian, is a consultant in Public Medicine with the Northern Ireland Public Health Agency, which is based in Belfast.

He became a member of the Royal College of Physicians of Ireland in 1976, and a Fellow ten years later. He succeeded another Belfast consultant, Dr Michael Scott, as the Dun's Librarian in 2004. Dr Darragh remarks:

> This is a fascinating role and I am deeply interested in the history of medicine, particularly the environment surrounding the development of medicine, and how it can be studied within the context of its times. The Dun's Librarian has oversight of the Heritage Centre, bringing together and safeguarding the College's collection of books, pamphlets, artworks, silverware, medical instruments and historical memorabilia.

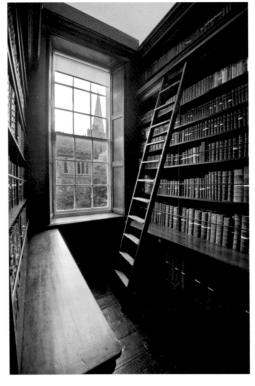

Marsh's Library was founded in the early eighteenth century by Archbishop Narcissus Marsh (1638–1713). Designed by Sir William Robinson (d.1712), the Surveyor General of Ireland, it is one of the very few eighteenth-century buildings left in Dublin that is still being used for its original purpose. Many of the collections in the Library are still to this day kept on the shelves allocated to them by Marsh and by Elias Bouhéreau, the first librarian, when the Library was opened.
The interior of the Library has remained largely unchanged since it was built three hundred years ago. It is a magnificent example of a late Renaissance and early Enlightenment library.
The Library is run as a charity.
MARSH'S LIBRARY, DUBLIN

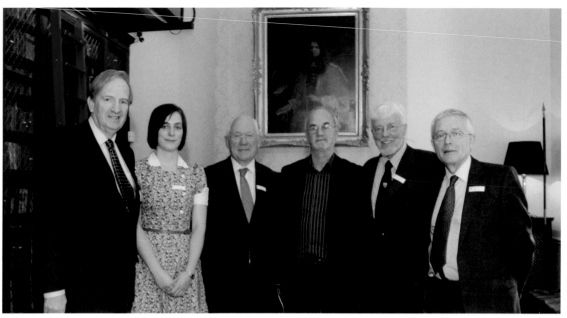

FROM LEFT: Current and past Dun's Librarians, Prof. Davis Coakley, Harriet Wheelock (Keeper of Collections), Prof. John Murphy, Robert Mills (former Librarian), Dr Michael Scott and Dr Paul Darragh. This photograph was taken in October 2013 during celebrations for the 300th anniversary of the library.

RCPI

These include the Kirkpatrick Index of obituaries of Fellows of the College and, most noteworthy, doctors of Irish origin from the seventeenth to the mid-twentieth century. The Heritage Centre acts as a central point of contact for enquiries about historical information, and promotes the study of the history of medicine on behalf of the College.

One of our main objectives is to remain relevant in the age of social media, and the Heritage Centre's blog and Twitter-feed have proved very popular and have helped to raise awareness of our collections. Our large archive collection, which was catalogued with support from the Wellcome Trust, has proved very valuable to researchers, and is frequently consulted by scholars.

It is very important to have an electronic catalogue of our holdings, so that medical historians and others can source material from the comfort of their home or office desk. When they spot something which they need, they are more liable to come and consult the 'hard copy' of the book itself.

When I took over, we did not have a catalogue online, but Harriet Wheelock, our Keeper of Collections, has carried out important work in this area. The overall size of Dun's Library is around 30,000 volumes, including pamphlets and journals, with half the collection stored on-site, and half in off-site storage. The online catalogue contains records for about half of the Library's collection.

Cataloguing of the rest of the Library remains a substantial challenge, and the lack of a complete catalogue is preventing the Library from being used to its full potential.

Given his role and personal interest in the history of medicine, Dr Darragh has a great appreciation of the value of the Dun's Library:

> One of our great strengths is in Irish medical history, particularly from about 1780 to 1900.

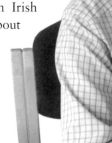

Dr Paul Darragh, Dun's Librarian

ALF McCREARY

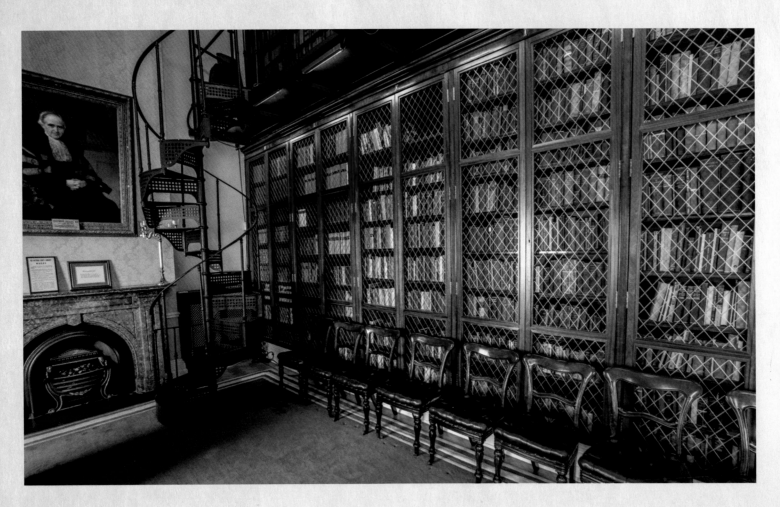

The Library at No 6 Kildare Street
RCPI

This represents a time when the Royal College of Physicians of Ireland was flourishing, and when Irish medical figures were among the world's leaders. Dun's Library also holds the personal libraries of several important figures from this period.

We have an extremely valuable asset in our possession, and the history of our past and that of Irish medicine is in good hands. However, in looking to the future, we face crucial decisions on what is the continuing purpose of the Dun's Library, what material needs to be retained, and what can be let go or used for other purposes.

The Dun's Library is and has been a brilliant acquisition, and physically the main room exudes knowledge, learning and grace. However it is our continuing challenge to preserve these qualities and also to remain relevant to the wider world in this all-consuming age of the internet and social media.

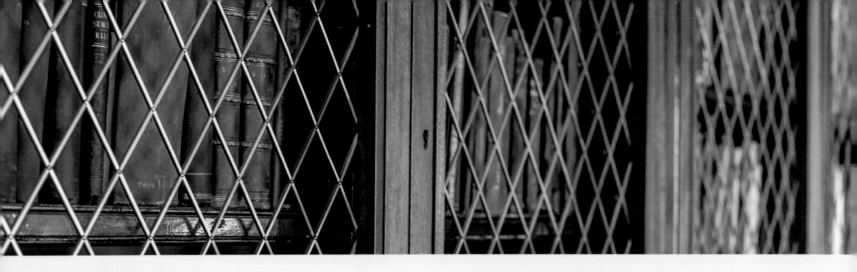

Dun's Librarians

Under the Will of Sir Patrick Dun, his personal library was left to RCPI, however as they had no permanent home the books were cared for firstly by his widow and then Fellows of the College.

Books in the care of

1713–26	Lady Dun
1726–43	Dr Henry Cope
1743–1756	Dr William Stephens
1756–1787	Dr Quin

In 1787 Dun's Library was moved to the Medical School in Trinity College and a Librarian was appointed from amongst the Fellows of RCPI.

Librarians

Sept 1787–May 1797	Dr Stephen Dickson
May 1797–Oct 1808	Dr John William Boyton
Oct 1808–Oct 1815	Dr Hugh Ferguson
Oct 1815–April 1819	Dr Peter Edward McLoughlin
April 1819–Nov 1819	Dr Francis Hopkins
Nov 1819–Oct 1826	Dr Edward Hill
Oct 1826–Oct 1833	Dr Thomas Herbert Orpen
Oct 1833–Oct 1840	Dr Samuel Litton
Oct 1840–Dec 1845	Dr John O'Brien
Jan 1846–March 1865	Dr George Alexander Kennedy

In 1865 Dun's Library moved to its current home in No 6 Kildare Street, and at the same time the College decided to appoint a non-medic as Dun's Librarian, to care for the library and carry out administrative work for the College. One of the Fellows was also appointed Honorary Librarian.

Honorary Librarian

Oct 1865–April 1869 Dr TW Belcher

Dr Belcher was the only Fellow to hold the title of Dun's Librarian. Dr TPC Kirkpatrick acted as the Honorary Librarian from c. 1910 until his death in 1954, although he never held the title.

Dun's Librarians and Clerks

Oct 1865–Oct 1883	HJ Fennell
Oct 1883–Oct 1884	TH Innes
Oct 1884–July 1894	SW Wilson
July 1894–Oct 1896	JC Benson
Oct 1896–Feb 1948	RGJ Phelps
Sep 1948–Oct 1979	Miss G Gardiner

In 1976 the first professional librarian was appointed to look after Dun's Library, and in 1980 the title of Dun's Librarian was given to a Fellow appointed by the College to oversee the running of the library.

Librarian

Oct 1976–May 1978	Miss M Ainscough
Sep 1978–May 2013	Robert Mills

Keeper of Collections

May 2013–present	Harriet Wheelock

Dun's Librarian

1980–1991	Dr Robert Towers
1991–1994	Prof Davis Coakley
1995–1997	Prof John Murphy
1997–2005	Dr Michael Scott
2006–present	Dr Paul Darragh

New Century,
New Challenges

The nineteenth century in Ireland was a
period of continued political turbulence
during which the 1801 Act of Union created a
new and radically different relationship
between the two islands. This in turn led to
yet more struggles for Irish self-determination
as the decades progressed.

O ne historian noted that through the Act of Union:

> The two countries were made one, the economy of Ireland was assimilated
> into the economy of England, the Irish Parliament at Dublin disappeared,
> and the Parliament at Westminster henceforth legislated for both countries.
>
> It was as if a marriage between England and Ireland had been celebrated,
> with the clauses of the Act of Union as the terms of the marriage settlement
> … The reality, however, was very different. The primary object of the Union
> was not to assist and improve Ireland but to bring her more completely into
> subjection.[1]

Be that as it may, another historian observed:

> After the excitement and the rapid changes of the later eighteenth century –
> the glittering pageant of the Volunteer movement, the high sense of national
> achievement in The Constitution of 1782, the hopes and fears aroused by
> the United Irishmen, the courage and terror in the insurrection, the bitter
> dispute and fiery eloquence amid which the legislative union had at last been
> carried – after all this, the political life of Ireland in the early 1800s seemed
> drab, and, at least to outward appearance, almost meaningless …
>
> It was not until the 1820s that the genius of O'Connell transformed …
> [the demand for Catholic Emancipation] … into a popular movement, and
> so gave, for the first time since the Union, a national character to Irish
> politics.[2]

The century also included the disastrous Great Famine in Ireland and continued
wars abroad, in which many Irishmen including doctors took part, as well as
the long reign of Queen Victoria.

The Victorian Era, which lasted from 1837–1901, marked the zenith of the
Empire and left its mark on so many aspects of British and Irish political, social

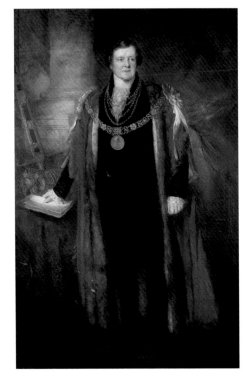

Daniel O'Connell, 'The Liberator'
Painting by Catterson Smith the elder,
RHA, 1841–2

and cultural life. It was against this rich and eventful background that the medical profession in Ireland gradually grew in stature.

Sir Patrick Dun's Hospital

However, one of the noteworthy developments of the early part of the century owed its origin to the past. The completion of the Sir Patrick Dun's Hospital in 1816 was the final chapter in the story of the long-deceased man who had done so much to make the Royal College of Physicians of Ireland a reality.

The foundation stone of Sir Patrick Dun's Hospital on Artichoke Road, which later became Grand Canal Street, was laid in 1803 by the Reverend Dr Kearney, Provost of Trinity College. The building was developed in stages, partly through a lack of funds; it was finally completed in 1816. Though Sir Patrick never intended that a hospital should be established in his name, its development is very much part of the story of the Royal College of Physicians of Ireland.

Although a number of voluntary institutions had been set up in Dublin in the eighteenth century, as described previously, there was an urgent need for a clinical hospital for teaching medical students.

One of the most distinguished members of the medical profession was Robert Perceval, a former President of the Royal College of Physicians, and also the Professor of Chemistry at Trinity College. He was acutely aware that if Dublin continued to lack a teaching hospital it could not hope to compete for students with places like Leiden and Edinburgh, and he persevered against considerable opposition to establish such an institution in Ireland.

There had been previous attempts to found a hospital in association with the Royal College of Physicians, but these ultimately proved unsuccessful. In 1788 the Royal College took over a house in Clarendon Street and fitted it up as a hospital. It had 16 beds and opened only during the winter months. However it was closed after two years due to the high cost of maintenance, compared to other Dublin hospitals, and directions were given that the equipment should be transferred to Mercer's Hospital or Dr Steevens' Hospital.[3]

In 1793 there was a further, but no more successful, attempt at providing a teaching hospital. A house was taken on Blind Quay, later known as Wellington Quay, and it was fitted-up with 31 beds. A Physician-in-Ordinary was appointed in February that year, under the patronage of the Royal College of Physicians.

By November 1793, over 250 people had been treated, mainly for contagious diseases, and each day there was a visit from at least one of the Medical Professors. However the running costs were too high, and only £96 had been received in public subscriptions over four years.

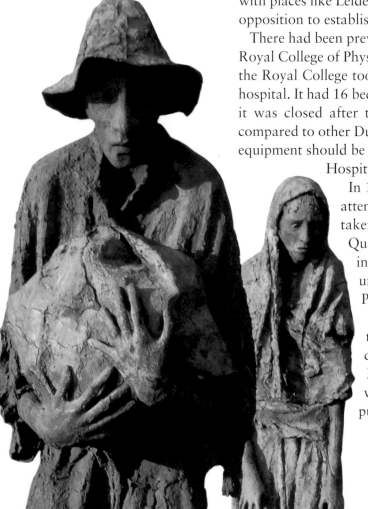

The Famine Memorial on Custom House Quays in Dublin, by Rowan Gillespie, 1997.
The sculpture is a commemorative work dedicated to those Irish people forced to emigrate during the Famine. Starving victims arriving in the city brought enormous problems of both disease and fever for the medical profession to cope with.
PHOTOGRAPH BY FINTAN MULLAN

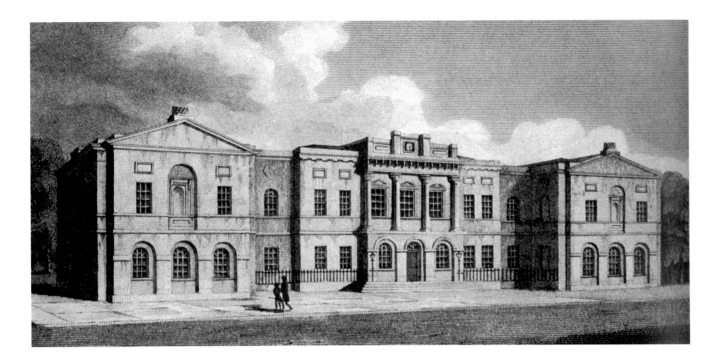

Sir Patrick Dun's Hospital, Dublin. The foundation stone was laid in 1803 and the building was finally completed in 1816.
RCPI

Despite the heavy expenditure, it appears that no clinical lectures were given at this hospital, and it closed in November 1796.[4]

Robert Perceval and his supporters had not only vision and persistence, but also political friends in high places, and as a result of their influence and persuasion, the School of Physic Act of 1 August 1800 stipulated that £1200 from the Dun's Estate would be used to build a new teaching hospital.

This was a significant step forward for the medical profession in Ireland. Clinical lectures were given earlier at Mercer's Hospital and in Dr Steevens' Hospital while the new teaching hospital was being built. The lectures were eventually transferred to Sir Patrick Dun's Hospital in 1808, and for more than 150 years the Hospital played an important role in the education of thousands of medical students; it made a key contribution in other ways too, including midwifery and nursing.

However it was continually short of money, until – with other institutions – it benefitted from the Irish Hospitals' Sweepstake from the mid-twentieth century.

Sir Patrick Dun's Hospital closed in 1986 as part of the redistribution of medical services in Dublin. Sir Patrick Dun would undoubtedly have been astonished at the way in which his vision had worked out in practical terms, so long after his death.

New Home

The establishment of Dun's Hospital in the early nineteenth century was also a timely bonus to the Royal College of Physicians of Ireland.

Significantly, the new hospital gave a permanent home to the College which hitherto had had a peripatetic existence since Lady Dun had closed the doors of her house. The building provided accommodation not only for Sir Patrick Dun's Library, but also a room for the Royal College, as well as one for the new hospital's governors.

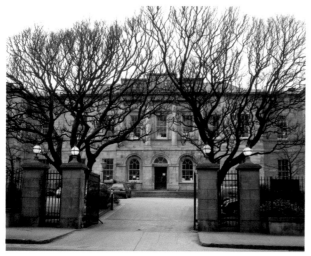

The former Sir Patrick Dun's Hospital on Grand Canal Street, now occupied by the HSE (Health Services Europe)
DUBHEIRE

However the physicians of the College found the new arrangement unsuitable, and in 1824 they prepared a petition for the Government in which they described the rooms as 'remote and unsuitable'.[5]

Part of their agenda was their failure to establish a state-of-the-art premises for the Royal College, despite a promise from the Government at the time of the 1692 Charter that they might obtain one of the houses confiscated from the supporters of the defeated King James II.

The physicians were also aware that the Royal College of Surgeons in Ireland had received around £30,000 in endowments and grants. The Royal College of Physicians would however have to wait for several more decades before

Dr Osborne
1794–1864

Dr Jonathan Osborne, who was President of the Royal College of Physicians from 1834–35, was Physician-in-Ordinary at Sir Patrick Dun's Hospital and also a physician at Mercer's Hospital. He wrote many scientific papers, and in 1840 he was elected Professor of *Materia Medica* and Pharmacy at Trinity College: a post he held until his death 24 years later.

Dr Osborne is considered to be Ireland's first nephrologist, and made an important contribution to nephrology, the study of kidney disease.

His first publication was *A Sketch of the Physiology and Pathology of the Urine* (London, 1820), and his name was associated with William Charles Wells, of St Thomas' Hospital, London, and John Blackall of Exeter, as well as Richard Bright, whose work led to the identification of 'Bright's Disease'. This is used in modern medicine to describe a kidney disorder associated with acute or chronic nephritis.

Osborne was an independent thinker who initially queried Bright's conclusion. However he wrote later:

> I was quite unprepared to admit its correctness, and I have become a convert to his opinion only by virtue of a long series of observations, many of which were instituted in the expectation of overthrowing it.[6]

Professor Brian Keogh, who was President of the Royal College of Physicians from 1997–2000, noted in a paper written with an American colleague Dr JF Maher in 1992, that Osborne's writings:

> ... were characterised by originality of thought, and by classical learning. His peers considered him an admirable teacher, with an original mind and an ardent thirst for knowledge. He was full of information, and none could communicate it more happily.[7]

Osborne also wrote *The Annals of Sir Patrick Dun's Hospital*, which was published in 1831. These contained a short outline of the life of Sir Patrick Dun as well as a review of the complicated events after his death, and the developments leading up to the establishment of Dun's Hospital.

Professor Osborne underlined importance of the hospital to the local community, and its geographical importance to Dublin port as the only hospital close to the river. This meant that a large number of patients suffering from fevers and other illness contracted abroad could be admitted to Dun's for treatment with the least possible delay.

In later life Professor Osborne was badly affected by rheumatism and he expressed the wish to be buried in the upright position as he did not want 'any fellow at the Resurrection' to have any advantage over him.

Whether or not Osborne was merely joking, his family and friends obviously took him seriously. His coffin was placed upright in the vaults of St Michan's Church in Dublin, where a number of other distinguished medical men were buried in a more conventional manner.

Death is a great leveller, but on this occasion the literally upright Professor Osborne had the last word ...[8]

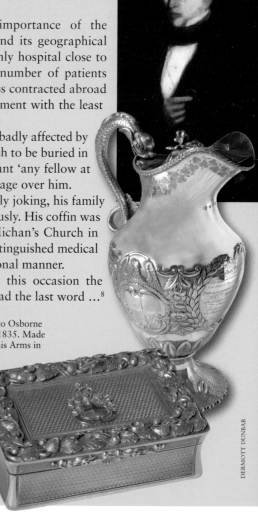

A large silver gilt snuff box, which was presented to Osborne by the College when he vacated the Presidency in 1835. Made in Dublin specially for the occasion, the lid bears his Arms in relief, edged by a border of oak leaves and acorns. The other object is a handsome silver flagon, with a handle in the form of a dolphin, also Dublin-made (1837), and given to Osborne by his pupils. Both items were collected by Dr Percy Kirkpatrick, and were presented to the College after his death by his sister, Miss Sybil Kirkpatrick.[1]
RCPI

DERMOTT DUNBAR

they could establish premises which they would regard to be commensurate with their professional status and social prestige.

One of the recurring problems was of course finance, and in the early years of the nineteenth century the College was hard up. Without significant help from the Government and other benefactors, the establishment of a new College Hall was out of the question, at least for the time being.

The worrying state of the financial situation was confirmed in 1816, when a Committee was appointed to inquire about the income from Dun's estate. It found that there was a balance of just over £110, and debts amounting to over £170, which was not a healthy state of affairs.

The Committee discovered that in 1792 the College had paid 30 guineas for a hogshead of claret for the retiring President. This extravagant practice was to last for another few years, but it was stopped between 1795 and 1802, and, in a period of strict controls on expenditure, the only annual outlay was a payment of two guineas to the Bedell.

However the President's gratuity for holding office had been reintroduced, and by 1808 it was raised to £50. This practice of paying for services rendered was then extended, and the Treasurer and the Registrar, who had previously been unpaid, began to draw 20 guineas each. It emerged that since 1802, over £1,087 in total had been paid to the President, Treasurer and Registrar, and more than £714 to the Censors in the course of carrying out their duties.

The Committee pointed out that if this not inconsiderable amount had been invested at a rate of simple interest, the total would, by 1816, have increased to £2,219. This would have been almost enough to build a College Hall, which was 'an object justly considered of the greatest importance to the profession'.[9]

A watercolour of the headquarters of the Royal College of Surgeons in Ireland, 1810. The College was established in 1784.
ROYAL COLLEGE OF SURGEONS IN IRELAND

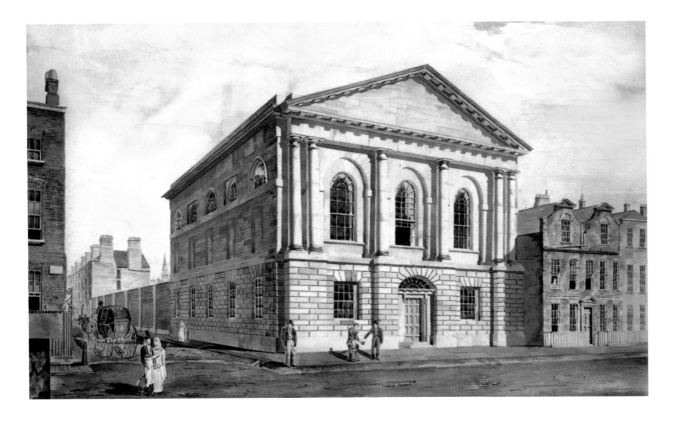

89

To add to the problem, the Royal College had an annual income from Licentiates of just £150 a year, because on average only three people were admitted annually.

Shortfall

It was clear to the Committee, and to anyone with even a rudimentary knowledge of accounting, that the College was spending more than it brought in, and that no financial reserves could be accumulated.

Very wisely, the Committee advised that expenditure should be reduced to the 1801 level, and it was recommended that no grant be given to any of the College officers in future out of the Dun's estate private funds.

However this was challenged by the then President, Francis Hopkins, who put forward a written case for continuing the honorarium, because the President:

> … not only furnishes a place of accommodation for the reception of the body, but by prescriptive usage incurs a positive expense for their gratification.[10]

However his appeal was unsuccessful, and the College decided to cut back its expenditure. The situation was so bad financially that in November 1816 Dr Batholomew Dillon, a Licentiate who had retired to Waterford, hearing about the difficulty of the College in collecting the money from Dun's estate in that same county, offered to organise a better way of doing so.

The Hibernian Marine School '… built as a nursery for orphans, and unprovided sons of seafaring men, where they are fostered, educated and reared for the sea-service in general. It is situated on the south bank of the river [Liffey] … half a mile further up the river, on the opposite, or north side, appears the Custom House.'
From Malton's *View of Dublin*
RCPI

With shipping from around the globe entering the docks, disease spread quickly if an epidemic had broken out, such as the Asiatic cholera of 1832. It left millions dead across India, China, Russia, Europe and England. In Dublin alone, cholera affected 11,000 with the death toll put at 5,273 people. There was another outbreak in 1849. The tenements in Dublin were fever nests for disease, and were never truly free from infection.

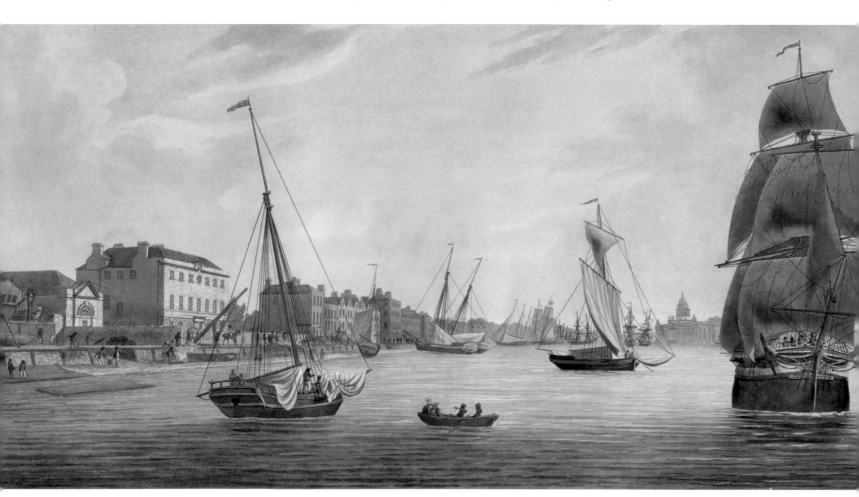

Dr Dillon even offered to put forward a large sum of his own money as security for the use of the College, as required. He may not have been aware of Sir Patrick Dun's unhappy experience of using his own money to help buy urgent medical supplies for the Kilmainham Hospital during the Williamite Wars. The generous and trusting Sir Patrick had fully expected to be re-imbursed later, but neither he nor his wife were paid one penny by the Government of the day, or thereafter.

Dr Dillon also had a contact, a P Walshe Esq., who had a portrait of Sir Patrick which had 'fallen into his hands by accidental circumstances', and if they did not already have a portrait of the great man, he would make it available.

The Royal College replied politely to Dr Dillon, pointing out that the office of agent for the Dun's estates was not vacant, but indicating that it would be grateful to receive Dun's portrait. So this was duly transported to Dublin in 1817, and the College Treasurer was ordered to collect it at the Grand Canal Harbour. He was also instructed to hand it over at the College's expense, to be placed either in the Library or the Lecture Room at Dun's Hospital.

A College Censor, Dr George Todderick, was entrusted with the portrait but before handing it over, he was required to find a properly qualified craftsman to retouch and varnish it, and to obtain a suitable frame. All of this was done at a cost to the College of 10 guineas, plus carriage expenses of 15s 2d. The portrait was eventually taken from Dun's Hospital to the present College Hall at No 6 Kildare Street where it is given pride of place to this day.[11]

More Challenges

The financial and other challenges facing the Royal College did not deter it from trying to fulfil its role as a medical body in addressing some of the major health problems of the day.

With the London College of Physicians and others, it attempted to address the vexed question of vaccination, and to deal with the various epidemics and other illnesses, including typhoid fever, smallpox and dysentery which so badly affected the population at large.

On 6 February 1805, a Royal Proclamation called for assistance from the medical profession in trying the prevent the spread of infectious fever, and the College met a fortnight later and stated that they 'were always ready to aid Government in such endeavours when called upon'.[12]

Despite its reputation and authority, the College was still small in numbers, and from 1801–6 the Fellows numbered only ten. The number of Licentiates varied from 25 to 31, so overall there were only 41 men at most who could legally describe themselves, according to the 1692 Charter, as 'physicians'.[13]

The College continued to adhere to its own high medical standards, and even in the first decade of the nineteenth century

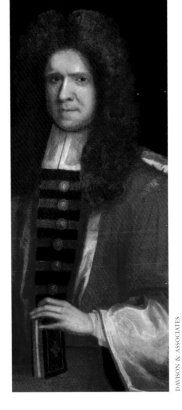

DAVISON & ASSOCIATES

When the portrait of Sir Patrick Dun was obtained by RCPI, it was believed to be by Sir Godfrey Kellner. However, when it was taken for restoration in the 1980s, it was found to be signed 'TP' – for Thomas Pooley. Pooley was the leading portrait painter in Ireland in Dun's time.

RCPI

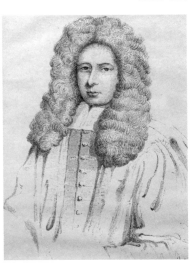

Engraving of Sir Patrick Dun

RCPI

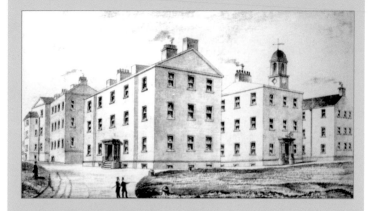

The Establishment of Cork Street Fever Hospital 1801

A number of public-spirited men including Arthur Guinness Jnr, Samuel Bewley and John David La Touche, helped to establish this hospital, and led a wide campaign against the spread of fever in the Dublin Liberties.

The Minutes of the first two meetings of the provisional Hospital Committee, which came together on 23 October and 28 October 1801 at the Royal Exchange Buildings, Dublin (now City Hall), show that those present had a clear idea of the nature and scale of health problems in a city where fever had been raging since 1798. The minutes state that:

> ... no adequate Hospital accommodation has hitherto been provided for the relief of the Sick poor of Dublin afflicted with fever (especially such as may be of a contagious Nature)... It has been found by experience that every exertion heretofore made for the relief of persons labouring under the above disorders at their own Houses has in great measure failed in producing the wished-for effect.

Committee members believed that the solution lay in the 'establishment of a House of Recovery, to which patients on the first appearance of Fever might be removed'.[16]

Just over two years later, on 14 May 1804, the first batch of female patients were admitted. The Fever Hospital consisted of two buildings: one for the sick, the other for convalescents.

The records from Cork Street Fever Hospital are held in the RCPI archive.[17]

Brú Chaoimhín Community Nursing Unit, formerly The House of Recovery, Cork Street Fever Hospital

declared themselves greatly disturbed by the number of people who practised without qualifications.

In an 1806 report they complained that:

> With regard to quacks, whose gross ignorance is notorious, though their number is not so great in this country as in England, yet they do much mischief by imposing on the credulity of the ignorant, and distributing their nostrums.

The College physicians also continued to jealously guard their status, and in the same report, they declared that medicine should be professed only by those suitably qualified, and stated firmly that 'the branches of Physic, Surgery and Pharmacy could be practised, as far as existing circumstances will admit, distinctly from each other'.[14]

Resentment

There was resentment among others in the medical profession who found the College stipulations restrictive, and one historian noted that:

> The Physicians, in their zeal, underestimated the competency of those Irish practitioners who practised medicine without obtaining a licence from the College, and overlooked the peculiarly enlightened views of the Irish surgeons'.[15]

The Royal College of Physicians was a conservative body, so much so that its physicians worried about the use of English, rather than the traditional Latin, when examining candidates for medical degrees. This, they believed, would eventually prove 'injurious' to the characters of members of the profession. This attitude may have been a mixture of respect for the Latin language which had served medicine well for so long, as well as a touch of elitism, and the anxiety (which assails most conservative groups in times of change) that new-fangled developments are not always for the better.

Accordingly, the King's Professors were told not to attend any examination for medical degrees if the questions and answers were to be spoken in English, and when acting as clinical lecturers they were 'to take the cases and make the report on the patient in Latin'.[18]

Changing Times

Nevertheless, changes were taking place within the profession at large, and the College had to keep in step with the times.

A Licentiates' group had been brought together in 1813 by Dr William Brooke, one of the most-respected and successful physicians of his era. He became a Licentiate of the College in 1793, and more than three decades later, his contribution to the profession, including his role as a lecturer in Medicine in Jervis Street Hospital Medical School, was recognised by the award of an Honorary MD from Trinity, and a Fellowship from the College.

Brooke was the obvious person to act as Chairman of the Licentiates' group, which hoped to give a more corporate expression of their views and interests. The problem had been that after the individuals had been granted their Licentiates, they had no further claims on the College, and no voice in running its affairs. In forming a group they could appoint delegates who hopefully could meet representatives of the College to discuss issues of mutual importance.

The Licentiates wanted to establish a Physicians' Hall, but the College made it clear that:

> ... there would be no backing for a College Hall, which the Fellows and Honorary Fellows wanted for themselves, but which they could not afford to acquire or to build.

Even though the agenda was therefore limited, an important meeting was held on 11 June 1816, roughly a year after the Battle of Waterloo, which helps to place in perspective the major political and international developments of those years during which the Irish physicians and their associates were trying to establish a greater corporate cohesion.

Incidentally it was a Licentiate of the College, Sir Fielding Ould, who had attended the Countess of Mornington in Dublin at the birth in 1769 of the Duke of Wellington, the victor at Waterloo.

During the meeting with the Licentiates on 11 June 1816, the College made it clear that it could

> ... in no respect whatever ... could it sanction the establishment of a Library or Reading Room, for the purpose of more intimately associating with the members of the College.[18]

However there was strong approval for the Licentiates' proposal to form an 'Association of the Members of the King and Queen's College of Physicians in Ireland', which would involve the 'individual co-operation of all the ... Fellows, Hon. Fellows, and Licentiates'.

The first meeting of the new Association, attended by 29 people, was held just over a fortnight later and, not surprisingly, Dr Brooke took the chair as President. This important development constituted Dublin's first Medical Society, but just like the Royal College of Physicians in its early days, it had no permanent home, and for years its members had to meet in the back area of a bookshop in College Green.

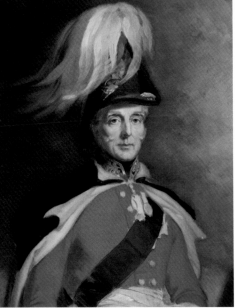

Portrait of Arthur Wellesley, 1st Duke of Wellington (1769–1852), by John Lucas
The Duke was delivered by Sir Fielding Ould. The Wellesley house was on Upper Merrion Street.

The Napoleonic Wars, and other major campaigns, created a huge and urgent demand for surgeons to help deal with the many injuries incurred on the battlefields and elsewhere.
NATIONAL GALLERY OF IRELAND

Dining Club

As with many professional bodies, where members like to relax in convivial company, the Association formed a dining club, and met bi-monthly six times

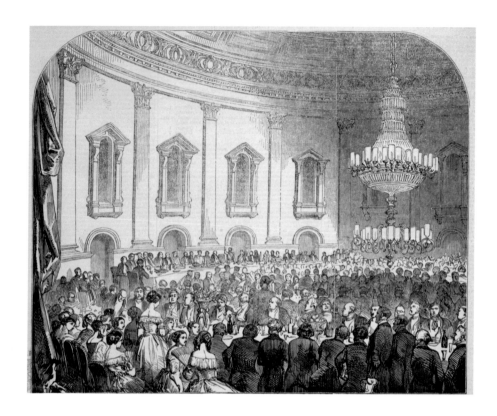

a year in a small room of the new Rotunda Hospital. Possibly to offset any suggestion that they would be accused of high-living, the members agreed that each meal would cost no more than 3s and 6d, and if wine was ordered, the total bill would be no more than seven shillings and, if possible, only six.

The meetings were to begin at 6 pm, according to the President's watch and in a subtle nod to the Almighty, any latecomer arriving after Grace would be fined sixpence, to be given to the cook. There is no record, however, of the cook encouraging members to arrive late!

The Association was however more than a gentleman's dining club. In the fourteen years after its establishment, the members produced five volumes of scientific papers. From 1832 onwards, further papers were published in the *Dublin Journal of Medical and Chemical Science.*

In 1864 the Association became the Medical Society of the College of Physicians, and in 1882 it constituted the Medical Section of the newly-founded Royal Academy of Medicine in Ireland.

Thus the development of the College and its associates into a more collective professional institution took a long time, and some people might argue that it took far too long.

Certainly in the early years of the nineteenth century the College appeared at times to be a faltering body with money problems, an inefficient administration, a conservative outlook, and a limited membership. It could also be argued, however, that, given the many tumultuous events Ireland had experienced since its earliest inception in 1654, it was something of a miracle that the College was still in existence at all by the start of the nineteenth century.

New Century – New Hospital

As mentioned previously, the foundation stone for Sir Patrick Dun's Hospital was laid in 1803. Several years later, the West Wing was opened, and ready for 30 patients.

Unfortunately, however, the Hospital's Commissioners ran out of money in completing the West Wing. The £1,200 from Dun's estate had been used up, and they applied for a grant from the Westminster Government which gave them £6200.

The central portion was finished in 1812, and the construction of the East Wing in 1816 completed the entire building, which had cost a total of around £4,000 – including £9,000 in Parliamentary grants.[19]

Architecturally Dun's was reminiscent of the grand style of the Royal Hospital at Kilmainham, but it had many of its own distinctive features. One of these was the height of the ceilings of the wards which were raised from eleven to thirteen feet. It was felt that the upward movement of air into the larger space would make the wards more hygienic, and thus help to lessen cross-infections. Other features included a spacious lecture theatre on the ground floor, and an imposing staircase. The lecture theatre, which underlined the Hospital's role in

The Rotunda Hospital

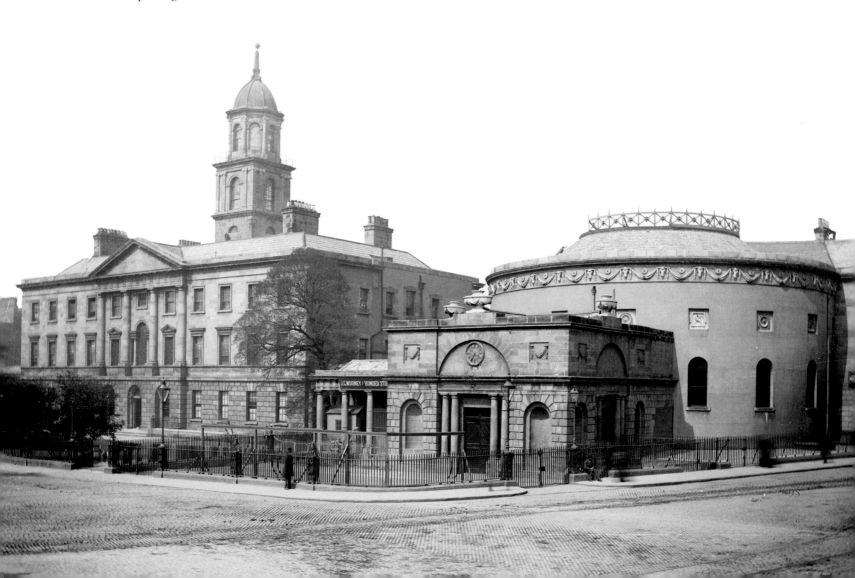

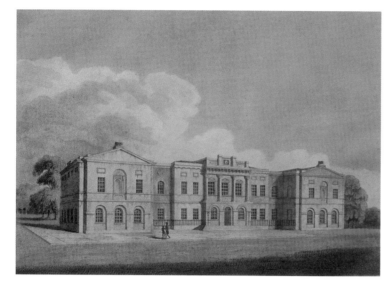

Watercolour of Sir Patrick Dun's Hospital
RCPI

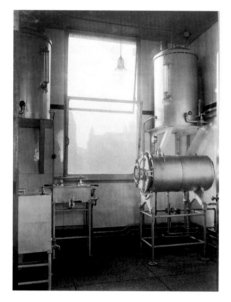

Dun's Hospital was one of the most
innovative of its time and had its
own distinctive features, including a
lecture room and operating theatres.
RCPI

teaching students as well as caring for patients, was replaced by an operating theatre in 1898, and by a newer operating block in 1930.

Spartan

The conditions for patients in the early hospital were spartan by today's standards, despite recurrent modern complaints about food and other issues. There were three diets – low, middle and full – which consisted of variations on the same ingredients, namely bread, milk and 'flummery', a starch-based sweet pudding.

Later on it was decided that treacle could be used as a sweetener for gruel, and that tea was to be dispensed with as an unnecessary luxury. Even half a century later, the physicians and surgeons in the Hospital were still strictly forbidden by the Board to alter these dietary arrangements.

Among the early admissions were large numbers of people who had risked drowning by falling into the nearby canal and canal basin. Many of these were workmen the worse for drink, who had unfortunately stumbled into the canal on their way home at night.

Cold baths seemed to be the norm in the early days, but in 1812 inquiries were made about the best place for the installation of a warm bath in the Hospital. However, little seems to have progressed on this front and three years later, in February 1815, it was reported that a fitting of a warm bath had not been done 'because the paint was not dry'.[20]

The Hospital was always short of money, as Dr TG Moorhead notes in his short history of Dun's:

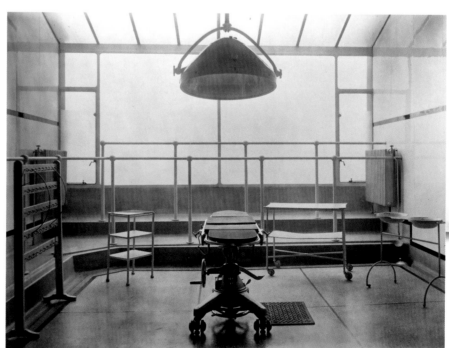

96

It is likely that the financial difficulties which the hospital experienced during many years partly arose from this fact – the public being unwilling to subscribe to a hospital whose primary object was to afford clinical instruction to medical students.

In addition, the public probably believed that the endowment arising from Sir Patrick's Estate was sufficient for the maintenance of the hospital, and believed it unnecessary to provide further funds.[21]

Despite all its difficulties, however, Sir Patrick Dun's Hospital provided a good medical education for generations of medical students, by the best practitioners of the day, and as Moorhead points out, for more than a century of its early existence, 'was always in the van of medical progress, and may be regarded as one of the most up-to-date teaching hospitals in the country'.[21]

THE STUDY OF ANATOMY

The importance of the study of anatomy for physicians as well as surgeons became apparent as time progressed, and the Scotsman Dr John Cheyne, who became a Licentiate and later a Fellow of the College noted as early as 1809 that Irish physicians had a good general training, but relied on their knowledge of symptomatology, paying little attention to anatomy.

The early nineteenth century however saw the emergence of a number of medical schools in Ireland which concentrated on the study of anatomy. This was principally precipitated by the Napoleonic Wars between Britain and France, where demand for surgeons outstripped supply. Around the same time, the proliferation of the small medical schools was seen as a challenge to the School of Physic at Trinity and also to the Royal College of Surgeons. However the appointment of Abraham Colles to the Chair of Anatomy and Physiology, and also Surgery at the Royal College of Surgeons in 1804, and the appointment of James Macartney from Armagh to the Chair of Anatomy and Surgery at Trinity almost a decade later, were important developments, as both men raised the teaching of anatomy to an international level.[22]

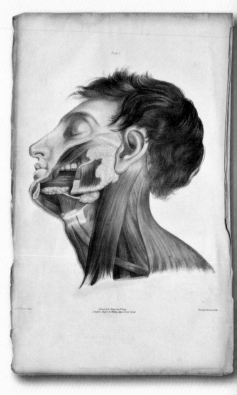

Plate from *Anatomical plates of the Viscera*, 1836, published by Jones Quain, a medical graduate from Trinity College. Artists J Walsh and W Bagg. RCPI

Anatomy and art

In Cork, a Dr John Woodroffe established a school affiliated to the South Charitable Infirmary, which was recognised by the Dublin College of Surgeons. Along with the medical students, Woodroffe lectured to local artists. It was one of these artist students who brought his school most fame. One of these was Daniel Maclise who is famous for his large figurative and symbolic compositions such as *The Marriage of Aoife and Strongbow* (1851), and for his great historical frescoes in the Houses of Parliament, Westminster.

Daniel Maclise

William O'Driscoll, a friend and biographer of Maclise, wrote:

... this early discipline of his hand and eye in the science of anatomy contributed very much to produce that marvellous facility and accuracy in delineating the human figure which imparts such a charm and grace to all his works.[23]

Daniel Maclise, self portrait, 1829
NATIONAL GALLERY OF IRELAND

A colleague of Maclise was the sculptor John Hogan, who went on to carve a life-size female skeleton from wood, so accurate that Woodroffe used it to illustrate his lectures.

Body snatching

Woodroffe experienced considerable hostility from the local population in Cork, who suspected his students were body snatching. It was reported in a local journal, *The Freeholder*, that some bodies had been found in a loft and that they were linked to Woodroffe's School of Anatomy.

Daniel Maclise recalled a sketching expedition with Samuel Forde to a ruined abbey at Kilcrea, outside Cork. It grew dark before they had finished, so they sought lodgings locally. During the night the cabin folk discovered that Forde had taken a skull from the abbey hoping to study it on his return to Cork. Forde and Maclise were assisted by some 'stout fellows ... flourishing blackthorn sticks' in returning the skull to the abbey.[24]

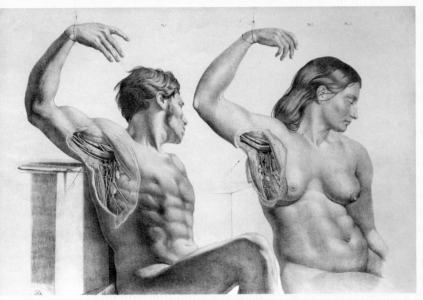

Joseph Maclise

Younger brother to Daniel, Joseph Maclise established his medical career in London along with fellow County Cork medics, Richard Bennett and brothers, Jones and Richard Quain.

Richard Quain was appointed Special Professor of Clinical Surgery at University College Hospital, London and became one of Queen Victoria's surgeons extraordinary. In 1844 he made a major contribution to the science of anatomy with the publication of a lithographic atlas entitled *The Anatomy of the Arteries of the Human Body*. Quain based the atlas on his experience of nearly one thousand dissections. In the introduction he thanked his friend and former student, Joseph Maclise for drawing the 87 illustrations in the volume.[25]

> To carry out my views as to delineations, I obtained the assistance of my friend and former pupil Mr Joseph Maclise. In reference to that Gentleman's labours, it may be allowed to say, that while I have had the cooperation of an anatomist and a surgeon, obviously a great advantage, the drawings will, I believe, be found not to have lost in spirit or effect.[26]

Joseph published his own *Surgical Anatomy* in 1851 and a second book in 1859, *On Dislocations and Fractures*. He drew the illustrations himself and based them on dissections made in Paris and London. The subjects were almost certainly obtained from local workhouses and infirmaries[26] and the illustrations are beautiful works in their own right, as well as displaying excellent anatomical detail.

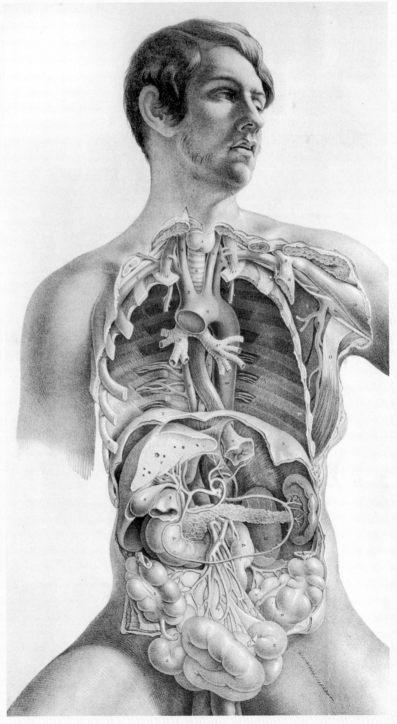

TOP: Male and female axillae compared, from *Surgical Anatomy*, 1851, by Joseph Maclise
ROYAL COLLEGE OF SURGEONS IN IRELAND
RIGHT: The thorax and abdomen, from *Surgical Anatomy*, 1851 by Joseph Maclise
ROYAL COLLEGE OF SURGEONS IN IRELAND

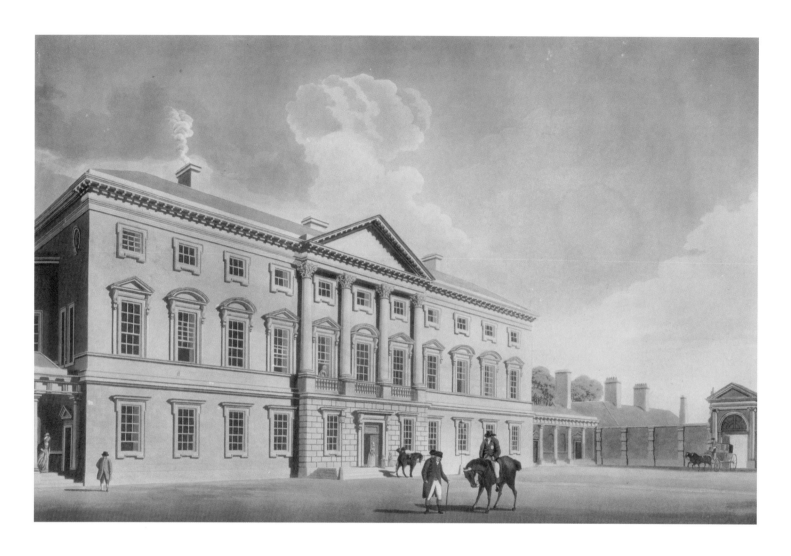

Laying the Foundations

Despite the evolution of the 'Golden Age' of Irish Medicine in the nineteenth century, the early 1800s were tough for some medical practitioners, due to the fact that many of the aristocracy who had found their niche in the Ireland of the eighteenth century had moved away.

In the early part of the nineteenth century, Dublin was:

> … now little more than a provincial city. One by one the mansions of the nobility were turned over to other purposes; and the Parliament House itself was sold to the Bank of Ireland, with the significant stipulation that the interior should be so reconstructed as to efface every visible reminder of its original function.[1]

Another historian noted:

> As for the civic culture of the Georgian Ascendancy, it declined along with the decay of Dublin – generally represented by early nineteenth-century observers and novelists as an echoing shell, full of grand but redundant buildings.[2]

Against such a background it was of little surprise that one medical historian observed:

> ... the truth was indeed that consulting physicians had very good reason to regret the Act of Union, and the passing of a resident aristocracy.
>
> Before 1800, the peers and greater gentry had maintained their town houses in Dublin, attended Parliament and Vice-Regal Courts, and thus contributed to the city's wealth. They had paid the consultant his traditional guinea fee. London had now become the centre of attraction for these families.[3]

'Charlemont House, the town residence of the Earl of Charlemont, is most cheerfully situated on a rising ground in the middle of a terrace called Palace Row, forming the north side of an elegant square, named Rutland Square. The square, which is well planted, is at the rear of a fine stone building raised for the reception of pregnant women, which, with publick music rooms adjoining, make the whole south side of the Square. From the door of Charlemont House is seen the Lying-in House or Hospital, with its portico and tower ... '

From Malton's *View of Dublin*

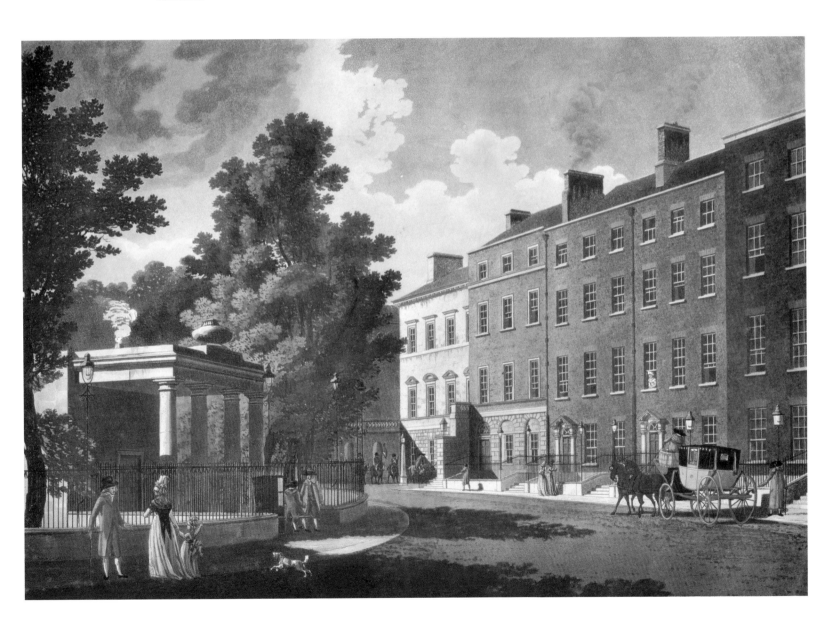

Splendour and Gloom

Despite the prevailing gloom, the College of could still rise to the occasion, and in July 1821 they were busy preparing for the State visit of King George IV to Dublin, shortly after his accession to the Throne.

George was widely and correctly regarded as self-indulgent and profligate, and the events of his colourful personal life would have kept today's tabloid newspapers endlessly supplied with material. These included the banishment of Queen Caroline from his Coronation ceremony by simply locking the doors of Westminister Abbey to keep her out – on the grounds that she had no ticket.[4]

Nevertheless the King was the King, and Dublin society – perhaps partly through gritted teeth – was preparing to give him a proper reception, as befitted the Monarch. A Committee formed by the College was instructed to draft an Address, and since the King was to receive it in person, the Fellows, Honorary Fellows and Licentiates would be summoned to a meeting to put on a proper costume for the occasion, before proceding to the appointed place to meet His Majesty:

King George IV's Triumphal Entry into Dublin, August 1821

Painting by Joseph Patrick Haverty

UK GOVERNMENT ART COLLECTION

The costume arranged for the Fellows, to be worn over full dress, consisted of a scarlet gown similar to that of Doctor of Physic, with an added margin of black velvet one inch deep, attached to the sleeves and front, together with a lace band.[5]

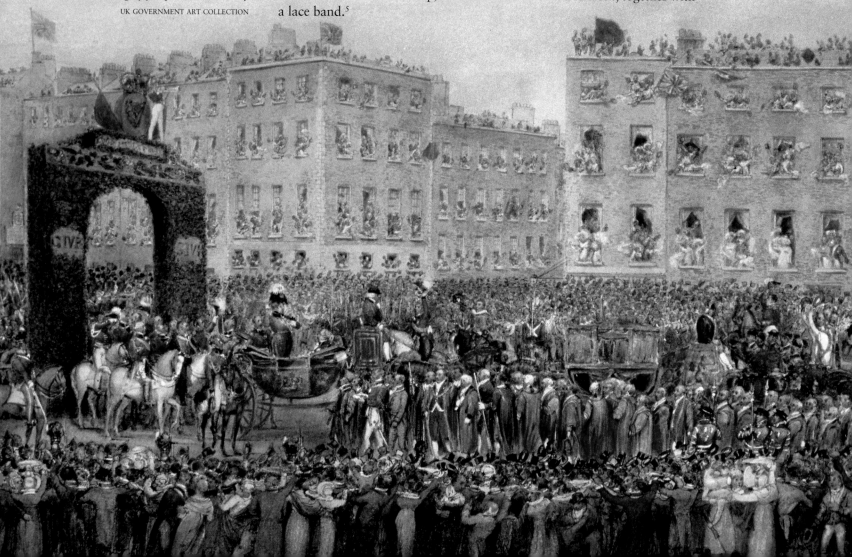

This dressing-up was akin to that undertaken by the Belfast Harbour Commissioners whose secretary Edmund Getty designed distinctive cashmere waistcoats for them to wear when meeting Queen Victoria at the port only 28 years later. Similar waistcoats are worn by the Commissioners to this day. In the elevated world of Royal audiences, presentation is all.

King George IV disembarked at Howth Harbour in August and later went to Phoenix Park to meet his subjects. Clearly he was on an extended visit, and eight days later he held a reception at Dublin Castle, which was attended by a large cross-section of society.

Representatives of the College travelled to the Castle in style, in two carriages. The President and Vice-President were driven in the first, and several Censors in the second. The carefully-prepared address was handed over to the King himself by the President, James Callenan, who had less than a month left in office.

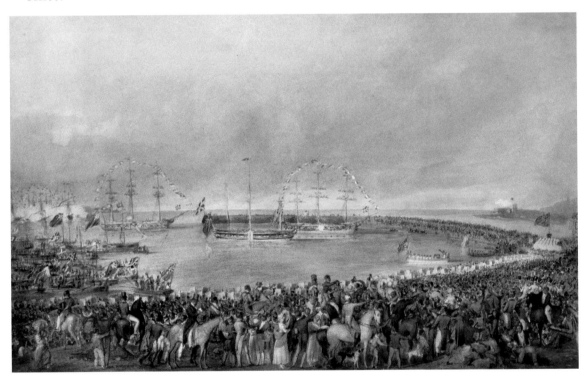

'Father of the Profession'

One of the important medical guests at the King's Reception was the ailing Dr Robert Perceval who had been the prime mover in promoting the all-important School of Physic Act of 1800. Because of severe pain in his hips, he had to use a crutch, but he attempted to approach the King without it. A contemporary report noted that he seemed so distressed without his crutch, that the King held out his hand to assist him.

Perceval had been a stern critic of the way in which the College had run its affairs for a long period in its early days, but time had mellowed the barbs of

King George IV's Embarkation at Kingstown, 3 September 1821.

Painting by Joseph Patrick Haverty
UK GOVERNMENT ART COLLECTION

his not entirely justified criticisms, and he had become a much respected figure with all members of the medical profession.

He had been one of the major promoters of the Royal Irish Academy and of a large General Dispensary at Temple Bar. He was also keenly interested in safeguarding the welfare of prisoners through the work of the Prison Discipline Society.

In his prime Perceval was reputed to have earned as much as £7,000 a year.[6] This most prestigious appointment was that of Physician-General, but he had had to relinquish this post after only a year due to ill-health. Despite his infirmities, he lived to the age of 83, and died on 3 March 1839.

On hearing of his death, the College immediately adjourned that day's activities, and paid their respects to the memory of 'a former President, and Fellow of this College, and Father of the medical profession in Dublin'. Incidentally, Perceval stipulated that any portion of his remains which might help the cause of science should be made available to the Pathological Society. Some five years after his death, a portrait of him was presented to the College by his friend, Dr Charles Philips Croker. It was given pride of place in the College Hall.[7]

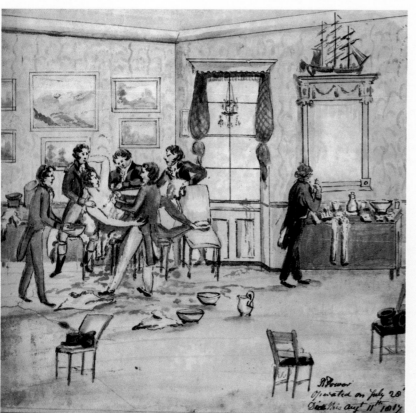

This vivid watercolour, of an operation being carried out in the drawing-room of a house in fashionable Merrion Square, Dublin, 1817, illustrates the pain and distress of early nineteenth-century surgery without the benefits of good hygiene and anaesthetics. The unfortunate patient died shortly afterwards.
MEATH HOSPITAL COLLECTION

More improvements needed

Men like Dr Robert Perceval had prospered personally during their careers, but they had also tried to further the practice and teaching of medicine generally. Despite the improvements however, much of the medical practice in the early nineteenth century remained primitive and dangerous, compared to that of today.

Surgery without anaesthetic was indescribably terrifying for the patient, and also stressful for the surgeons and those tasked with holding down the struggling body of a person suffering excruciating pain.

One of the most graphic illustrations of such trauma is depicted in a painting of a messy operation on a patient with a tumour, which was carried out in a drawing-room in a Merrion Square residence on 20 July 1817. The surgeon was Rawdon Macnamara, and the man holding the patient's shoulder was Sir Philip Crampton, who was wearing a hunting jacket and riding boots. Sadly, but hardly surprisingly, the patient died within a couple of weeks.

Crampton, incidentally, was a forceful and colourful character who was President of the Royal College of Surgeons on four occasions, and also a founder member of Dublin's Zoological Gardens.

Body snatching

Getting valuable opportunities to practise surgical skills depended greatly on a liberal supply of corpses. Unfortunately, it was difficult to obtain bodies for dissection purposes, partly because the legal authorities only allowed such procedures to be practised on criminals who had been executed for murder.

As mentioned earlier, the alternative was 'bodysnatching', the illegal practice of digging up corpses for mercenary gain. Quite often enterprising medical students engaged themselves in this nefarious business, but there were also professionals who would provide bodies for dissection, at a price. They were known as grave robbers, resurrectionists or 'sack 'em up' men, and among the the most famous were Burke and Hare, two Irish navvies who robbed graves in Edinburgh and even resorted to murdering hapless lodgers in Hare's guest-house.

The practice also flourished in Ireland, in places such as Kilmainham and elsewhere, and also in the North.

For dissection in the teaching of anatomy bodies could not be stored, so it was a race against time to work on the corpse before putrification set in. Dissection was a grim business carried out under the cover of darkness, with a premium being paid for fresh bodies.

In the nineteenth century doctors were taught anatomy after the discovery that surgery involving the limbs could be life-saving, by preventing the outset of 'gas gangrene'. Surgery at that time generally meant the amputation of limbs, and this persisted right up to the end of the First World War as the most effective treatment of infected wounds. A skilled surgeon could amputate a limb in three minutes.

DR PAUL DARRAGH, RCPI

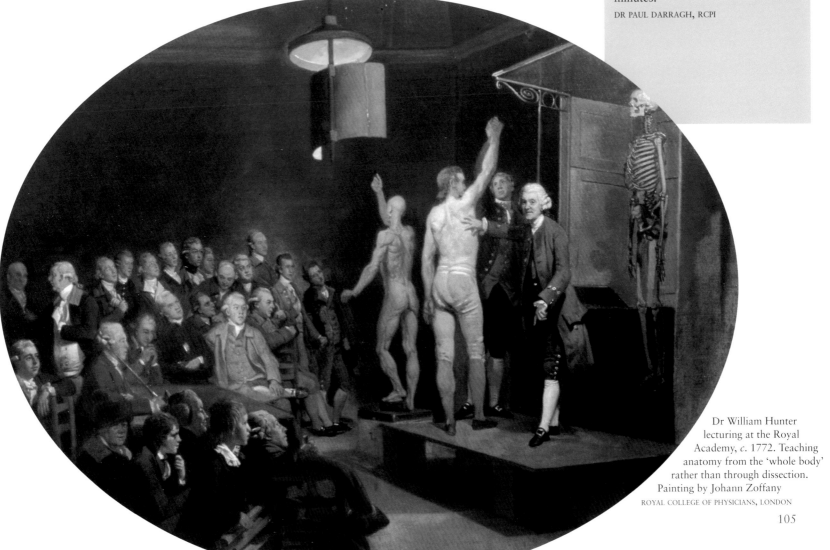

Dr William Hunter lecturing at the Royal Academy, *c.* 1772. Teaching anatomy from the 'whole body' rather than through dissection. Painting by Johann Zoffany

ROYAL COLLEGE OF PHYSICIANS, LONDON

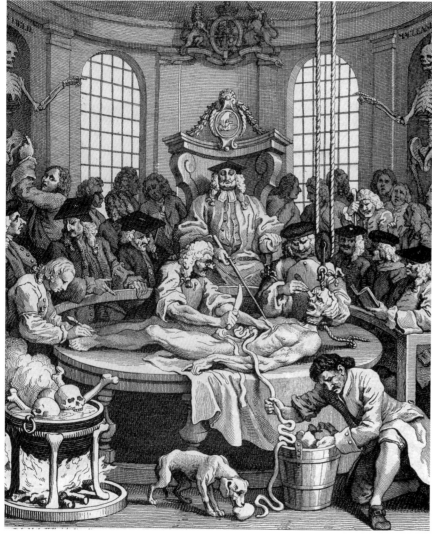

The Reward of Cruelty, 1751, by
William Hogarth, 1697–1764
The body of the fictional Tom Nero is
dissected after hanging.
NATIONAL GALLERY OF IRELAND

Relatives were naturally anxious to protect the dead bodies of their loved ones, and at St John's Church in Donegore, near Antrim, there is still a well-preserved burial mound with strongly barred gates to protect corpses from body snatchers. This relic of a barbarous practice still stands near the grave of the celebrated Irish poet and antiquarian, Sir Samuel Ferguson.

The arrest of Burke and Hare in 1825 put paid to the practice of body snatching. Hare turned King's evidence, but Burke was publicly hanged. The details of body snatching revealed at their trial led to widespread outrage, and in 1832 the British Government passed the Anatomy Act, which stipulated that bodies for dissection should be of those who had died and remained unclaimed for burial, or those bequeathed as voluntary donations for medical research, provided that the relatives also consented.[8]

Dr John Cheyne

Physicians, as a body, still regarded themselves as the elite of the profession, much to the annoyance of surgeons, apothecaries and others. However, they too had much to learn, and they based their practice largely on the study of symptoms and information from patients, rather than the pathology and scientific study of diseases.

The physicians still relied largely on long-established and rudimentary practices, such as blistering, dry-cupping, bleeding and the use of leeches, as well as the use of various medications, including laxatives for purging the body. The benefits of leeching are still appreciated today.

Despite fewer rich pickings for doctors in early nineteenth century Ireland, as noted above, there were still prospects for a skilled and socially and professionally enterprising physician to make a good living.

Such a man was Dr John Cheyne, who had a foot in both pre- and post-Union Ireland. Like some of his most distinguished forebears in the College, he had arrived in Ireland as a surgeon with an army unit, and later settled in Dublin to make an important contribution to Irish medicine, as well as prospering financially.

Born in a medical family, Cheyne qualified as a medical student in Edinburgh in 1795. Three years later he was sent to Ireland as a surgeon with a horse

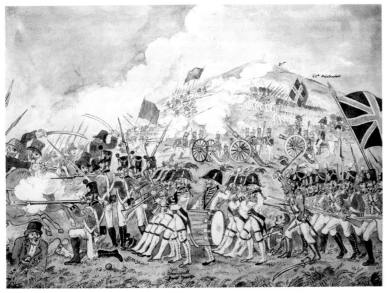

artillery unit and was present at the vicious Battle of Vinegar Hill which ended the '98 rebellion in Wexford.

The drama and slaughter of such an encounter aside, Cheyne decided that he was not suited for the life of an army surgeon, in which he had too much time on his hands for merely shooting game and playing billiards. He therefore returned to Scotland, where he was put in charge of the Leith Ordnance Hospital.

He also shared in his father's general medical practice and worked closely with Sir Charles Bell, an expert on facial paralysis. Cheyne demonstrated great methodology, keeping detailed records and performing autopsies where possible. He developed an interest, too, in fever and children's diseases.

During this period in Scotland, he published three works, and two of these were particularly important. His *Essay on Hydrocephalus Acutus, or Dropsy in the Brain* (1808) includes the first detailed description of acute hydrocephalus, and his *Pathology of the Membranes of the Larnyx and Bronchia* (1809) is concerned with the lesions of croup.

Canny Scot

Cheyne was a canny Scot whose ambition was to have a prosperous practice in a large city. He was shrewd enough to note that such opportunities were limited in England, and so returned to Ireland in 1809, just eleven years after his savage introduction to the Irish at the Battle of Vinegar Hill.

On arrival, Cheyne cast a shrewd eye over medical practice in his newly-adopted country:

> I soon discovered that the field was extensive, and the labourers liberally rewarded. The physicians whom I found in the confidence of the public were mostly of the School of Cullen: they were possessed of good general information, but chiefly relied on the accuracy of their symptomatology; they had paid but little attention to morbid anatomy.
>
> Much of the purely medical practice of Dublin was passing into the hands of the surgeons, who, although certainly less skilful in the treatment of acute diseases, were better acquainted with the nature and tendency of organic lesions.
>
> In this state of things, I discerned a good ground of hope. I was sufficiently well acquainted with acute diseases, and, thanks to Sir C Bell, I had acquired a taste for pathology.[9]

The Queen's Own Royal Dublin Militia going into Action at Vinegar Hill, with the Light Company advancing and firing and covering the Road, 1798.

Original pen sketch by William Sadler, 1879

NATIONAL LIBRARY OF IRELAND

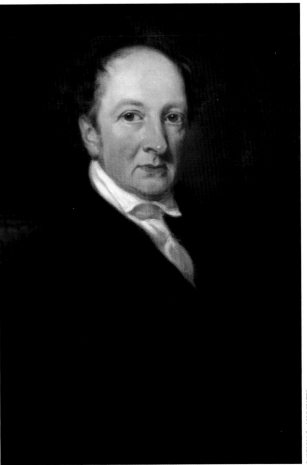

Dr John Cheyne, 1777–1836
Cheyne was a leading physician who eventually became Physician General to the army in Ireland. He became a Licentiate of the Royal College of Physicians in 1811, and 23 years later, a Fellow.

Portrait of John Cheyne attributed to William Deeny

RCPI

DAVISON & ASSOCIATES

Cheyne's observations were highly pertinent, as was reflected in the appointment of two outstanding anatomists to key positions around that time – Abraham Colles to the Chairs of Anatomy and Physiology, and Surgery, at the Royal College of Surgeons in 1804, and James Macartney to the Chair of Surgery at Trinity in 1813.

Slow start

Although John Cheyne was professionally ambitious, he started off his practice as a physician in Ireland slowly, and his income for the six months from November 1810–May 1811 was just three guineas. He had married Sarah Macartney, a daughter of the Vicar of Antrim, the Reverend Dr George Macartney, and he had wisely advised her to stay in her father's house in the North until he established himself in Dublin.

Cheyne persevered, and in 1811 he became a Licentiate of the College, and was elected a Fellow some 23 years later. In 1811 he was also appointed a physician at the Meath Hospital, and in 1813 he became the first Professor of Medicine at the Royal College of Surgeons' Medical School.

In 1815 he was appointed Physician to the House of Industry Hospitals – Richmond, Whitworth and Hardwicke – and he resigned from his role at the Meath. In this new post he concentrated on acute diseases, including fevers. By 1816 his annual income had risen to £1,710.

Shortly afterwards however, Cheyne resigned from the House of Industry and from his professorship at the Royal College of Surgeons. This was partly due to his desire to maintain a high income from his own practice, at a time when consultants had to rely on private work for their livelihood, and Cheyne had to provide for a large family of sixteen children.

Despite a marked interest in making money, he decided not to carry out consultations outside Dublin because of his failing energy. This cost him – by his own estimate – some £1,500 a year. He suffered from fatigue for a long time, and when working at the House of Industry, he said that he invariably came home exhausted.

Cheyne-Stokes respiration

This fatigue cannot have been diminished by Cheyne's output as a medical writer, and in 1815 he launched a periodical entitled the *Dublin Hospital Reports*, in association with Abraham Colles and Charles Hawkes Todd.

In the second edition of this publication, Cheyne made his name with his contemporaries and succeeding generations of doctors. In his report on a *Case of apoplexy in which the fleshy part of the heart was converted into fat*, he described a patient's irregular breathing, and some 28 years later the outstanding cardiologist, William Stokes, referred to a similar breathing

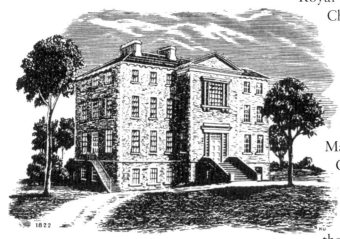

Meath Hospital
The Meath Hospital was founded in 1753 to provide health care for the poor of Dublin's Liberties. Funded entirely by voluntary subscriptions and donations from prominent citizens of the day, the hospital would attract some of Ireland's most celebrated physicians and surgeons and become an internationally recognised centre for the advancement of medical science.

In 1998, along with the Adelaide and the National Children's Hospital, the Meath moved to the new Hospital at Tallaght, now known as Tallaght Hospital.

The Meath Hospital, Dublin, Dr Peter Gatenby, Vol. 58, No. 2, Autumn 2005, pp122–8, Old Dublin Society and Meath Hospital and Adelaide Website

disorder. This distinctive respiratory condition eventually became known internationally as 'Cheyne-Stokes Respiration'.

Despite his complaints about fatigue, and a busy professional schedule, Cheyne felt strong enough enough in 1820 to accept the highly prestigious post of Physician General to the Army in Ireland. There he was able to use his previous military experience to deal with malingering among soldiers, which he described as an 'intolerable nuisance'.

He also had to deal with the prevalence of consumption in the army, which was a common cause of soldiers' deaths. Cheyne would have known about the recently developed and somewhat primitive form of a stethoscope, and other instruments and procedures, for the diagnosis of would-be recruits with poor breathing.

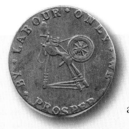

Token from the Workhouse
www.workhouses.org/DublinNorth/

The House of Industry and its Hospitals: the Richmond, Whitworth and Hardwicke

When the House of Industry opened, facilities for the sick, infirm and insane were totally inadequate, especially since it also had to cope with a large population of destitute children. The house was originally intended to be have been funded by voluntary contributions, however these soon proved insufficient and from 1777, it received a parliamentary grant, initially of £4,000 per annum. By 1839 this government support increased to over £20,000 per annum, at which time the House contained 1,665 inmates.

A large complex of buildings subsequently evolved around the new House of Industry, including:

An asylum for aged and infirm poor
An asylum for incurable lunatics
The Bedford Asylum for the reception of children
The Hardwicke Fever Hospital
The Whitworth Hospital for chronic medical patients
The Richmond Surgical Hospital
The Talbot Dispensary, which provided medical and surgical relief to the extreme poor of the north-west quarter of the city, numbering over 300 a week.[10]

In 1798 the Governors had petitioned the House of Commons to build a proper infirmary, and construction of the Hardwicke Fever Hospital had begun in 1803. The Richmond Surgical Hospital was opened in 1810 to care for the 'ruptured poor'. The distinctive red-brick building now functions as Dublin Metropolitan Court. The Whitworth Hospital for chronic patients was built in 1814, just south of the new House of Industry.[11]

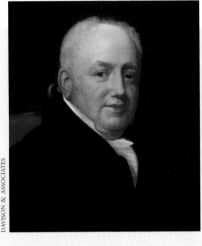

Portrait of Alexander Jackson
RCPI

DAVISON & ASSOCIATES

'Curable' lunatics might be placed in the Richmond Lunatic Asylum, immediately adjacent to the House of Industry, and opened in 1814. This institution provided treatment for pauper lunatics from all over the country. It was under the influence of Alexander Jackson, a Licentiate, who, according to Professor John Widdess, was 'after Jonathan Swift … the pioneer of what is now termed psychiatry in Ireland'.

Jackson believed in the segregation of various types of mental patient, as he believed that 'the unhappy maniac who is constantly roaring' would deter the recovery 'of a patient who is convalescent in an adjoining cell'.[12]

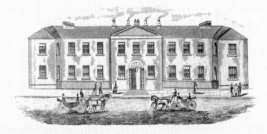

The Whitworth Medical Hospital
RCSI

Dr John Cheyne became Physician to the House of Industry in 1815 when Jackson resigned the position to become first medical officer of the Richmond Lunatic Asylum (later to become Grangegorman). It is reported that Cheyne was able to complete his daily visit in 'little more than an hour, by virtue of experienced and well-trained sick-nurses, who allowed nothing to escape their observation'.[13] Cheyne was noted as one of the pioneers of the training of nurses in Ireland.

109

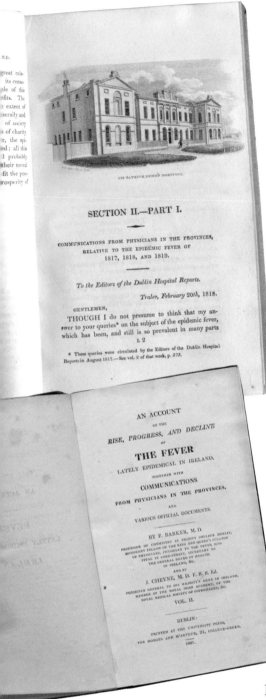

Two volumes published in 1821 by Barker and Cheyne on fever in relation to epidemics in Ireland, together with communications from physicians in the provinces.

RCPI

Departure

From about 1825 John Cheyne began to suffer from depression, and by the age of 49 his health started to fail. In 1831 he retired to Sherrington in Buckinghamshire. There he helped to look after a number of sick villagers, and he also continued to write.

Prior to his departure from Ireland, Cheyne received a glowing tribute from the College, which was signed by 45 of Dublin's most distinguished doctors. In it, they praised him for his faithfulness, his medical knowledge and his sound practical judgement. They also asked him to reconsider his decision to leave, but their plea was unsuccessful.

John Cheyne died in 1836, and seven years later his final book was published: *Essays on Partial Derangement of the Mind in supposed Connection with Religion*. It is a topic that has a curiously modern connotation. The book had an introduction by his colleague and friend Abraham Colles, and contained his short autobiographical sketch.[14]

Like another of his distinguished colleagues, Richard Helsham, who died almost a century earlier, Cheyne had left clear instructions about his burial. His Will stated that his body, attended only by his sons, should be carried to his grave very early on the fourth or fifth day after his death:

I would have no tolling of bells, if it can be avoided. The ringers may have an order for bread, to the amount usually given on such occasions; if they get money, they will spend it in the alehouse, and I would have them told, that in life or death I would by no means give occasion for sin.

My funeral must be as inexpensive as possible; let there be no attempt at a funeral sermon. I would pass away without notice from a world, which, with all its pretensions, is empty.[15]

Despite Cheyne's melancholy at the end of his life, he had much about which he could be proud. He is regarded as one of the founders of Irish medicine, and though some clinicians might conclude that he was not among the highest-fliers of the Golden Age, his methodical approach to medical practice and his voluminous writings have safeguarded his reputation as one of the most significant figures in the history of the Royal College of Physicians.

His contribution to Irish medicine is well-summarised by Professor Davis Coakley, who stated that the papers which Cheyne wrote for the Dublin Hospital Report's periodical:

… set the standard for the subsequent famous work of the physicians and surgeons who would form the Irish School of Medicine. William Stokes described these papers as models of clinical observation, presented with both accuracy and clarity.[16]

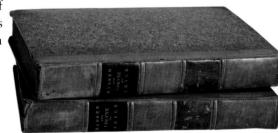

110

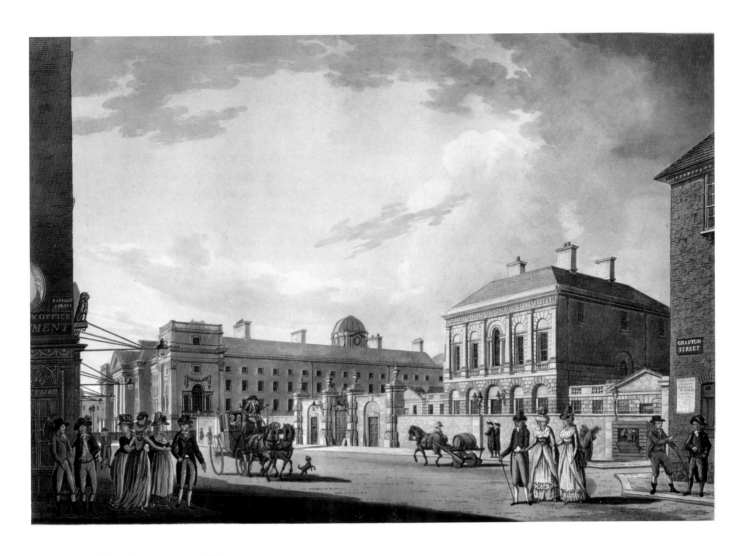

Robert Graves
and William Stokes

The so-called 'Golden Age of Irish Medicine', which flourished in the nineteenth century, has been summarised expertly by a number of people, including the late Professor John Feely, a distinguished Clinical Pharmacologist and a former Registrar of the College of Physicians from 1989–96.

He noted that:

> With the decline of the system of hereditary physicians in Ireland, those wishing to study medicine had to travel to Britain, France and the Netherlands, particularly Leiden, where the impact of Boerhaave's clinical approach subsequently influenced teaching in Vienna and Edinburgh.

'The Provost's House, as it is called, is an elegant mansion, is the residence for the Provost of the University. It is situated to the south of the west front of the College ...'
From Malton's *View of Dublin*
RCPI

He continued:

> We find that those who were to play such a pivotal role in nineteenth-century medical education in Dublin travelled widely to these centres. It was the founding of the voluntary hospitals, the bedside teaching and the emphasis on the study of pathology, together with the broad and enlightened approach of gifted practitioners such as Graves, Stokes and Corrigan that brought about the great era of Irish medicine in the last century.[1]

The Dublin School

The Golden Age of Irish Medicine was synonymous with the establishment and achievements of the 'Dublin School'. This included the contribution of a number of outstanding doctors, and in particular the work of three of its most eminent members – Robert Graves (1796–1853), Dominic Corrigan (1802–80) and William Stokes (1804–77).

Robert Graves

Robert Graves was an outstanding teacher and physician, whose name is associated in medical circles worldwide with a disorder of the thyroid gland known as 'Graves' disease'. He is also associated with revolutionising the treatment of fevers. Graves was a Fellow and Censor of the College, and President from 1843–45.

Born in Dublin on 28 March 1796, he was the youngest son of Dr Richard Graves, the Dean of Ardagh and a Professor of Divinity at Trinity College Dublin, and his wife, Elizabeth Mary Drought, the daughter of another TCD Professor of Divinity, James Drought.

In 1811, at the age of 15, he gained first place in the entrance examination for Trinity. Where he was greatly influenced by the outstanding teacher, James Macartney and developed a wide knowledge of anatomy, which was unusual for an aspiring physician in those days.[2]

After graduating from Trinity, Graves took the path well-worn by many of his predecessors, in leaving Ireland to gain experience further afield. He went to London, and then to Europe where he visited a number of excellent medical schools in Holland, Denmark, Germany, Italy and France. In Berlin he was particularly impressed by their methods of bedside teaching, and this experience helped him to introduce new and radical approaches to clinical teaching on his return to Ireland.

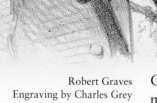

Robert Graves
Engraving by Charles Grey
RCPI

More Challenges

Graves returned to Ireland after a short time in Edinburgh, and was admitted as a Licentiate of the College in 1820. The next year he was appointed Physician of the Meath Hospital. A pupil Arthur Young, later described Grave's arrival on the premises and how he was surprised one morning at seeing this lithe, dark-haired, eagle-eyed, and energetic-mannered gentleman come in:

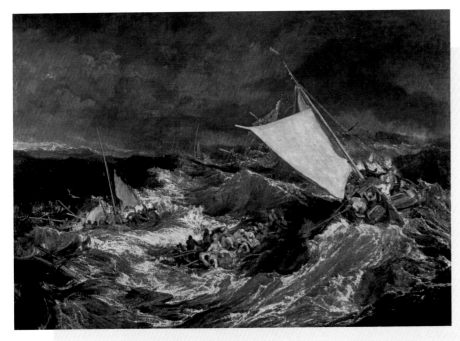

The Shipwreck
by Joseph Mallord William Turner, 1775–1851
TATE IMAGES

European Adventures

Graves was not only a demonstrably bright young man, but also the kind of fulsome Irish character who seemed to attract adventure everywhere he went.

He was reportedly imprisoned in Austria for a short time on suspicion of being a spy, because the authorities did not believe that an Irishman could speak German so fluently. The situation might have been resolved more speedily if Graves, who was also fluent in French and Italian, had brought along his passport.

On another occasion off the coast of Italy on his way to Sicily he was swept up in a storm, and the brig in which he was travelling was soon in great difficulty. The crisis was not helped by members of the Sicilian crew who, in Graves' opinion, were ill-found, ill-mannered and ill-commanded. The vessel's sails were rent asunder by the howling gale, the brig sprung a serious leak and the pumps stopped working.

The situation became so dire that the captain and crew prepared to abandon ship. When Graves' sole fellow-passenger, a Spaniard, broke the bad news to him, he reacted with characteristic vigour, despite the fact that he was lying in a cabin suffering from a painful, though undisclosed malady.

In a story of derring-do that would make a suitable adventure for the pages of *Boys Own* magazine, Graves reputedly grabbed an axe from outside his cabin and confronted the captain, who was about the lower the lifeboat and make off with his crew – but without Graves and the Spanish passenger.

Undeterred, Graves faced up to the captain, who was wielding a knife, but now backed off – no doubt impressed by the coolness and courage of this remarkable stranger. Graves then rallied the crew, repaired the pumps with leather cut from his own boots and managed to control the leaks in the vessel. The ship made it safely to port.

Happily Graves and all those on board survived. Even if the tale may have increased in the telling over the years, it has an almost Biblical quality reminiscent of the survival of St Paul on his difficult sea-journey in the Mediterranean, many centuries earlier.

> I was told that this was Dr Graves … and the facility with which he answered the many questions put to him, and the amount of information he conveyed, so clearly and in such charming language, made a very strong impression on my mind as a youngster; and, as I observed him in later life, each succeeding year increased my admiration of his learning, his assiduity, and his depth of professional information.[3]

Courage

Shortly afterwards, Graves encountered another major challenge which demonstrated his courage once more, also leading him to an important discovery in terms of his profession.

In 1822 he had interrupted his busy routine to go to Galway, where many people were dying from a typhus epidemic in the wake of a famine in the west

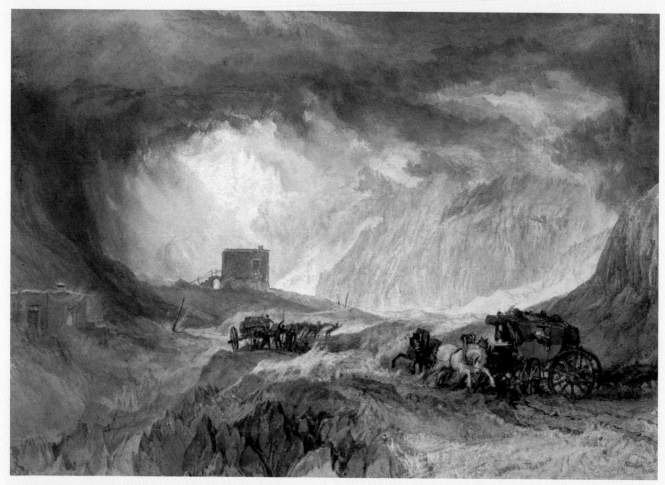

The Passage of Mount Cenis
Painting by Joseph Mallord William Turner, 1775–1851
BIRMINGHAM MUSEUMS AND ART GALLERY

Famous Painter

As if all of Grave's other adventures were not enough, he also had a remarkable tale about an encounter with a stranger on his travels in Italy. In the autumn of 1819, he was crossing the Alps through the Mont Cenis Pass, when he noticed that his somewhat taciturn companion was making sketches in a notebook. As Graves also had a talent for drawing, they began to discuss their mutual interest.

They sketched together as they passed through Turin, Milan and Florence, before eventually reaching Rome. During their time together they did not share their identities, though Graves noticed that his companion had a remarkable proficiency in sketching cloud-formations. It was only when he arrived in Rome that Graves discovered the identity of his fellow traveller. He was the celebrated English painter Joseph Mallard William Turner.

Graves said later:

> I assure you there was not a single stroke in Turner's drawing that I could see like nature; not a line nor an object, and yet my work was worthless in comparison with his. The whole glory of the scene was there.[4]

Again this story may have been embellished in the telling, but few people can boast that they shared a sketching journey through the Alps and Italy with one of the world's most renowned artists. By the time the young Graves had returned to Dublin to embark on his distinguished medical career, he had, it seems, experienced more adventures than others in their entire lives.

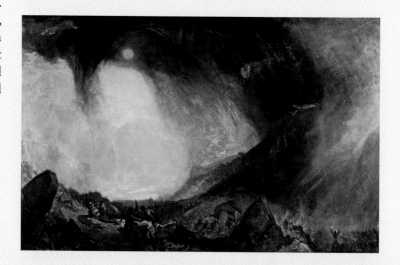

114

Snow Storm, Hannibal and his Army Crossing the Alps, 1812
Painting by Joseph Mallord William Turner
TATE GALLERY, LONDON

of Ireland. A large number of doctors were trying to contain the disease and many of them also died. In desperation the Government had appealed for volunteers, and Graves and five other doctors had come forward.

The young Graves was appalled by the scenes of suffering and distress which he encountered. He later wrote that the terror of contagion among the local inhabitants was so great, that in some cases sick people were turned out of their family cabins, or left in isolation inside.

This inspired Graves to look more deeply into the treatment of fevers. Whereas the contemporary medical approach was to virtually starve the patient, Graves took a very different view, and recommending that patients needed good nourishment to build up their strength and help them recover. In one of his famous ward rounds, as recalled by his pupil, William Stokes, he pointed out that a fever patient who had been well fed on his instructions was looking much better.

Graves had turned to his students and in characteristic style, he provided them with his own epitaph. He pointed to the patient and said:

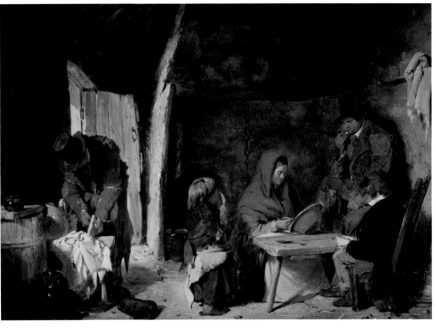

A typical dwelling in rural Ireland where disease spread quickly through poor living conditions and malnutrition.

Scene in an Irish Cabin
by Erskine Nicol, 1851
MUSEUMS SHEFFIELD

> This is all the effect of good feeding, and lest when I am gone, you may be at a loss for an epitaph for me, let me give you one, in three words – 'He Fed Fevers!'[5]

Clinical Teacher

One of Robert Graves' most significant contributions was his innovative approach to clinical teaching, by which he drew widespread attention to the cutting edge of medical education in Ireland in the nineteenth century.

In 1824 Graves, and others, founded the Park Street School of Medicine. In his 'Clinical Lectures On the Practice of Medicine', he would begin by outlining with admirable clarity what he expected from his students:

> You come here to convert theoretical into practical knowledge; to observe the symptoms of diseases previously known to you only through the medium of books or lectures; to learn the art of recognising the symptoms, and of appreciating their relative importance and value; to study their connection with morbid alterations of internal organs; and, finally, to become acquainted with the best method of relieving your patient, by the application of appropriate remedies…
>
> Remember, therefore, that however else you may be occupied – whatever studies may claim the remainder of your time, a certain portion of each day should be devoted to attendance at an hospital, where the pupil has the

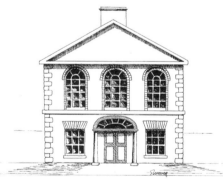

Park Street School of Medicine
Drawing by Eamon Sweeney

advantage of receiving instruction from some experienced practitioner.[6]

Graves' students had to work hard to keep up with their gifted but demanding teacher. He insisted that a greater number of students should be responsible for the care of patients. Significantly, he moved the focus of clinical instruction from the lecture hall to the patient's bedside. In doing so he underlined the importance of hands-on medicine, as opposed to purely theoretical learning from lecture-room dissertations.

It seems scarcely credible to modern readers that students in nineteenth-century Ireland, and previously, were able to gain a degree in medicine without having to examine a patient.

Until this point any practical training had been much more impersonal. Medical students visited hospital wards, partly to gain brownie points for good attendance and partly to try to pick up valuable information from their clinical teacher, who would be moving quickly around the room – no doubt *en route* to another important medical appointment.

Big Changes

Under Graves students were encouraged to develop their own powers of observation, and to make sure that mistakes in clinical judgments, if and when they occurred, were swiftly corrected.

They were also taught to think carefully about the medication they described, and the likely cost to the patients. In other words, the sick person was to be at the centre of concern, and his or her well-being was more important than the assembly of a plethora of statistics, or the need to meet government targets – a system which devalues national health provision in some countries to this day.

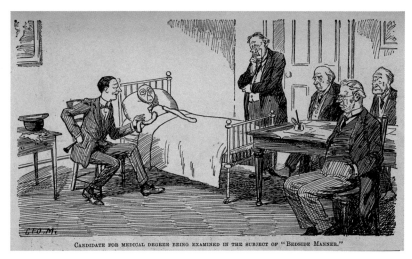

CANDIDATE FOR MEDICAL DEGREE BEING EXAMINED IN THE SUBJECT OF "BEDSIDE MANNER."

A medical student being examined for his bedside manner by a group of senior doctors.
Wood engraving by G. Morrow, 1914. Robert Graves was a pioneer in emphasising the need for students to work directly with the patients.
WELLCOME LIBRARY, LONDON

Physician and Lecturer

Robert Graves had a busy working day, and his ward rounds at the Meath Hospital began at 7 am. Arthur Guinness, a member of the famous brewing family, described the atmosphere:

> As he had a very large practice, he used to come in winter time, when I was a resident, about seven o'clock in the mornings when it was quite dark in the wards, and many a time I walked round with the clinical clerk, Hudson and often carried a candle for Doctor Graves.

Graves had a deep-toned voice, which caused 'Old Parr' the apothecary, who was a regular joker and punster to say: 'Graves always speaks in a sepulchral tone'.[8]

Napoleon, Sir Frederick Conway Dwyer and the RCPI

Sir Frederick Conway Dwyer was born in Dublin in 1860; he was educated at Trinity College and worked as a surgeon at several of the leading hospitals in the city. He was actively involved with the Royal College of Surgeons in Ireland, serving on their council for many years, and acting as Professor of Surgery and President of the College. He died on 10 October 1935 at the Pembroke Nursing Home in Dublin.

Given Dwyer's obvious association with the College of Surgeons, it is perhaps surprising that the College of Physicians holds some significant items of his, but events following his death led to a posthumous connection with the latter. As the *Irish Independent* and *Irish Times* both reported, Conway Dwyer left the majority of his fortune (over £36,000, the equivalent of over £1.5 million in today's money) to his friend, Mrs Mary Tyrell. She is described in the articles as the daughter of his great friend, Thomas O'Kearney White, and also the owner of the nursing home in which Conway Dwyer died. His Will seems to have caused a bit of a stir, and there was a certain amount of speculation about Mrs Tyrell. Within the volume of cuttings, held on archive – there is a printed apology from one newspaper;

> We are informed that Mrs Tyrrell is not and never was a nurse and that she did not nurse Sir Frederick either during his last illness or at any time … We apologise to Mrs Tyrrell for the inaccuracies which occurred in the reports of our Dublin correspondent.

Amongst the possessions that passed to Mary Tyrell was Conway Dwyer's collection of Napoleonic artefacts. This collection, which includes Napoleon's toothbrush and snuff box, had been put together by another Irish surgeon, Barry Edward O'Meara (1789–1836). O'Meara acted as Napoleon's doctor while he was on St Helena, and published an account of his experience, *Napoleon in Exile: A Voice from St Helena* (1822). Mrs Tyrell presented the items to the Royal College of Physicians following Dwyer's death. Why she decided to give them to the College of Physicians rather than the Royal College of Surgeons is unclear.

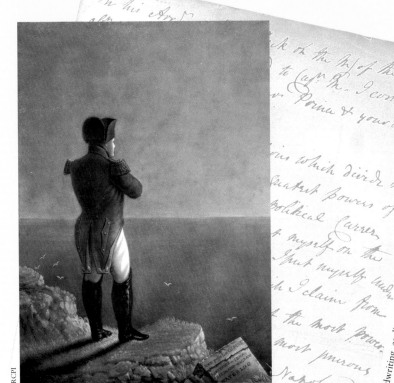

Napoleon on St Helena

RCPI

Letter from Napoleon to the Prince Regent, 1815. In O'Meara's handwriting, as dictated by Napoleon
WELLCOME LIBRARY

The opinion traditionally held within the College of Physicians is that during Dwyer's life, the College of Surgeons had disapproved of his friendship with Mrs Tyrell and she had not been invited to attend College of Surgeons' events. So that after her friend's death she was not very well disposed towards them! Whatever the reason Conway Dwyer's Napoleonic collection remains at the College of Physicians, as one of the more unusual collections.[7]

St Helena is an island in the South Atlantic Ocean, about midway between South America and Africa. It acquired fame as the place of Napoleon Bonaparte's exile, from 1815 until his death in 1821.

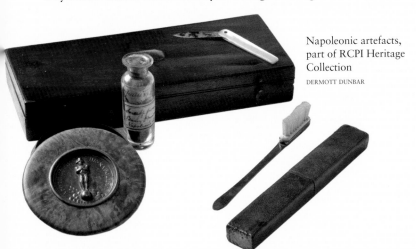

Napoleonic artefacts, part of RCPI Heritage Collection
DERMOTT DUNBAR

117

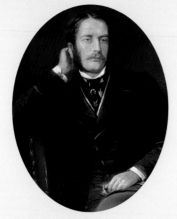

Portrait of Lord Ardilaun
by Francis Sargent

Arthur Guinness, Lord Ardilaun
1768–1855

Arthur Guinness was a member of
the famous Dublin brewing family.
A philantropist, and a member of
the Cork Street Fever Hospital for
many years, he was on the Boards
of a number of other Dublin
hospitals.

Guinness was also well-known in
business circles, and was a
Governor of the Bank of Ireland,
and President of the Dublin
Chamber of Commerce.

On one occasion it seems that Graves examined a patient suffering from a
serious wasting condition, who told him that he was 'poorly'. Graves briskly
replied 'You are doing well, my poor fellow,' but then he turned to his pupils
and said, 'Gentleman, moribundus', and walked on.[8]

Given Graves's knowledge and style, it was little wonder that students flocked
to hear him, and soon after his return to Dublin he had as many as 130 people
at his lectures – more than any other teacher of that time.

In 1827 Graves was appointed King's Professor of the Institutes of Medicine
in the School of Physic, covering pathology, physiology and therapeutics. Every
weekday during term, he lectured at 4pm in Sir Patrick Dun's Hospital, where
medical students were trained.

The timing of the lecture indicates the length of Graves' working day, which
began with an early ward round, and continued probably long after the lecture
finished. It was also a long day for students, and a 4 o'clock lecture can be one
of the most tiring of the day for teachers as well as students.

Nevertheless, Graves' lectures were so popular that when he entered the
lecture hall, a frisson of excitement went round the room. This was described
by William Wilde who recalled in 1842:

> Then all weariness was forgotten – all languor vanished; the notebooks were
> again resumed – the attention that had already flagged at an earlier hour of
> the day, was aroused by the absorbing interest of the subject, and the energy

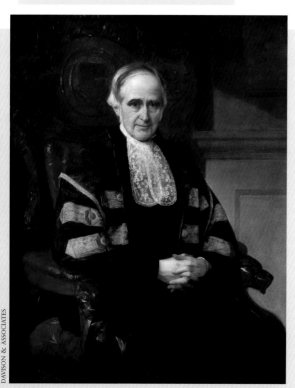

Fleetwood Churchill
Portrait by Sir Thomas Alfred Jones
RCPI

Ould, Churchill and Obstetrical Instruments

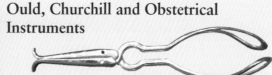

In his *Researches on Operative Midwifery*
(1841), the Dublin-based Fleetwood Churchill
(1808–78) stated that:

> the greatest triumph of surgery is to
> diminish the frequency of operations … the
> invention of the forceps, and their
> employment in practice, is the greatest
> improvement recorded in the annals of
> operative midwifery.

The obstetrical forceps were invented by the
Chamberlen family in the seventeenth century,
who managed to keep their design a secret into
the early eighteenth century. In common with
many other obstetricians, Churchill produced a
range of his own obstetrical instruments,
including forceps, crotchet and craniotomy
forceps. The latter two items were used for still
births, or:

> … where one life is sacrificed to secure the
> other: the mother's safety being purchased by
> the destruction of her child, in cases where
> both would be lost if no interference.

In a review of craniotomy instruments,
Churchill comments on an instrument designed
by another Dublin obstetrician: the *Terebra
Occulta* of Sir Fielding Ould (*c.* 1710–89) which
its designer described as:

> being a piercer, to perforate the head of an
> infant, in order to lessen the size of it, by
> evacuating part of the brain.

Although Churchill agreed that the design, with
the piercer concealed within a sheath, would do
less damage to the mother, he stated that:

> it must have been nearly useless, from the
> small opening it made.

of the lecturer; nay more, the noisy bustle usually attendant on the breaking up of a lecture was exchanged for discussions upon the subjects treated on, or eager enquiries of the Professor for the solution of difficulties – and the freshness of morning again came over the exhausted student's mind.[9]

Robert Graves medical reputation soared in the English-speaking world, and Dublin became the focus for many distinguished medical men from Europe and the United States.

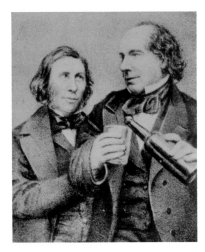

William Wilde with William Stokes sharing a bottle of beer.
RCPI

Best Known

Hermann Boerhaave had championed clinical bedside teaching a century earlier both in Leiden and German medical Schools.
RCPI

In 1843 Graves published his best-known work *A System of Clinical Medicine*. It sold out quickly, with a second edition being published five years later. The book was later translated into German, French and Italian. The book underscored Graves' pre-eminence in medical theory and practice, and his distinguished reputation in medical circles remains intact more than 170 years later.

Professor Davis Coakley, in his excellent account of Graves' career, stated:

> There can be few, if any, other single-author books on clinical medicine with a similar wealth of original observations on so many different conditions.[10]

Personal and Later Life

In the year that Graves published this *magnum opus*, he also resigned from his beloved Meath Hospital, although he remained as a consultant to several other medical institutions.

Despite his remarkable professional success, he experienced tragedy and loss in his personal life. In 1825 his first wife died, and their young daughter also died six years later. He married his second wife in 1826, but she died a year later, and their daughter also died in childhood.

His third wife, whom he married when he was 33, was said to have expensive tastes which undoubtedly put pressure on his earning capacity and made it necessary for him to sustain a large private practice. This might, to some extent, have influenced his decision to resign from the Meath Hospital at the age of 47.

He retired to an estate in the west of Ireland, and died years later, on 19 March 1853, from the effects of an abdominal tumour. In his last hours, he rather touchingly asked his family, who had gathered by his bedside, to recite some of the prayers he had shared with his father as a child.[11] Some 24 years after his death, a statue of Graves was unveiled in the home of the College in Kildare Street, where it still stands in the room named after him. His effigy is captured for posterity in the marble, but his legacy to medicine is timeless.

Professor T Joseph McKenna, a former President of the College, and a recipient of the Stearne Medal, has offered a modern and fascinating perspective of the man who is possiby best known for his association with 'Graves'

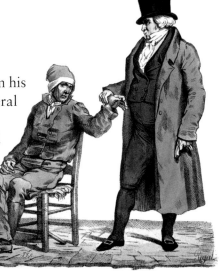

The rich doctor to the poor patient, 'You are very well'.
Pulse-taking was the common way to make a diagnosis, with the pulse being the only part of the body that the physician could freely touch.
Encouraged in particular by Robert Graves, the ancient art of pulse-taking moved from the purely qualitative to include a quantitative note.[12]
WELLCOME LIBRARY

Disease'. Writing in *The Lancet*, Professor McKenna summed up Graves' career as follows:

> That his name is the most revered today does justice to his many contributions to the development of clinical teaching, his original observations, and his prolific authorship of medical papers, which were the most respected of their time – as recognised then by Trousseau in Paris and subsequently by Osler.
>
> One of these papers, 'Newly observed affection of the thyroid gland in females', was published in the *London Medical and Surgical Journal* in 1853. It was in this that he detailed the clinical features now recognised as Graves' disease – even though it had been described earlier, by Caleb Hillier Parry in 1825. It is remarkable that it is for this contribution that Graves is best remembered, although it was arguably one of his lesser achievements.[13]

Engraving of William Stokes, from a painting by Frederic Burton
RCPI

William Stokes

The dawning of Ireland's Golden Age of Medicine was attracting international attention, but as noted earlier, this period of growth was the work of a number of men, of whom Graves was one of the most eminent. His name is most often associated with William Stokes, a former pupil, and also with Sir Dominic Corrigan, whom we shall meet at some length in the next chapter.

William Stokes, who was born in 1804, was part of the tightly-knit world of Dublin medicine. He was the son of Whitley Stokes, a physician in Meath Hospital, who himself had succeeded John Cheyne as Professor of Surgery at the Royal College of Surgeons, and had later become Regius Professor of Physic at Trinity.

Stokes followed in his father's footsteps as a doctor, but his path into medical practice took some time. He did not go to Trinity, but in 1822 took a course in anatomy at the Royal College of Surgeons. He then studied chemistry in

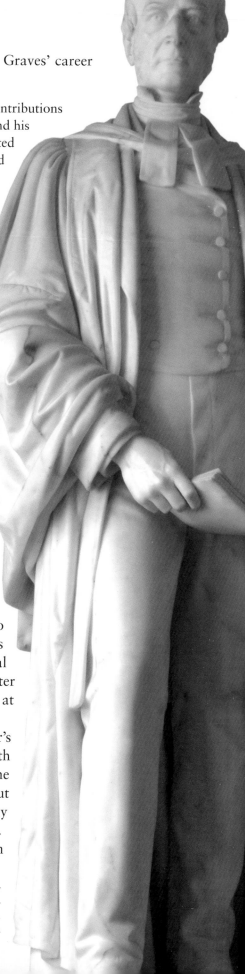

Statue of Robert Graves, started by JH Foley and completed by Albert Bruce-Joy, which stands in Graves' Hall, RCPI.

DERMOTT DUNBAR

MY DEAR GRAVES,

Permit me here to inscribe your name with that of my father. To him we owe, in a great measure, the founding of clinical instruction in Dublin ; and to you, the signal advancement of it by the introduction of the practical method. Accept this book in testimony of the kindly intercourse that for many years has passed between us, and as a mark of gratitude for benefits which can never be forgotten nor repaid.

WILLIAM STOKES.

AN

INTRODUCTION

TO THE

USE OF THE STETHOSCOPE;

WITH

ITS APPLICATION TO THE DIAGNOSIS IN DISEASES
OF THE THORACIC VISCERA;

INCLUDING

THE PATHOLOGY OF THESE VARIOUS AFFECTIONS.

By WILLIAM STOKES, M.D.

EDINBURGH:

PRINTED FOR MACLACHLAN AND STEWART;
BALDWIN, CRADOCK, AND JOY, LONDON;
AND HODGES AND M'ARTHUR,
DUBLIN.

M.DCCC.XXV.

Glasgow, and later, at his father's request, read medicine in Edinburgh, and graduated in 1825. The next year he joined Robert Graves in the Meath Hospital. They formed a strong professional partnership, and also became close personal friends – an occurence which is not as common as it might be assumed among high-powered professional people.

Stethoscope

Stokes had been so impressed by the work of the French doctor, René Laënnec, who had invented the stethoscope, that he wrote a book on the use of this relatively new instrument, which was looked on with suspicion – and in some cases, hostility – by many doctors, with the notable exception of Robert Graves.

Stokes, like his mentor Graves, had an early personal experience of fever which he developed in 1827, at the age of 23 and he almost died from the illness. Nevertheless he recovered sufficiently to cooperate with Graves later that year in writing a short book on fever, *Clinical Reports of the Medical Cases in the Meath Hospital*.

This was based on their own clinical experience, and was aimed mainly at their students. It was dedicated to John Cheyne as a tribute to his earlier contribution to medicine.

William Stokes had a reputation as a very compassionate physician, and the story is told that during an epidemic in Dublin, he treated a refugee and penniless French priest. Some years later Stokes

Dedication to Robert Graves from his pupil William Stokes in his publication *The Diagnosis and Treatment of Diseases of the Chest*
RCPI

An early stethoscope
RCPI COLLECTION

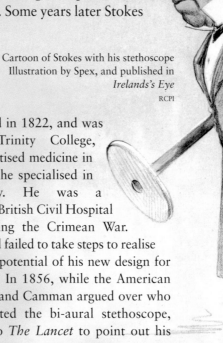

Cartoon of Stokes with his stethoscope
Illustration by Spex, and published in
Irelands's Eye
RCPI

Stokes, Leared and the Stethoscope

René Laënnec (1781–1826) invented the stethoscope in 1816 as an aid to diagnosing chest conditions, and to avoid the embarrassment of having to put an ear to the chest of female patients. Based on experiments with a rolled-up tube of card, Laënnec's stethoscope was a simple long wooden tube.

In 1825, while a medical student in Edinburgh, William Stokes (1804–77) published the first treatise in English on the use of the stethoscope. Returning to Ireland, he fought an uphill battle to introduce new methods of physical diagnosis, for which he was ridiculed, satirised and caricatured in the process.

In 1851 Arthur Leared (1822–79) exhibited the first design for a bi-aural stethoscope at the Great Exhibition, which used gutta-percha tubes. Leared was

born in Wexford in 1822, and was educated at Trinity College, Dublin. He practised medicine in London, where he specialised in gastroenterology. He was a physician at the British Civil Hospital at Smyrna during the Crimean War. However, Leared failed to take steps to realise the commercial potential of his new design for the stethoscope. In 1856, while the American doctors, Marsh and Camman argued over who had first invented the bi-aural stethoscope, Leared wrote to *The Lancet* to point out his prior claim.[14]

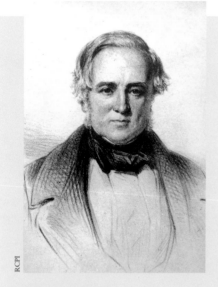

Robert Adams
1791–1875

Robert Adams was a leading surgeon and cardiologist, whose work on disorders of the heart led to the term Stokes-Adams Syndrome.

His earlier work, on the connection between a slow pulse and a loss of consciousness, was an important contribution to cardiology, and some two decades later the distinguished physician William Stokes would make further observations on this condition.

Adams was a President of the Royal College of Surgeons in Ireland and of the Dublin Pathological Society on three occasions. In 1862 he was appointed Surgeon in Ordinary to the Queen in Ireland, and also Regius Professor of Surgery at Trinity.

He was interested in many other subjects which were within the wide professional spectrum of physicians, and his work focused on respiratory, vascular and joint diseases, as well as cardiology.

Adams was highly regarded by William Stokes, and by the medical profession in general.[16]

was on holiday on the Rhine when his steamer docked at a small port.[15] Stokes noted the preparations being made for the embarkation of an important passenger, who turned out to be the French priest he had treated free of charge in Dublin. The priest had obviously prospered, because he was now Chaplain to the Empress Eugenie.

However he did not forget the man who had helped him in his distressing illness, and as a token of his thanks, he gave Stokes his ring, which later became a family heirloom.

Physician, Teacher and Author

Stokes rapidly made his name in Dublin, and he was a noted lecturer, researcher, and author. In 1838 he was one of the founders of the Pathological Society of Dublin, which was the first of its kind in the British Isles.

His highly-regarded lectures were printed in the *London Medical and Surgical Journal*. They were also edited and published in Philadelphia in 1840 under the title, *Clinical Lectures on the Theory and Practice of Medicine*, and became a standard American medical textbook.

With his background knowledge of the stethoscope on which he continued to carry out research, Stokes became an expert on respiratory conditions. One of his major works was his book, *The Diagnosis and Treatment of Diseases of the Chest*. It was published in 1837, and was translated into German.

Cardiologist

Following this study, Stokes concentrated on heart disease, and made a major contribution to the study of cardiology.

His work was published in the *Dublin Quarterly of Medical Science*, and his acknowledged *magnum opus* was his book, *Diseases of the Heart and the Aorta* (1854), which contained descriptions of the medically well-known Stokes-Adams syndrome, and the Cheyne-Stokes respiratory condition which has been mentioned earlier.

This publication was so advanced for its time that it became extremely well-known throughout the medical world, and helped to earn him the award of the Order of Merit from the German Emperor, Wilhelm I.

Despite his remarkable successes, Stokes remained modest, and he constantly paid tribute to the work of other doctors. This in turn helped to enhance the international reputation of the Dublin School of Medicine.

Stokes received a wide range of awards and honorary doctorates, and he was also President of the College. He was undoubtedly one of the most distinguished men to hold that post, and again, his reputation helped to enhance that of the College itself.

Stokes had been made a Licentiate of the College in 1825 but he had to wait another

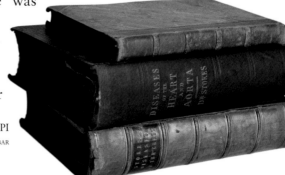

Publications by William Stokes, RCPI

DERMOTT DUNBAR

fourteen years to become an Honorary Fellow. This was because he had not graduated in Arts, and his medical degree was from Edinburgh – and not from Trinity, Oxford or Cambridge, which the College of Physicians's Charter required.

However Trinity came to the rescue, possibly because its members did not wish to repeat the debacle over Fielding Ould, as mentioned earlier. The Trinity Board said it would confer an Honorary MD on any six Licentiates nominated by the College. Stokes was included, and he was subsequently made an Honorary Fellow. He became President in 1849. The only other candidate that year was his old mentor Robert Graves, whom he rather embarrassingly defeated by eighteen votes to one.

Wide Interests

Outside the field of medicine, William Stokes had wide interests. He had many friends, and his home in Merrion Square was regularly frequented by the leading cultural figures of the day. He was deeply interested in history and archeology, and in 1874 was elected President of the Royal Irish Academy.

Stokes was also sustained by a long and happy marriage and close family. One of his sons, William Stokes became a very distinguished surgeon, and wrote a book about his father.

Stokes' later years, unlike those of other distinguished physicians like Cheyne, were relatively untroubled, and he continued working beyond the age of seventy – which was no mean achievement in those days.

He died in 1877 at his home in Howth, and he was widely remembered and respected as a great doctor and a good human being.

A statue of William Stokes also stands in the Royal College's home in No 6 Kildare Street, in the same room as that of his illustrious colleague Robert Graves.

In an address given during the tercentenary celebrations of Trinity Medical School in 1892, the Rector of the University of Amsterdam, Professor Stockvis, spoke glowingly of both Graves and Stokes. He said:

> The history of medicine is proud of these men. They are not national, they are international glories; and so long as human suffering shall be relieved by medicine, so long will be the names of Graves and Stokes be honoured all over the world.[17]

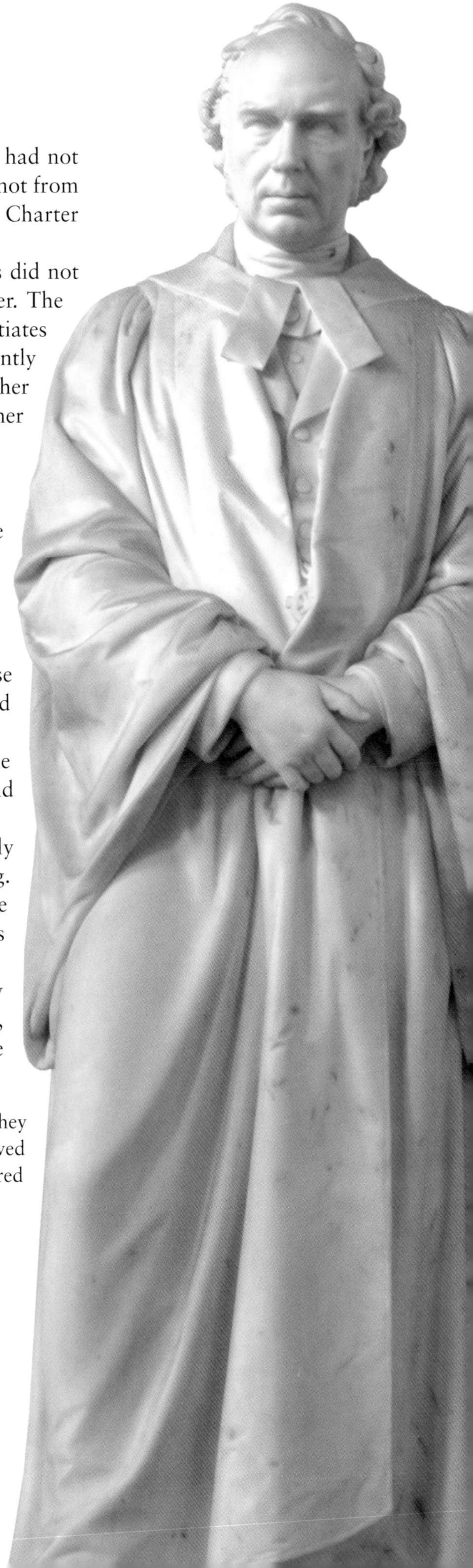

Statue of William Stokes
by John Henry Foley
stands in Graves Hall, RCPI

DERMOTT DUNBAR

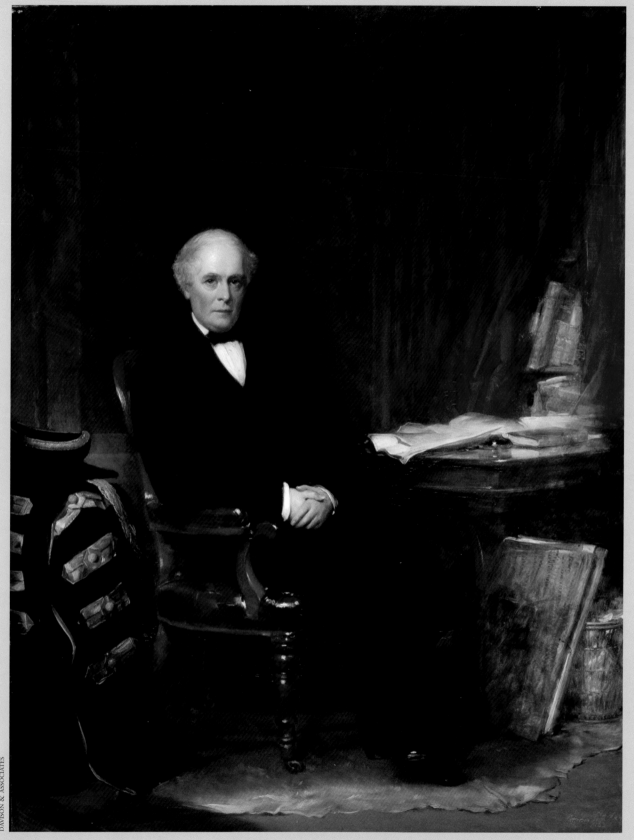

Dominic Corrigan
Painting by Catterson Smith the Elder
RCPI

Sir Dominic Corrigan

One of the most distinguished figures in the history of the College was Dominic Corrigan, who served as President for five successive terms, from 1859–64.

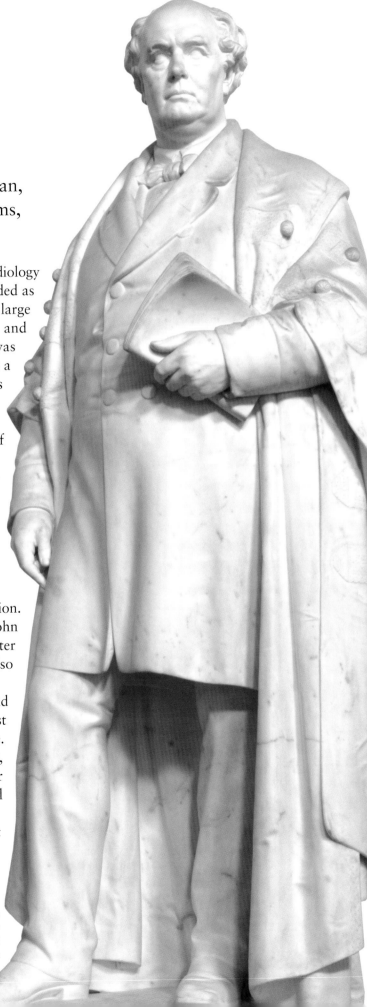

Dominic Corrigan made a significant contribution to cardiology and other branches of medicine. He was widely regarded as one of the most effective Presidents of the College; he had a large and lucrative practice, he had a wide circle of cultured and professional friends; he was a skilled politician who was honoured with a Baronetcy by Queen Victoria. He was also a Vice Chancellor and a Senate member of the Queen's University of Ireland which was established from the three constituent Queen's Colleges founded by Queen Victoria in Cork, Galway and Belfast under the Government of Sir Robert Peel in 1845.

Most significant of all, unlike the majority of his high-profile medical predecessors, Dominic Corrigan was not a Protestant. Through his natural ability and achievements however, he became one of the most upwardly mobile and successful Catholics of his generation.

Early Days

Corrigan belonged to a family which had no medical tradition. Born in 1802, he was the son of a Catholic merchant, John Corrigan who lived in Thomas Street Dublin (which later became the site of an Augustinian Church). The family also had a small farm at Kilmainham.

Dominic John Corrigan was the second of six children, and he was brought up at a time when the Penal Laws against Catholics in Ireland were becoming more relaxed in practice. With the passing of the Catholic Emancipation Act in 1829, the way was open, in theory, for an ambitious and clever young Catholic to make his mark within the professional and social life of nineteenth-century Ireland.

The reality, however, was different, and even the bright and ambitious young Corrigan had to strive very hard to succeed, because of his religious background.

Statue of Dominic Corrigan
by John Henry Foley
in Graves Hall, RCPI

DERMOTT DUNBAR

Maynooth

Corrigan was educated in a lay college associated with St Patrick's College in Maynooth, which had been established in 1795. It was during this time that he attracted the attention of two important mentors – Dr Edward O'Kelly, a local medical practitioner and Physician to the college, who taught him some of the basics of medicine, and also Dr Cornelius Denvir, later the Catholic Bishop of Connor in the North, who taught him mathematics and physics, which would help him in his study of medicine in later years.

Following his training at Maynooth, Corrigan went to Trinity College, where he came under the influence of the legendary Professor of Anatomy and Surgery, James Macartney, an Armagh man who was one of the most influential figures in early Irish medicine and scholarship.

As a medical student he took part in the ward rounds at Sir Patrick Dun's Hospital; he also attended lectures given there by many of the leading doctors of the day.

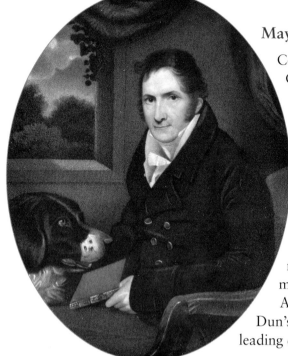

Matters of Life and Death

James Macartney
RCPI

Corrigan was a lively student, who allowed himself to become involved with the shady but essential practice of body snatching. This has been mentioned earlier, but in Corrigan's case it was described vividly from his first-hand experience.

It was a ghastly business of which Corrigan did not approve, but in his old age he reflected upon some of those body-snatching adventures of his youth. Writing anonymously in the *British Medical Journal* of 11 January 1879 – shortly before his death – he published a piece entitled, 'Reminiscences of a Medical Student prior to the passing of the Anatomy Act'.

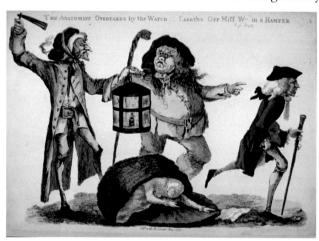

'The Anatomist Overtaken by the Watch'.
WELLCOME LIBRARY

He described how he and his companions moved with their bare hands, the clay and stones that had recently been covering a coffin. Then a rope with a grappling hook was lowered, and the lip of the coffin was broken open.

The corpse was lifted by the neck with a rope, and the whole body was smuggled to a transport waiting nearby, to be taken to a dissecting theatre as quickly as possible. Corrigan was particularly appalled by the fact that the corpses were stripped naked because a body snatcher caught in possession of a shroud was liable to be prosecuted. The practice of body snatching was a crime, and not something to be taken lightly.

Corrigan was evidently sensitive to the plight of the relatives of the person whose dead body was so ignominiously raised up, stripped naked and hurried away for dissection.

He also described how, on a hazy night in one graveyard, he and his companions saw a white floating object or shroud, apparently waved by an unseen hand, at a grave from which they intended to steal a body:

> … two of us approached to examine the object, when we found it was the white skirt of a poor woman's dress, who was rocking herself to and fro over the grave.
>
> She was the widow of the poor man buried beneath, who had died on his way home from working the harvest in England, and the poor woman had remained to watch over his remains.
>
> It need scarcely be added, that we pledged ourselves to respect the remains for her sake, that we kept our word, and that we made up a small collection to afford her some aid.[1]

In this short passage Corrigan revealed the harshness of the times, and the anguish of a woman, who without a husband to earn money in order to stave off chronic hunger and illness, faced untold suffering.

Edinburgh Graduate

The young Corrigan received a good medical education in Dublin, but finished his course in Edinburgh, where he graduated with an MD in 1825, the same year that William Stokes also graduated there in medicine.

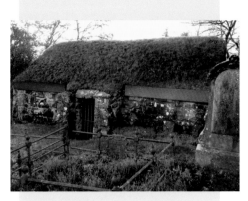

The remains of a protected burial house at St John's Church, Donegore, County Antrim.
ALF MCCREARY

Watchtowers and watchhouses were built in some graveyards for the prevention of bodysnatching. Some graves were also surrounded by a framework of iron bars, constructed in an effort to protect the newly deceased. Iron coffins too were used and finally bodyguards could also be employed to keep watch over the grave until the body had decomposed enough to be of no use to an anatomist.

In a letter to a friend, written shortly afterwards, Corrigan underlined how nervous he had felt during the process, despite his considerable ability. Many modern students can take comfort from knowing that one of the most distinguished members of their profession felt just as nervous as they do when sitting their final examinations.

Corrigan was a young man in the relatively foreign environment of Edinburgh, and he was being examined as a student who had done much of his training in Dublin. He wrote:

> Coming before the professors here, a perfect stranger to them, I dreaded that they might be more strict, and reasonably so, on me than on one of their pupils.
>
> This had, at least, the effect of making me study more than otherwise I might. My examination lasted about two hours, and was, I think, as fair as if I had studied under themselves.[2]

Corrigan also paid a fulsome tribute to one of his old tutors, Professor Devlin at Maynooth, who had taught him chemistry:

> This pleased the professor of chemistry here, and (each professor thinking his own branch the most important) when announcing to me the result of the examination, he told me it would be very pleasing to all the professors if my countrymen came as well-prepared before them.

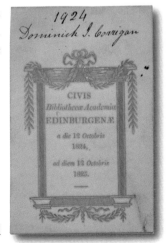

ABOVE AND OPPOSITE: Corrigan's lecture and library cards for Edinburgh University
RCPI
OPPOSITE: University of Edinburgh, Medical School, New Building, Teviot Place
CANMORE IMAGES

University of Edinburgh.
13 MAY, 1825
LECTURES on BOTANY.
ROBERT GRAHAM M.D.
Au. D. S Corrigan
No. 102
RCPI

127

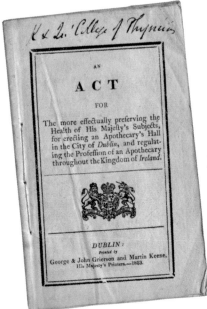

Corrigan's annotated copy of an Act to create an Apothecary's Hall in Dublin and regulation of the profession, 1823. He practised at a local dispensary after graduation.

Under the Apothecaries' Act no apothecary could take an apprentice who had not been examined by the Hall, and apprentices were required to serve for seven years. Under the Act also, no one could open an apothecary's shop without a certificate from the Hall, and there were restrictions on the sale of poisons. Appeals against the Hall decision could be made to the King and Queen's College of Physicians in Ireland. The Hall also had the right to impose a fine on those who broke the terms of the Act.[3]

RCPI

I thanked him for the compliment. And never before, I believe, thanked a stranger so sincerely, for during the short interval that lapsed between the termination of my examination, and the verdict being made known to me, I suffered anxiety that I would not again experience for any consideration.[2]

In this letter Corrigan showed his shrewdness in dealing with people, and this quality would stand him in good stead during his long and successful career.

First Appointments

When he returned to Dublin, Corrigan practised for a short time at a local dispensary, as did his contemporary Stokes, in the tradition of young doctors gaining a toehold on the ladder of professional advancement.

In 1825, Corrigan began his practice at 11, Upper Ormond Quay. He had a wide range of patients including some from the merchant-classes and also the poor, many of whom were living in the most appalling and distressing of circumstances. Crowded into insanitary and disease-ridden accommodation, they were prey to various kinds of fevers, including rheumatic fever. This was an unfashionable area in which to work, well away from the mainstream medical practice of the successful and well-to-do, but Corrigan was determined to succeed.

In his definitive and elegant biography of Corrigan, *Conscience and Conflict*, the author Eoin O'Brien writes:

Corrigan's ambition to succeed arose, not from necessity as much as from pride – a pride that was in its origins Irish and hence rebellious and stubborn.

He determined early on in his career that he would reach the top of his profession regardless of what the obstacles might be. His personality was well-suited to adversity, and his spirit was stimulated by controversy, all the more so when he was at the centre of it.

His capacity for work was, even by Victorian standards, voracious. Failure did not discourage him, or if it did, it certainly never deterred him; in fact, the greater the reverses, the more determined he became to succeed.[4]

O'Brien also describes Corrigan's physical attributes and temperament thus: 'In appearance he was tall, erect, of commanding figure, not, it was said, unlike Daniel O'Connell.' He was a man of great physical energy, and a splendid horseman. 'In temperament his distinguishing traits were kindness and tenderness towards the sick, and the ability to make a bold decision.'[5]

Further Advancement

Corrigan did not have long to wait for preferment, and in 1826 he was appointed as a physician at the Sick Poor Institution of Meath Street.

Even at this early stage, he had begun to make a name for himself with a series of papers in *The Lancet*, the first of which appeared in

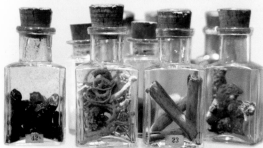

Dispensary bottles

RCPI

1828. In some of which he criticised the accepted medical norms of his day. One of his most important contributions was an article on aneurism of the aorta and on systolic heart murmurs.[6]

In 1831 Corrigan, then aged 29, was appointed Physician to the Charitable Infirmary, Jervis Street, which was arguably the most significant break-through of his career. It was here that he published some of his most important papers, and carried out much of his outstanding clinical work.

In his new post he continued to enhance his reputation by working with cases of aortic incompetence. One of his important early papers, *On permanent patency of the mouth of the aorta, or inadequacy of the aortic valves*, appeared in the prestigious *Edinburgh Medical and Surgical Journal* in 1832. This condition was to become known universally as 'Corrigan's disease'. Also coined was the term 'Corrigan's Pulse', which gives a clear indication of a patient suffering from aortic incompetence.

Although he was not the first physician to describe the aortic valve incompetence condition, Corrigan's description was so clearly written that it drew the attention of physicians worldwide, and the condition was henceforth associated with his name.

In 1838 he made another important contribution to cardiology, with a paper, *On Aortitis, as one of the causes* of *angina pectora, with observations on its nature and treatment of.*[7]

Certificate of attendance by Corrigan of clinical lectures for six months at Jervis Street Infirmary, 1834.
RCPI

Dominic Corrigan's medical interests ranged widely however, and in 1838 he presented another significant paper to a meeting of the College, in which he described the condition known as 'cirrhosis of the lung'. This was later published in the *Dublin Journal of Medical Science*, and contained some original observations on a lung condition known as 'pulmonary fibrosis'.

Inventor

Corrigan was also noted for his inventions, which included a bed for immobilised patients, an inhaler, the design for a stethoscope, and an ingenious device known as 'Corrigan's Button'. This was a small metal plate with a handle which was heated, and then placed along the sciatic nerve to help alleviate pain.

Detail from a drawing by Corrigan for an 'Economical bedstead prepared for the Central Board of Health, Ireland'.
RCPI

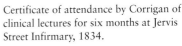

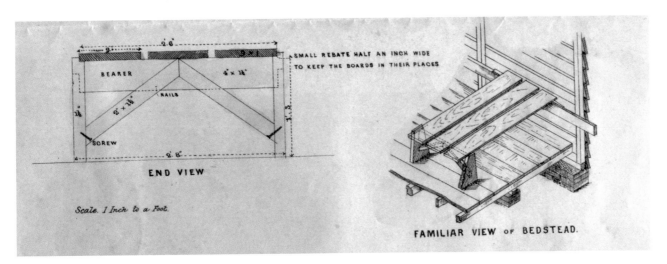

129

No doubt Corrigan's ingenuity would have earned him a fortune today in the treatment of this widespread condition.[8]

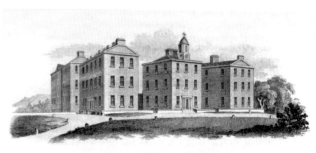

FEVER HOSPITAL, CORK STREET.

Cork Street Fever Hospital
RCPI

Outstanding Lecturer

Corrigan was a good bedside teacher, and an outstanding lecturer. He taught in the Dublin School of Anatomy, Surgery and Medicine from 1833 to 1846, and his lectures brought him widespread acclamation. His course opened with the important topic, 'The abnormal sounds of the heart and arteries', and his lectures were well-illustrated. His popularity was reminiscent of Robert Graves who also filled his lecture halls with enthusiastic audiences.

In 1846 Corrigan transferred his lectures to the Richmond Hospital, where he had been a physician for several years. He remained on the staff there, until his resignation from the House of Industry Hospitals. He made a strong impression in the Richmond, which he liked and which, in his opinion, compared well with the major hospitals in Europe. From 1837–40 he had been a physician at the Cork Street Fever Hospital; he was also appointed as Lecturer to the Apothecaries' Hall in 1837.

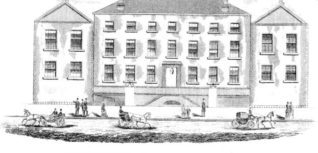

RICHMOND SURGICAL HOSPITAL

110 BEDS

One of Corrigan's gifts as a physician was his keen observation of patients. He once advised a young colleague not to look at his watch when treating patients, but suggested that he should have a clock discreetly placed in the room which he could view, unknown to the patient. The story is also told of how Corrigan noticed, to a husband's surprise, that his wife 'was on the mend'. Corrigan said that he had deduced this by, 'an infallible system … the handle of a looking-glass peeping from under her pillow'![9]

This was another example of the astuteness and, in Oscar Wilde's words, the 'uncommon common sense' which stood Corrigan so well throughout his career.

The Richmond Surgical Hospital, North Brunswick Street, from a hospital certificate. Originally built as a Benedictine Convent in 1688, it was used as a surgical hospital from 1811–1900.
RCSI

The 'new' Richmond Hospital, built 1894, is now a Court House.
DENIS HUTCHINSON

Dublin School

Corrigan had much in common with Stokes and Graves. They all shared the same attitude to clinical teaching, encouraging students in making their own observations, and placing the patient at the centre of medical provision.

As we have seen Corrigan and Stokes were colleagues from the time they had graduated together from Edinburgh University, and even though Corrigan had come from a less privileged background, he had demonstrated the skill and tenacity to enable him to take his place among the front-ranking men in the medical world of his day. As he progressed, he moved to ever more salubrious addresses. He eventually lived in the fashionable Merrion Square, and rode each day on horseback to the Richmond.

Sadly, however, a large number of his medical contemporaries lived in much less fortunate circumstances, particularly in the rural areas, and this was exacerbated by the Great Famine.

The Great Famine

There were many famines and epidemics in Irish history, but the Great Famine of 1845–50 was a catastrophe of the greatest magnitude. Its origins and outcomes are still controversial, and many books – indeed entire libraries – have been written on the subject.[10]

Within the confines of this publication, however, we will focus on how the Great Famine affected the medical profession in Ireland, as far as is known, and also how it impacted on a number of its leading members, including Graves, Stokes and Corrigan.

In several successive years, from 1845 onwards, a blight destroyed the potato crop, on which the vast majority of the population depended for sustenance. Ireland was not able to cope with such a massive natural disaster.

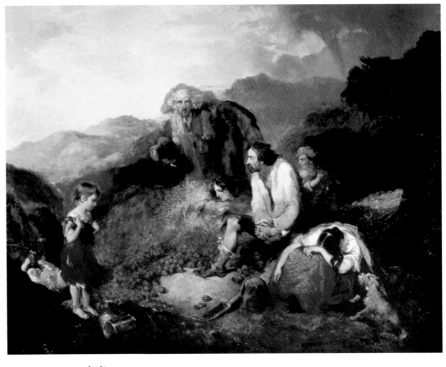

Discovery of Potato Blight
by Daniel McLeod
DEPARTMENT OF FOLKLORE, UNIVERSITY COLLEGE DUBLIN

'Ireland is threatened with a thing that is read of in history and in distant countries, but scarcely in our own land and time – a famine. Whole fields of the root have rotted in the ground, and many a family sees its sole provision for the year destroyed.'
The Spectator, 25 October 1845

Hospitals were overwhelmed by the sheer volume of people needing help, and poor, hungry wretches were crammed into specially-erected tents and fever sheds, often situated outside the main hospital buildings. Hunger and illness were rife, and it is virtually impossible to calculate the huge numbers of people who died. As one historian noted:

> Hospitals and work-house records were often imperfectly kept; and even if they were complete, it would still be necessary to take into account the unknown thousands who perished in their own homes, or by the wayside, untended and almost unnoticed.[11]

HARDWICKE FEVER HOSPITAL
120 BEDS

Historians generally agree that over one million people perished during the Great Famine from hunger and illness, and that another million left Ireland to escape malnutrition, disease, poverty and death, and to start a new life in North America and elsewhere.

Despite the huge challenges and the inadequate medical and other resources available, there was an attempt by a hastily-appointed General Board of Health to develop an improvised nationwide network of temporary fever hospitals, between 1846 and 1849. Sadly, however, in the words of one historian:

> The attempt came too late to avert a major disaster, but it did something to mitigate the effect of the epidemics: and the high death-rate among hospital and dispensary doctors is evidence that, whatever the shortcomings of the medical services as a whole, individual medical practitioners did not shirk their duties.[12]

The Hardwicke Fever Hospital played a major role in controlling the epidemics of the Great Famine. Dominic Corrigan, who was a member of the General Board of Health, was in charge of the Hardwicke Fever Hospital and from there directed relief operations for the country.
BELOW: One of Corrigan's case books from the Royal College of Physicians' archive.
RCPI

There was a significant death-rate among city doctors, and particularly dispensary doctors in rural areas, who faced enormous hardships at the best of times.

This point was taken to heart by William Stokes, who described the arduous life of the country doctor when he and a colleague, Professor James Cusack, the President of the Royal College of Surgeons, gave evidence in London prior to the drafting of the 1843 Medical Charities' Bill.

They had compiled a report on the conditions for rural dispensary doctors, and their findings were published in an article, *On the Mortality of Medical Practitioners from Fever in Ireland*, published in the *Dublin Quarterly Journal of Medicine* in 1847.[13]

They discovered that in the quarter-century prior to 1843, nearly 25 per cent of Irish medical practitioners had died while carrying out their duties. Most had died from typhus, and in that period the mortality rate among physicians was well over twice that among Army officers in combat from January 1811–May 1814.

Stokes and Cusack pleaded for better salaries for country physicians, and emphasised that there was no relief provision for the families of those who had died carrying out their duties.

Unfortunately the proposed 1843 Bill was dropped, and nothing was done until 1851, when the Medical Charities Act was passed.

Nevertheless, the graphic description by Stokes and Cusack of the hardships facing country physicians in Ireland makes for grim reading:

> ... the medical practitioners in Ireland are placed in a position very different and far more serious than that of their brethren in Great Britain: for while the latter have only to contend with infectious fever occasionally – and, rarely indeed, in the rural districts – the Irish physician has to combat it in all situations, and at all seasons ...[14]

As Stokes told a Parliamentary Committee in 1843 that the situation was so bad that:

> Such a number of my pupils have been cut off by typhus fever as to make me feel very uneasy when any of them take a dispensary office in Ireland. I look upon it almost as going into battle.[14]

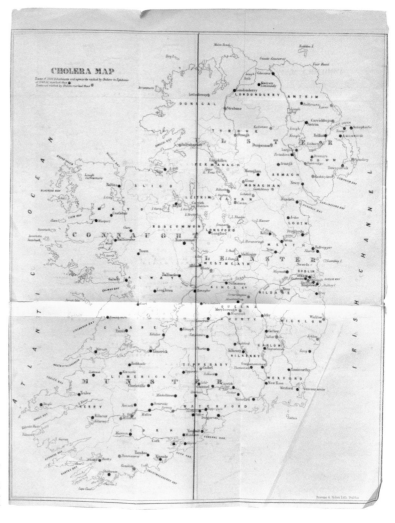

Cholera Map, 1866
Towns of 2,000 inhabitants and more which were affected by cholera in the epidemic of 1848–50 are marked with a black spot. The cholera-free towns are marked in red.

Significantly, Dominic Corrigan believed that cholera was spread by a miasma rather than through contagion, and this led to an important change in the treatment of the illness.[16]
RCPI

During the Great Famine period Stokes and Cusack produced another survey of the death-rate among doctors. They reported that, in 1847 alone, a total of 178 doctors 'exclusive of pupils and army surgeons', died and the great majority of these from a disease 'contracted in the discharge of public medical duties'.[15]

It requires little imagination to visualise the extra hardships facing doctors during the unmitigated disaster of the Great Famine.

Stokes and Cusack in their 1848 report in the *Dublin Quarterly Journal of Medical Science* painted a vivid picture of the challenges facing a rural doctor:

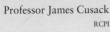

Professor James Cusack
RCPI

> labouring among the poor in wild and thinly-populated districts, where the medical man has often to ride or drive for many hours, exposed to cold and wet, and frequently at night, suffering great fatigue, and then becoming exposed to concentrated contagion in some of the wretched, isolated hovels of the peasantry.[17]

Exact figures for medical mortality in those years are not available. The 1851 Census, conducted in March of that year, recorded that there were 6,811 people

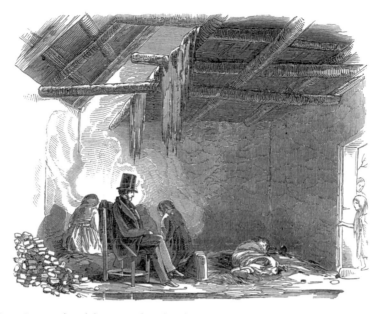

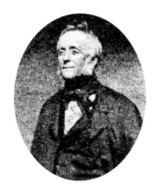

Dr Dan Donovan was appointed Medical Superintendant to the Skibbereen Dispensary, he was the first medical officer at the new Skibbereen Workhouse in 1839.
In 1846 and 1847 Dr Donovan wrote *A Diary of a Dispensary Doctor* which was published in Cork's *The Southern Reporter*. Some of his detailed descriptive accounts and harrowing reports were reproduced in *The Illustrated London News*.
SKIBBEREEN HERITAGE

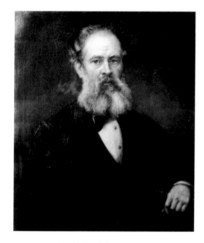

David Hadden, 1817–78, was a licentiate of the Apothecaries' Hall in Dublin. He practised as a dispensary doctor in Skibereen which experienced some of the worst effects of the famine – poverty, hunger, disease and death. The gratitude of the survivors in Skibbereen and the esteem in which they held their doctor can be judged by the various gifts they presented.[18]
Painting by James Butler Brenan

'ministering to health' in Ireland. There is no doubt however that these figures would have been much higher, but for the ravages of the Great Famine.

Concern and Conflict

The almost unending litany of death and misery was naturally of the utmost concern to everyone, including the founders of the Dublin School of Medicine, but the issues arising from the Great Famine led to a serious difference of opinion between Robert Graves and Dominic Corrigan, who was a member of the General Board of Health.

In many ways, the Great Famine of 1845–50 was a national disaster waiting to happen. Corrigan had already warned in a pamphlet that the utter dependence of the Irish population on potatoes as their staple diet would leave them vulnerable to famine and fever if that source of food was no longer available.

The General Board of Health tried to do its best in the appalling circumstances. However one of its most controversial measures was the decision to pay dispensary doctors the paltry sum of only five shillings a day, as a supplement to their already low salaries.

The medical profession was outraged at what it regarded as a derisory fee for doctors who were putting their lives on the line in dealing with famine victims; many had died already. However the authorities were deaf to any protests, replying that the five shillings daily was a just reward. The press largely took the doctors' side, and the issue quickly became a major public debate.

Unfortunately for Corrigan, who was a high-profile member of the Board, a great deal of the hostility was directed against him personally, and not least by his eminent colleague, Robert Graves. Graves wrote an extraordinarily long, and in parts rambling, letter to *The Dublin Quarterly Journal of Medical Science*, which was published in its August/November edition of 1847 – incidentally the same journal had published the first report by Stokes and Cusack on mortality among doctors.

In the letter Robert Graves reflected on the shortcomings of the General Board of Health, and also stated:

John Oliver Curran, 1819–47, was a general practitioner and one of Stokes' favourite pupils. Curran died of typhus contracted from a patient in his care. This event inspired much of the opposition to Corrigan and the treatment meted out to the dispensary doctors.[19]

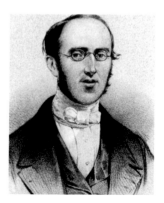

... Dr Corrigan certainly deserves much praise for his diligence; but surely the Government did not act wisely in so constituting the Board that it became a nonentity the moment he ceased to attend.

Now when we call to mind that Dr Corrigan's numerous avocations as a lecturer, a hospital physician, and a practitioner of considerable repute, must ingross a great deal of his time, we begin to tremble for the very existence of the Board of Health; but we need be under no apprehensions on the subject, for it appears to be *proven*, that the learned Doctor, no matter wherever else he may be, *is always there*, in virtue of a miraculous *ibiquity*! (sic).[20]

Such comments must have been hurtful to Corrigan, whose high profile on the General Health Board was partly down to his hard work and sense of duty. He may have felt like retaliating to Graves' personal criticisms, but wisely he chose to remain silent.

However it was also around this time that Corrigan, rather unwisely in medico-political terms, decided to seek support for an Honorary Fellowship from the College. As one of the outstanding members of his profession, his acceptance should have been automatic. Unfortunately, however, he was 'blackballed', and his attempt to receive an Honorary Fellowship failed. It was thought that his election was blocked by Robert Graves because he disapproved of Corrigan's membership of the General Board of Health which had, in Graves' opinion, awarded dispensary doctors such a derisory daily fee for their work during the Famine.

History, of course, has recorded many similar situations where people quickly apportion blame to the most obvious target, but quite often the real culprit is

The ballot-box used in the blackballing of Corrigan.
RCPI

Letter to Lord Clancarty from Corrigan, 1846
RCPI

In this letter Corrigan outlines some of his views on the sick poor in Ireland, in the knowledge that Lord Clancarty (William Thomas Le Poer Trench, 3rd Earl of Clancarty) had read his pamphlet on Famine and Fever. The Earl and his predecessors were considered good landlords who made efforts to alleviate some of the extremes of suffering of their tenants.

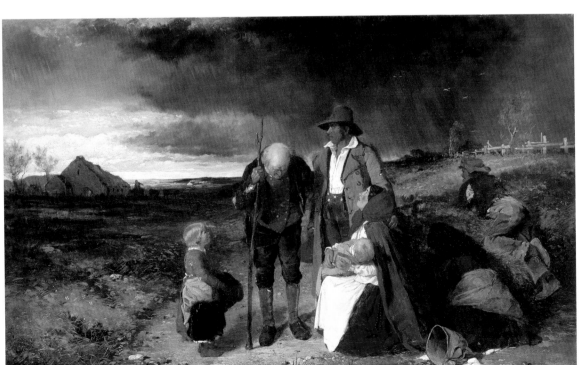

During the Famine tens of thousands were expelled from their homes. Landowners claimed that they had no option but to evict tenants who failed to pay their rent, but many saw the Famine as an opportunity to clear the land for more profitable uses.[21]

An Ejected Family
by Erskine Nicol
NATIONAL GALLERY OF IRELAND

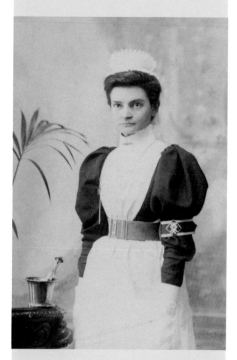

Blanche Thompson, a nurse at the Hospital for Women, Birmingham, was the granddaughter of Henry Hill Hickman, a pioneer of anaesthesia.
WELLCOME LIBRARY, LONDON

The second half of the nineteenth-century saw two major developments in medicine – anaesthesia and vaccination. Nursing also underwent a revolution around this time – 'the work of Florence Nightingale had changed nursing from a despised branch of domestic service into a respectable profession for middle-class women. Her designs for airy, well-ventilated hospitals were followed by hospital builders for half a century'.[23]

a different person altogether. Whatever the rights or wrongs of the 'blackballing incident', it was unfortunate that Graves criticised Corrigan personally, rather than focusing his attack on the Board, or the Government itself.

Graves may have been annoyed because at the time of his appointment to the Board, Corrigan was not a member of either the Royal College of Surgeons or the Royal College of Physicians. Yet even with the benefit of hindsight, it is difficult to understand why Graves felt compelled to criticise Corrigan so publicly.

However, Professor T Joseph McKenna points out that while Graves was a brilliant clinician, he was not as astute politically as Corrigan, and that therefore he was not as able to advance himself as far within the social fabric of their time:

> I have the impression that Graves thought of himself as something of a failure in comparison to Corrigan, whose star was shining.
>
> Graves ran for the Presidency of the Royal College of Physicians in 1849, but was roundly defeated by Stokes, who was not only his colleague but also a former pupil. Graves also ran for the Chair of Medicine at Trinity, although he was already the Professor of Physiology. Again he was defeated by Stokes, and around the same time he retired from the Meath Hospital, which he loved.
>
> Robert Graves was the kind of man who believed that excellence would be rewarded for its own sake, but Corrigan had a different concept. He believed that being astute politically was just as important as being brilliant professionally. Both men were brilliant but some people argue that Corrigan achieved much more in his lifetime, both for himself and the Royal College of Physicians, and for Irish medicine in general.[22]

Whatever psychology or political nuances were involved in this matter, both Robert Graves and Dominic Corrigan, as well as their esteemed colleague William Stokes, made a huge contribution to the Dublin School, and to the Golden Age of Irish Medicine. These achievements were well summarised by Professor Sir Peter Froggatt, a former Vice-Chancellor of Queen's University, and a former Pro-Chancellor of the University of Dublin.

> Ireland's great literary tradition is highly acclaimed, but it is only doctors for the most part who know of her equally proud medical one.
>
> Rooted through the centuries, it reached its finest flowering during the nineteenth century when Dublin became a medical Mecca, and Ireland could boast an unusually comprehensive system of medical care, which was the envy of the wealthier countries.
>
> Few areas of medical science have failed to benefit from an often eponymously-commemorated Irish pioneer, whether home-based, or from the extensive Irish diaspora.[24]

Difficult Times

There is no doubt that the first half of the nineteenth century in Ireland was difficult and demanding. There

Robert Graves in his later years
RCPI

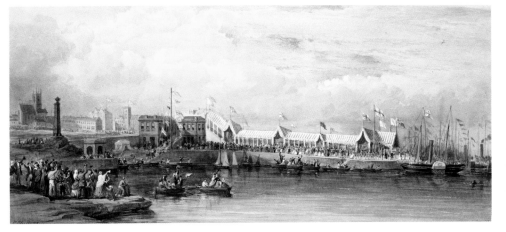

Queen Victoria's flotilla leaving Kingstown Dock. The Queen's visit to Ireland marked a symbolic end to the famine.
Watercolour by Philip Phillip, 1849

were important developments within Irish medicine, and the description of 'the Golden Age' was thoroughly deserved – though this has to be tempered by the reality that general medical provision was severely limited at that time in a country where so many of the population were still living in dire poverty.

In many senses the Great Famine from 1845–50 is seen by historians as an immensely tragic watershed, and as a dividing line in the history of modern Ireland.

Professor JC Beckett, writing nearly a century later, noted astutely:

> When, in August 1849, the queen [Victoria] made her first visit to Ireland, she was welcomed with enormous popular enthusiasm; but it would be a mistake to regard this enthusiasm as a true indication of Irish feelings toward Britain, and it certainly had no lasting effect on British feelings towards Ireland.
>
> As the two countries approached the end of a half-century of parliamentary union, they were, perhaps, more completely estranged from one another than they had ever been before.[25]

The sense of isolation in the early years after the 1801 Act of Union developed into a period of growing Catholic self-assertion, which in turn helped to lay the foundations for a strong movement towards national self-determination.

It was against this difficult and complex political background that the story of the College continued in the latter half of the nineteenth century.

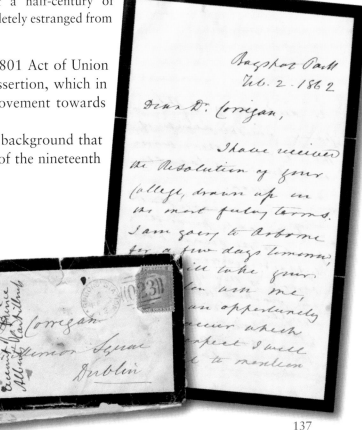

A letter to Corrigan from Sir James Clark, 1862, Physician-in-Ordinary to Queen Victoria. Sir James thanks Corrigan for the resolution of the College on the death of Prince Albert, which he promises to present to the Queen. He also gives Corrigan details of Prince Albert's last illness and death.
RCPI

6 At home, No 6 Kildare Street

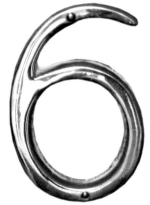

The second half of the nineteenth century witnessed substantial progress by the Royal College of Physicians of Ireland, which at last was to establish for itself a permanent home in Dublin.

The College also continued to play an important role in the medical life of the country, and not least through the continued contribution of outstanding physicians, including Sir Dominic Corrigan and others.

Such progress was made against a background of ongoing political uncertainty and sporadic strife, with the Westminster Parliament unable to devise a system of government that would bring peace to the long-troubled island of Ireland.

New Developments

Despite the disaster of the Great Irish Famine and its aftermath, the business of the College progressed steadily. In 1849 William Stokes was elected President. In the process, as has been mentioned, he defeated his former teacher and colleague Robert Graves, by eighteen votes to one.

This was a sad rebuff for his old mentor and friend. Assuming that the single vote for Graves was cast by the man himself, it was clear that in medico-political terms Graves was becoming yesterday's man. From today's perspective however, his contribution to Irish medicine remains unsullied, and his reputation is still bright as one of the chief instigators of 'the Golden Age' of Irish medicine.

Medical historians are divided as to when this golden era began to recede, but one medical writer has summed up some of the innovations towards the end of the century which help to set it in context.

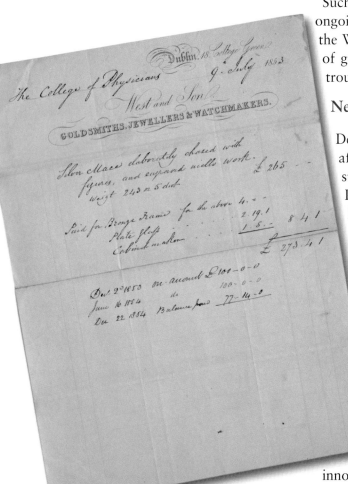

Invoice for the Mace from West and Son

The Mace
RCPI

The resolutely clinical rather than laboratory focus of the Dublin School was to remain a characteristic of Irish medicine. By the middle of the twentieth century, the individualised, personal approach had become a doctrine. Unfortunately for the fame of the Dublin School, it was not one which was shared by the rest of the world.[1]

Nevertheless, by the mid-nineteenth century, the reputation of the leaders of Irish medicine remained high, and there were a number of people in the profession who believed that the Royal College of Physicians should put in place some of the formal trappings commensurate with its growing stature.

New Mace

In March 1850 a physician named James Foulis Duncan (who was later to become President from 1873–5) proposed that the College should have gowns as resplendent as those of the University graduates. Only a week later, Dr Aquilla Smith proposed that a new mace should also be provided. No doubt this was to set off the splendour of the new gowns.

A committee was quickly formed to advise on the cost of the proposed new garments and mace. Within only three weeks the College had accepted the grand design for a new mace from a noted Dublin portrait painter Frederick William Burton, RHA, who was a friend of Stokes. He subsequently became the Director of the National Gallery in London, from 1874–94.

The estimated cost of the new mace was £50, but – not surprisingly – this sum was in the final event grossly inadequate. In all ages the price of institutional pride cannot be measured precisely in financial terms however, and when a prestigious body needs a symbol of its importance, the money will be found from somewhere.

However the College determined that while the President should also have a splendid gown made from black tabbinet (a poplin fabric), with gold lace. The Registrar would not be required to

Engraving of Aquilla Smith, based on a drawing by FW Burton
RCPI

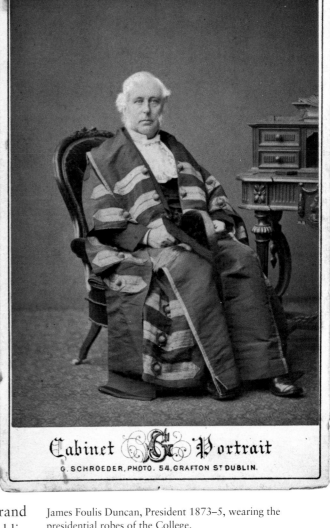

James Foulis Duncan, President 1873–5, wearing the presidential robes of the College.
RCPI

An invoice for the supply of a new gown
RCPI

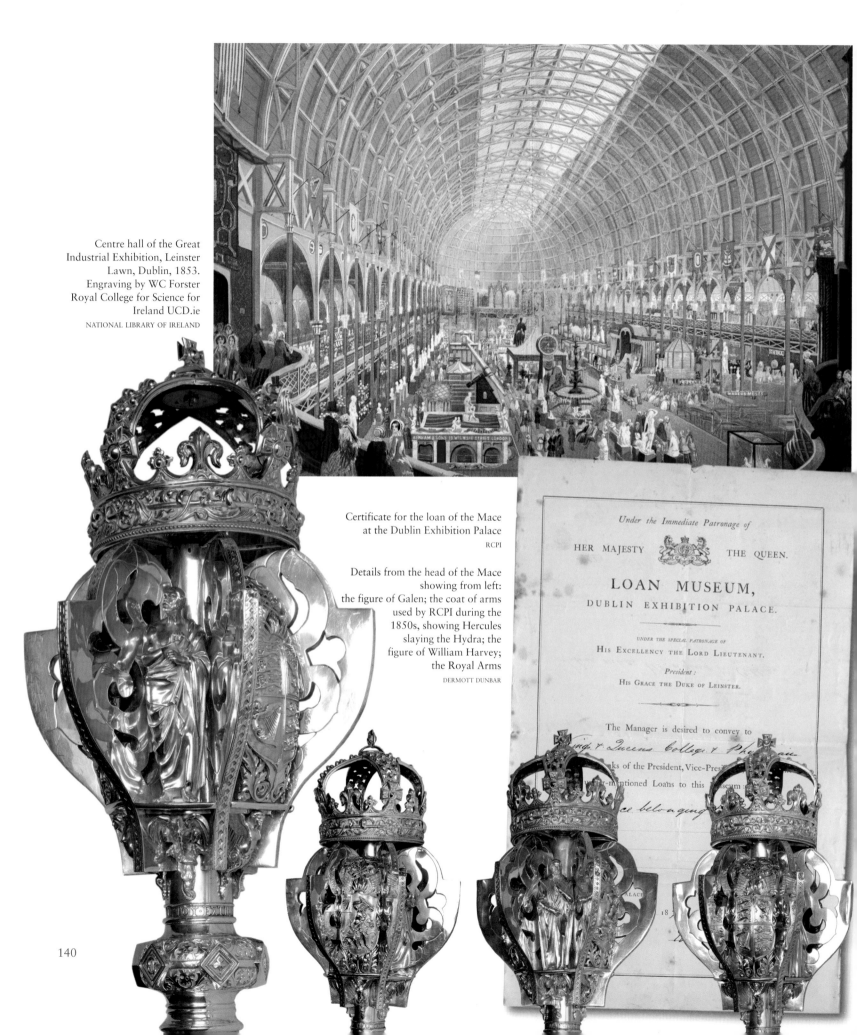

Centre hall of the Great Industrial Exhibition, Leinster Lawn, Dublin, 1853.
Engraving by WC Forster
Royal College for Science for Ireland UCD.ie
NATIONAL LIBRARY OF IRELAND

Certificate for the loan of the Mace at the Dublin Exhibition Palace
RCPI

Details from the head of the Mace showing from left: the figure of Galen; the coat of arms used by RCPI during the 1850s, showing Hercules slaying the Hydra; the figure of William Harvey; the Royal Arms
DERMOTT DUNBAR

Under the Immediate Patronage of

HER MAJESTY THE QUEEN.

LOAN MUSEUM,

DUBLIN EXHIBITION PALACE.

UNDER THE SPECIAL PATRONAGE OF
HIS EXCELLENCY THE LORD LIEUTENANT.

President :
HIS GRACE THE DUKE OF LEINSTER.

The Manager is desired to convey to

~~King & Queens College & Physician~~

~~thanks~~ of the President, Vice-Pres~~ident~~

~~the under-~~mentioned Loans to this ~~Museum~~

~~Mace belonging~~

18

140

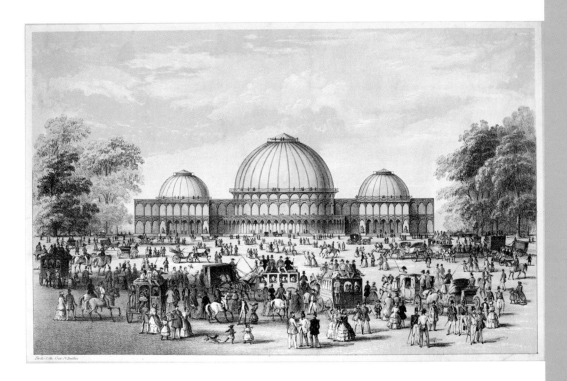

wear any such academic costume, and that the question of gowns for the Examiners (Censors) should be put on the long finger.

The Dublin firm West and Son, of College Green supplied the College with a beautiful new mace, at a cost of £265 – more than five times the original estimate. They also provided a bronze case for the comparatively trifling sum of £8 4s 1d. The College exhibited their splendid new acquisition at the Great Industrial Exhibition of 1853.

No 6 Kildare Street

However the real status symbol for the College would be the completion of its permanent base in central Dublin in the mid-nineteenth century.

The College had tried unsuccessfully on several occasions before this to find a permanent home, after before unceremoniously ejected by Lady Dun from her house in the eighteenth century.

A particularly sore point was that the Royal College of Surgeons had received a large amount of Government money since their establishment in 1784, and had completed their impressive new building on St Stephen's Green.

In 1824 the physicians asked the Government for a £10,000 grant to construct a new building. There had been continuous complaints from all quarters about their accommodation in the new Sir Patrick Dun's Hospital; the way in which Dun's Library was being housed was also judged wholly inadequate.

The then Dun's Librarian, Dr Hugh Ferguson stated bluntly:

> I beg leave to inform the College of Physicians that there are
> several things wanting in the library room at Sr Pat. Dun's

William Dargan – entrepreneur

The 1853 Great Industrial Exhibition in Dublin, which was funded by the Irish roads and railway engineer, William Dargan, proved a popular attraction, but it left him with a deficit of £21,000. This was a huge sum at that time.

His contemporaries were so grateful for his generosity that they formed a Dargan Testimonial Committee which set up a fund to create the Dargan Industrial College, and later an Art Institute. Ultimately, however, the project became the National Gallery of Ireland, which was opened in 1864, roughly six months before the Royal College of Physicians of Ireland moved in to their new home at nearby No 6 Kildare Street. A statue to Dargan was erected in front of the National Gallery, which has a Dargan Wing, on the site where the exhibition was held.

Dargan's company was also employed by the Belfast Harbour Commissioners to cut through the dense mudbanks in the River Lagan and to open up the port to much larger international shipping. The thick silt, referred to by Dargan as 'the stuff', was dumped at the eastern side of the Lagan. It became known as 'Dargan's Island', and later as 'Queen's Island' where the ill-fated *RMS Titanic* was built.

William Dargan declined a Baronetcy from Queen Victoria. He died in 1867 following a riding accident. Dargan's funeral was one of the biggest seen in Dublin for many years, and his remains were interred in 'the O'Connell Circle' at Glasnevin Cemetery.

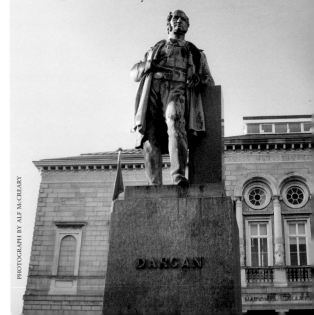

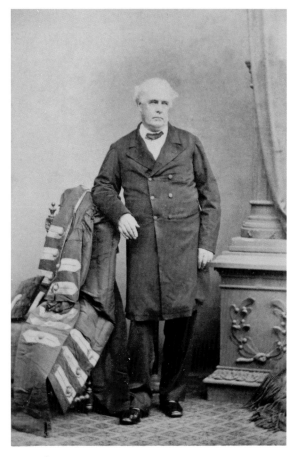

Photograph and signature of the elderly
Dominic Corrigan

The Racket Court

There's Adams with his temper mild
And Mavis oft with temper riled
There little Todd, who dodges so
And Dandy Rooke, make a nice show
There's Sidney in an old red shirt
Blue trews, old shoes, all over dirt,
Who's with fright pale – with terror grim
If hard hit balls fly closer.
There's Dr Ellis – if his play you take,
The game and his temper, he'll forsake.
There's the mighty Pat, the great M.P.,
Who thinks no player so great as he.
There's Guinness with his mincing walk,
And Tim O'Brien, of mighty talk.
There's Corrigan hitting hard and wild,
Browne the reverse – just like a child.
There Corballs too, makes mighty strokes,
And Sidney's funk, plainly evokes.
There's Dr Smith and Vickers too,
Shortsighted and stumpy what can they do?
There's Thompson too, who plays
right well
And Monaghan too, the Registrar, swell.

Hospital, viz, a mat for the floor, some chairs, perhaps a table, fire irons and a ladder, the presses being higher than in the other room. There are several such articles of furniture in the apartment [at TCD] at present, but old, not worth removing, and the floor mat would not fit.[4]

Nevertheless, the College of Physicians had to make do with their unsatisfactory accommodation at Dun's Hospital, and once more the Government turned a blind eye to all their entreaties for help. This may have been partly because the policy-makers valued more highly the well-being of surgeons, who were indispensible to the Armed Forces in the many wars of that period, and partly because the surgeons may have been better political lobbyists than the physicians, and therefore had more friends at court.

In the first half of the nineteenth century there were a number of properties which might have seemed suitable for a new College Hall for the physicians, and several proposals and schemes were put forward. None of these came to fruition.

However in 1860 there finally was a breakthrough when the Kildare Street Club offered its building to the College at a sum of £6,000. What was needed now was a strong figure to lead the physicians into a new, permanent home, and the money to pay for it.

Top Man

'Cometh the hour, cometh the man', as the saying goes, and that man was Dominic John Corrigan who had recovered from his earlier rejection by the College for an Honorary Fellowship, and had been elected President in 1859, for the first of five terms of office.

A reference to this has been made in the previous chapter, but it is important at this stage to flesh out Corrigan's story and underline his remarkable achievement in becoming the first Catholic President of the College in mid-nineteenth century Ireland.

His rejection for an Honorary Fellowship in 1847 was in stark contrast to his treatment by the Royal College of Surgeons of England several years earlier. After sitting his examination for a surgical diploma in 1843, the only question asked of him by the Board of Examiners was whether he was 'the author of the essay on the patency of the aortic valve'.[5] This was similar to asking a

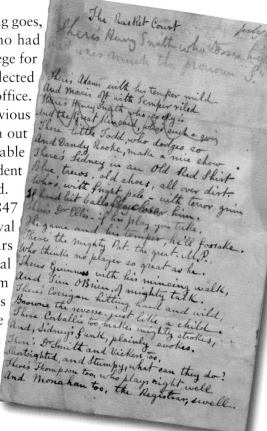

A poem (with transcription, left) written by Dominic Corrigan in 1858, in which he pokes fun at his colleagues on the racquet court in Kildare Street.

mathematician if 'two and two make four'! The question from the London examiners was an acknowledgement of Corrigan's eminence in England as well as in Ireland.

Corrigan, however, did not give up on the Royal College of Physicians of Ireland. In 1849 he was awarded an Honorary MD from Trinity, and six years later, successfully sat the examination to become a Licentiate of the College – a test which at that stage would have been more appropriate for his students rather than the distinguished teacher that he was. However he had made his point. After obtaining the Licentiate in 1855, he became a Fellow one year later.

It seemed only a matter of time before Corrigan would become President. He did so in 1859 when he was proposed for office by his colleague, William Stokes. The election of a Catholic President of what had been generally perceived as the very 'Protestant' College of Physicians was noted at all influential levels of society. It was clear that Corrigan, who had been honoured by his appointment as Physician-in-Ordinary to Queen Victoria, had really arrived, as one of the most influential and successful Catholics of his generation.

There is no doubt also that Corrigan had the ability and the authority to push through the plans for a permanent home for the College, one with the prestige and central location to reflect the status of its Licentiates and Fellows.

Pressing Ahead

The Kildare Street premises consisted of two houses, and a committee of four, led by Corrigan, inspected the property, and decided that it would be suitable for a College Hall.

Their offer of £5,000 for the property was accepted, and possession would be given on 1 July 1861. The Fellows, Honorary Fellows and Licentiates of the College were invited to subscribe to £50 debentures, with interest at 4 per cent.

Two of the largest subscribers, Dominic Corrigan and John Moore Neligan, showed the way by each taking ten debentures at an individual cost of £500. Sir Henry Marsh contributed £200, and William Stokes £150, while Fleetwood Churchill gave his single debenture to

Sir Henry Marsh
1790–1860

Sir Henry Marsh was a distinguished Irish doctor, who originally studied to be a surgeon. Sadly, however, he suffered the loss of a right forefinger in a dissection mishap, and consequently concentrated on becoming a physician.

He rose to the forefront of his profession, and was also a leading figure in Dublin society. Marsh was a dashing figure who kept handsome horses and carriages, and was often seen speeding in style through the streets of the city. His superbly-carved statue by JH Foley stands in the home of the College at No 6 Kildare Street, along with those of the three major figures from the Dublin School of Medicine – Graves, Stokes and Corrigan.

Sir Henry Marsh was President of the Royal College of Physicians of Ireland on three separate occasions: from 1841–43, 1845–47, and from 1857–59. He received many honours, including a Baronetcy from Queen Victoria in 1839, having been Physician-in-Ordinary to Her Majesty in Ireland since 1837.

He was related to Archbishop Narcissus Marsh, the founder of the celebrated Marsh Library, and he came from a privileged medical background.

Henry Marsh was a founder, in 1821, of the Institute of Diseases of Children, which was the first of its kind in the British Isles. It provided free treatment to parents, as well as clinical teaching for medical students, and education for mothers in the care of their children. It later merged with the National Orthopaedic and Children's Hospital to become the National Children's Hospital in Harcourt Street.

Marsh served in several of the main hospitals of the day, and he was also a founder, in 1824, of the Park Street School of Medicine. He was Professor of the Practice of Medicine there from 1824–28. He was one of the founders of the Pathological Society of Dublin, in 1858, and he was a noted teacher and lecturer. In general he was respected 'for his profound knowledge, accuracy and diagnosis, and gentleness'.[6]

Statue of Sir Henry Marsh, *c.* 1860 by John Henry Foley, RCPI

DERMOTT DUNBAR

The design brief for No 6 Kildare Street, 1860

The College's building committee recommend that the expenditure shall not exceed for the present a sum of £5,000 but that plans may be received, the cost of which when complete may be £8,000. The plans must include:

a principle Hall to be about 60 feet by 30 feet Museum & Library with room for several offices viz, Reading Room, Registrar's Office, Committee Room & Beadles Room, &c &c. Building to be two floors high, of any style but Gothic. Front of cut stone wither limestone or Granite or mixed.[7]

The Building Committee managed to successfully conclude an architectural competition and secure a design that suited the purpose and image of the College. William Murray Junior's winning proposal encapsulated the College's great history and the aspirations of the physicians. Other proposals, such as McCurdy's, were too flamboyant and did not portray the conservative image which the College desired. Not only did the College successfully rebuild its premises but it also gained the approval and admiration of the *Dublin Builder* in its choice of architects and winning proposal.

This building not only represents an aspect of high Victorian Irish architecture but the actions, preferences and failings of an institution in its attempt to provide a suitable premises for its everyday needs.[8]

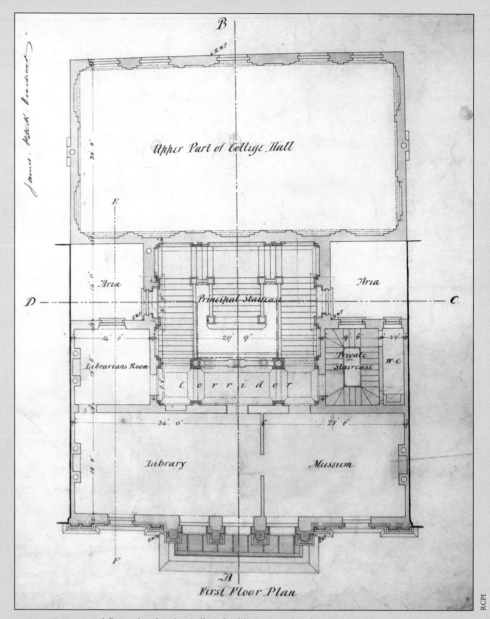

ABOVE: 1861 ground floor plan for the College building, completed in 1864

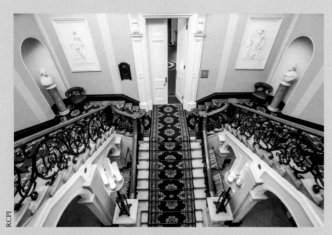

ABOVE: The stairwell looking down from the library, 2014
RIGHT: 1874 section plan for the extension to No 6 Kildare Street by McCurdy

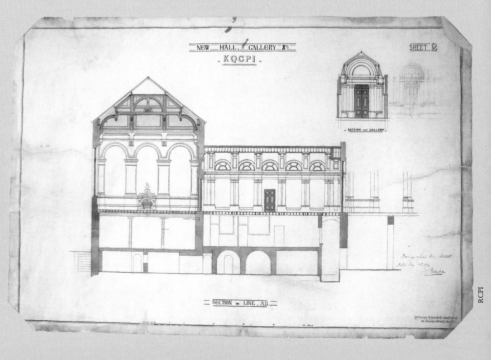

144

the College. Such generosity was commendable, but it also indicated that the leading physicians had lucrative practices.

Just as it seemed that everything was going according to plan, however, the Kildare Street premises were gutted by a huge fire on 11 November, 1860.

Nine fire-engines, 200 soldiers of the 96th Regiment, the Lord Mayor and the Chief Commissioner of the Dublin Police rushed to the scene. The drama was well captured by one medical historian, who recounted that:

> To everybody's horror, a man, with two screaming women, appeared at one of the top front windows. None of the fire services had an escape ladder. The man, James Wilson Hughes, the Club steward, got through the window and assisted the women on to the roof, over which they escaped.
>
> There were in the house a staff of fifteen, of whom twelve were women. All but three climbed to safety over the roofs: the housekeeper, a housemaid, and a barmaid fell into the flames and perished. One of the maids who survived was, embarrassingly, surprised in the bedroom of one of the male servants.
>
> Apart from the human survivors, two others were found by labourers who were clearing the debris in search of the victims' bodies – the pet pigeons which belonged to a boy who cleaned cutlery, and had them in his room near the kitchen. They were found alive and uninjured, though much exhausted.[9]

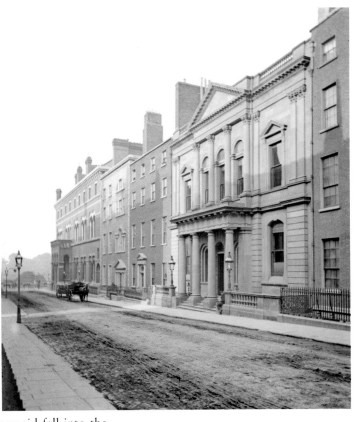

Photograph of Kildare Street *c.* 1860–83, from the Stereo Pairs Photograph Collection
NATIONAL LIBRARY OF IRELAND

The fire was a tragedy, and destroyed almost the whole building. However it also proved to be a blessing in disguise. The College was swiftly reimbursed by its insurance companies to the tune of £6,000, which was quickly and wisely invested in Government stock, and the Physicians could design a new building, from scratch.

The Building Committee decided to hold a competition, and they invited six architects to submit plans based on a list of requirements for accomodation in 'any style but Gothic'. All the designs were displayed in Sir Patrick Dun's Hospital, and the architect John McCurdy was awarded the £50 premium for second prize. However, his plan for a building displaying elements of classical Greek and Italian architecture was rejected as being too costly to implement.

In the end, the contract was won by William Murray, whose father had designed the alterations to the Royal College of Surgeons' building in St Stephen's Green in 1825.

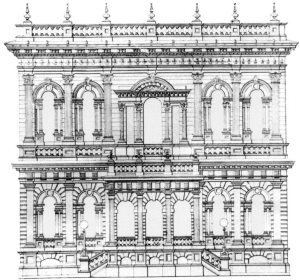

A lithograph of John McCurdy's design, which was rejected as too ornate. Published in the *Irish Builder*, 1862

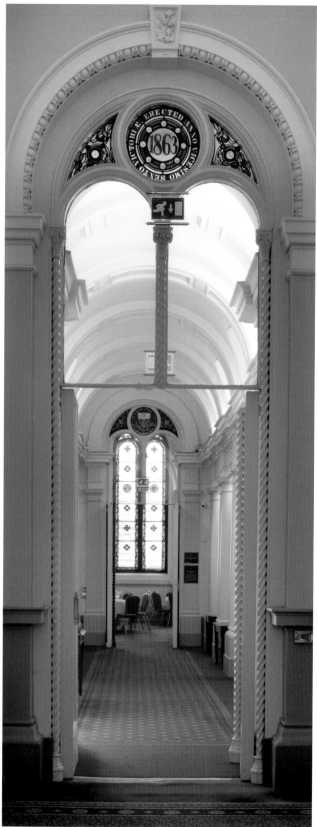

The 1863 stained glass above the doorway in Graves' Hall, looking through to the Corrigan window.

DERMOTT DUNBAR

Seven contracting firms applied to build the Hall, and the tender of £6,100 from William Beardwood was accepted.[10]

On 7 July 1862 the foundation stone of the new College Hall was laid, amid much pomp and circumstance, by the Lord-Lieutenant the Earl of Carlisle, with the aid of a silver trowel which had a handle of Irish bog oak and what the newspapers described as 'an elegantly-finished mallet'.[11]

The building work started almost immediately, but there were serious delays, and the College Hall was not opened until 1864, although one of the attractive stained-glass circular windows high up in the Graves Hall, and part of the plasterwork, is dated '1863'. Even the best-laid plans of élite physicians do not always work out as anticipated!

At one stage the workmen had been withdrawn from the site because the builder, according to the architect, was suffering from 'a dangerous and protracted illness'. William Murray also claimed that the time allowed for the completion of the building had been too short.[12]

In April 1864, several months before the College Hall was completed, the then President, Corrigan, announced that a stained-glass window would be installed in the main room of the new building at his own expense.

The Fellows and Licentiates responded by expressing their 'warmest thanks' to the President 'for the additional proof of the kind of interest in originating and carrying out the erection of the new Hall in a manner worthy of the College'.[13] The new building was finally completed in June 1864. It has since undergone several additions. An important early development in 1874, was the refurbishment of the additional Hall and a corridor, at a cost of £2,000, linking to the site of the old racquet court.

One of the most distinctive features of the Hall is the stained-glass window commissioned by Corrigan from Banff of Dublin, which depicts *inter alia* Corrigan's armorial bearings and those of his wife's family, 'Woodlock', with the inscription 'Ex Dono DJ Corrigan. Praesedis, MDCCCLXIV'. It was originally installed in what became the Graves' Hall, and was moved to its present position in 1874, when the Corrigan Hall was refurbished.

The completion of the College Hall on a prime site in the heart of Dublin was a triumph for Dominic Corrigan, particularly after so many decades of somewhat feeble efforts by the institution to establish a home for itself.

The College held their last meeting in Sir Patrick Dun's Hospital on 1 July 1864. The first official meeting in the new College Hall was held several days later. All those attending paid tribute to Corrigan and passed a resolution stating that:

> ... we cannot permit the present occasion of meeting for the first time in our new Hall to pass by, without expressing the satisfaction we feel at the altered circumstances in which the College is now placed from what it has been for so long a period, and the obligation we are under to our President, for having initiated the movement which has led to this result, as well as for the deep interest he has taken at all times in carrying out the undertaking.[14]

Corrigan was extremely conscious of the standing of his profession and of the College of which he had become President. It is recorded that, when he attended the Lord Mayor's inaugural dinner in the nearby Mansion House in 1864, he turned on his heel and left immediately when he discovered that he was not seated at the High Table, where he felt that a man of his eminence and professional representation should have been given his place.

An English publication, *The Globe*, had some fun by reporting that:

> Corrigan took the affront in high dudgeon and he wheeled about incontinently on his well-booted heel, gave himself a spin of indignation,

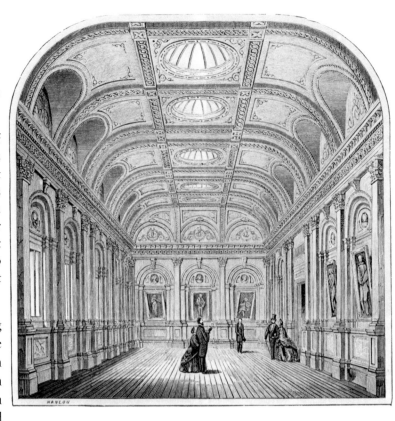

The Great Hall, now Graves' Hall, from an illustration published in the *Irish Builder*, 1862

Graves Hall today
RCPI

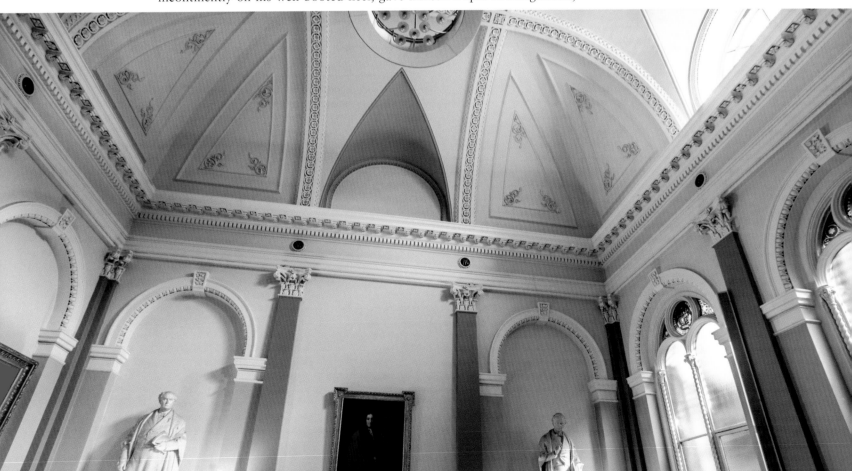

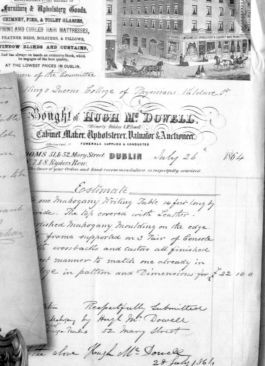

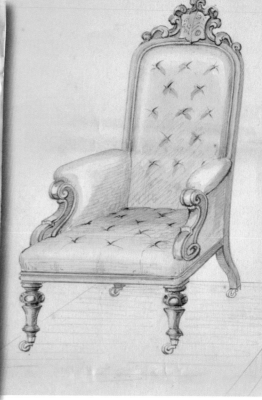

and trotted off, unimpressed by the unsavoury odours which might have tempted a weaker appetite to stay.[15]

Whatever the contemporary Press or others might have written or thought, Corrigan had once again made his point.

Later Career

Corrigan's career continued to flourish. In 1866 he was made a Baronet by Queen Victoria. Only four other doctors in Ireland had received such an honour – Thomas Molyneux, Edward Barry and Henry Marsh, (all from the Royal College of Physicians), and the eminent surgeon Sir Philip Crampton.

A strong supporter of medical reform and of dispensary doctors, Corrigan was also a long-time member of the General Medical Council. This necessitated many visits to London, in the days when travelling across the Irish Sea and back again required considerable time and stamina.

He also took an active interest in politics, and in 1870 stood successfully as a Liberal candidate for a Dublin seat in the Westminster Parliament, where he championed interdenominational education and temperance, among other issues. He retired from politics in 1873.

In 1875 he became President of the Pharmaceutical Society of Ireland, and even in his later years he continued to contribute to learned journals.

The President's Chair, dating from 1866, now sits in the Stearne room of the College.

DERMOTT DUNBAR

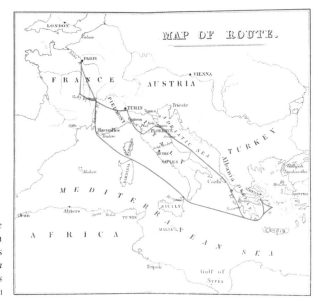

A map of the route taken by Corrigan in 1862, from his book, *Ten Days in Athens*

RCPI

Despite the pressures of his professional and public life, Corrigan had a wide range of interests, including the Royal Zoological Society of Ireland. He was also a leading member of the Royal Irish Yacht Club and an accomplished sailor, with a slipway at his magnificent seaside home, Inniscorrig in Dalkey, where he held a regatta in August every year. He also had an aquarium at Inniscorrig.

Corrigan was also widely-travelled, and wrote about his travel experiences in many publications. His record of a visit to Greece became an 1862 book, *Ten Days in Athens with Notes by the Way*. The trip was partly a 'busman's holiday': in Greece he visited a military hospital, and on the way home, he spent time in Florence where he visited several hospitals.

Despite his professional success, Dominic Corrigan experienced personal family tragedy with the death in the 1850s of his daughter Joanna, aged 17, and the loss of his eldest son John, a soldier, in Australia in 1866.

Last Days

Dominic Corrigan suffered a stroke on 30 December 1879, and died on 1 February 1880.

According to one report, his funeral was one of the largest which Dublin had ever witnessed:

> Following the Chief Mourners were the carriages of the President and Fellows of the College of Physicians, and a carriage conveying the College Mace, draped in crepe, borne by the beadle. After leaving the House at Merrion Square, the procession made a detour through Kildare Street, past the College of Physicians, opposite to which it halted for a few seconds and then proceeded to round by St Stephen's Green and Merrion Square to St Andrew's Church on Westland Row.[17]

It was a fitting tribute to a remarkable man and a devoted servant of the Royal College of Physicians. There were a number of fine obituaries of Corrigan, including one in the *Freeman's Journal*, which noted that:

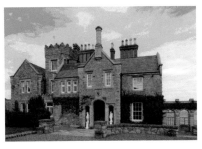

CORRIGAN.CA

Inniscorrig is a magnificent, solid-granite castle, dating back to 1847. With its own quay on Coliemore Road, the house is truly striking and one of Dalkey's finest.

It was built as a summer retreat by Sir Dominic Corrigan, who was based in No 4 Merrion Square in Dublin. According to the *Irish Times*, Corrigan was fond of entertaining on a large and lavish scale – King Edward VII is reputed to have been a guest at the house, and this 'was commemorated by a crown and stars in pebbles set into the patios on either side of the front door'. A replica of Corrigan's head is set into a granite bust above the front door.[16]

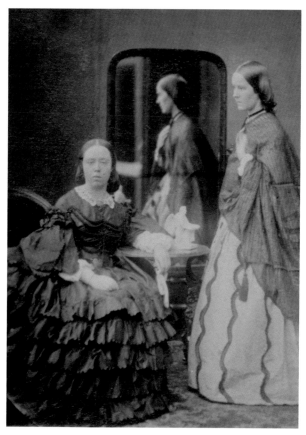

Two of Corrigan's three daughters, Mary and Cecilia. He also had three sons.

The people of Ireland regarded his career with peculiar interest, and his success with gratified pride. This feeling was in no wise sectarian. It was rather racial and national. They felt that intellectual triumph was their best and noblest vindication against the contumely which had fallen on them, in consequence of the ignorance enforced upon the nation by the Penal Laws.[18]

One of the most noteworthy tributes was published by *The Lancet*, which stated:

By the death of Sir Dominic Corrigan, the medical profession loses one of its most conspicuous members … Though a perfect Irishman, Sir Dominic was as much at home in London, as in Dublin, and though a Catholic in religion, he had too much humour, and too much humanity in his constitution, to be a bigot.[19]

Corrigan's death occurred some 20 years after he had first become President of the College but he had left his indelible mark on the institution which continued to play an important, and in one area in particular, a visionary role in medicine during the latter part of the nineteenth century.

Perhaps one of the most striking reminders of Corrigan's eminence and breadth of vision is a quotation from a speech he made to the British Medical Association in 1867:

… among the bonds that unite the three divisions of this our kingdom together, there are none stronger than those of our profession, soaring in its exercise above all sectarian discords. We know no difference of race, or creed, or colour, for everyone is our neighbour.[20]

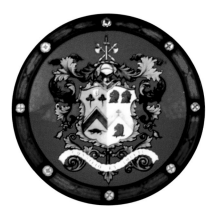

Detail of Corrigan's family crest from the stained glass window in the Corrigan room, at No 6 Kildare Street

Reform, Recognition, Revolution ...

The latter half of the nineteenth century brought important changes for the College in terms of new legislation, including the Enabling Act of 1876, which paved the way for women to practise medicine – a development in which the College would play a major and innovative role.

This era also saw a significant name-change for the College with the official adoption of the title of 'Royal' in 1890, and the implementation of a new Supplemental Charter to update the previous Royal Charter of 1692.

This period also witnessed important political changes including a growing sense of Irish nationalism and a deepening frustration with government from Westminster. This developed into a strong impetus towards Home Rule, an aspiration which was fiercely opposed by the Unionists in Ulster and which brought the threat of civil war.

By the end of the century, the seeds had been sown for outright rebellion in Ireland, and events moved swiftly and dramatically towards the partition of the island early in the twentieth century. These were stirring times indeed, but the positive work of the Royal College of Physicians continued despite such an uncertain and often violent backdrop.

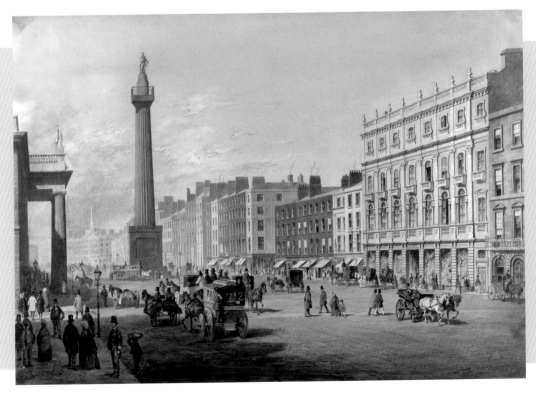

Sackville Street, Dublin, c.1853
Michael Angelo Hayes, 1820–77

This view of Dublin's main thoroughfare, now known as O'Connell Street, offers a glimpse of how the city looked in the 1850s. The street abounds with activity, as people bustle amidst carts, carriages and omnibuses. Dominating the scene is the 40-metre high landmark, 'Nelson's Pillar', erected in 1808. The pillar, made of Portland stone and topped with a statue of Admiral Nelson, was partially destroyed by a bomb in 1966, to be demolished two days later by Army engineers. In its place, the stainless steel Spire of Dublin (120 metres) now stands as a symbol of hope and progress.[1]
NATIONAL GALLERY OF IRELAND

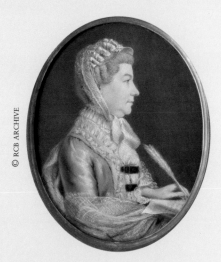

Although unable to qualify as medical practictioner in Britain prior to the Enabling Act of 1876, women were fundamental to many medical institutions.

Lady Arabella Denny

Arabella Fitzmaurice's maternal grandfather was Sir William Petty and, as was usual for a wealthy young lady, she performed acts of charity towards the tenants on her father's estate. She also ran an 'apothecary's shop', a basic dispensary.

When her husband, Colonel Arthur Denny died suddenly in 1742, Arabella lost her position at Wisnaw Castle, Tralee. With a reduced income, she moved to Dublin and became heavily involved with the Dublin Foundling Hospital, even to the extent of funding extra staff.

In 1766 she opened the first of the Magdalene Asylums for 'fallen women', employing Dr Robert Emmett as long-term medical advisor to the institution. She fundraised tirelessly using her many connections.

By the time of Arabella's retirement from the direct running of the Asylum in Leeson Street, Magdalene Asylums had been established across Ireland.[2]

New Moves

The regulation of practitioners of medicine in Ireland had long been a matter of contention between physicians, surgeons, apothecaries and others. In 1830, for example, a 'great meeting' of physicians and surgeons was held in the Royal College of Surgeons, with the idea of combining the entire medical profession in Ireland into one Faculty.

There were large numbers present, and no fewer than seventeen resolutions were passed unanimously. It seemed that an agreement had been reached. Richard Carmichael, a leading surgeon, who chaired a splendid dinner afterwards, waxed lyrical and noted that:

> … the unanimity, the friendly harmony, the undisguised good fellowship which prevailed, were truly refreshing and served as a happy omen of that better state of things, that sunshine of the profession, which we have no hesitation in predicting, which is likely to arise from this felicitous reunion.[3]

However, nothing came of this. The Royal College of Physicians and Trinity College were not persuaded by the arguments put forward for a single Faculty, and the Apothecaries were left out entirely.[3]

It then took more than 30 years to make significant progress. Meanwhile, in the 1850s, there was a marked increase in the number of candidates for the Licentiate of the Royal College of Physicians, and, as one medical historian points out:

> The concept of the General Practitioner was becoming established, and evidence of both medical and surgical education was being demanded for posts such as those of dispensary medical officers.[4]

Breakthrough

There was a breakthrough, however, with the 1858 Medical Act which provided for the regulation of the qualifications required by practitioners in medicine and surgery. Under this Act, the College was named as one of the recognised awarding bodies. A medical register was set up, and a General Medical Council was established.

The College was authorised to obtain a new Charter, under which it could change its name and assume for the first time the official title of the 'Royal College of Physicians of Ireland'. This would have allowed it to assume the 'Royal' title, in line with the practice of its sister colleges in London and Edinburgh.

However the Irish College did not act on this matter until 1890. Several years after the 1858 Medical Act was passed, Dominic Corrigan referred to this subject in his speech at the laying of the Foundation Stone of the new

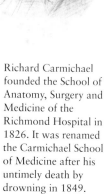

Richard Carmichael founded the School of Anatomy, Surgery and Medicine of the Richmond Hospital in 1826. It was renamed the Carmichael School of Medicine after his untimely death by drowning in 1849.
RCPI

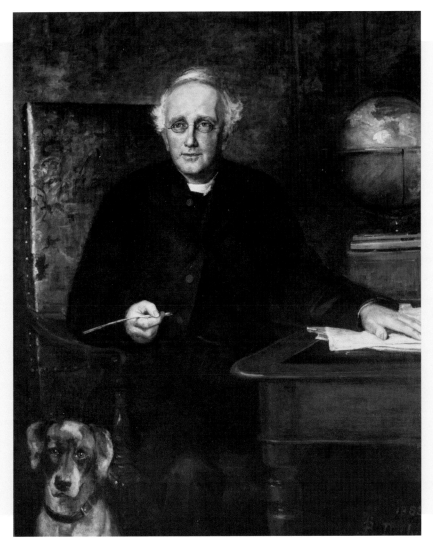

Rev Dr Samuel Haughton
1821–97
Victorian Polymath

Haughton was born into a well-known Quaker family and later ordained by the Church of Ireland. He was already Professor of Geology at TCD when he decided to study medicine, and he then combined his knowledge of anatomy and geology to show that many animal fossils had been distorted by geological processes.

In 1866, Haughton invented a new 'hangman's drop'. He realised that a longer drop was needed to break a person's neck swiftly during hanging, thus minimising their pain and suffering.

As well as the hangman's drop, Haughton developed the first reasonable estimate of blood pressure, based on how far blood spurted from a severed artery (the experiment was performed on a dog). He also calculated the age of the Earth using various approaches, including considering rates of sedimentation and cooling. At a time when most people were suggesting an age of, at most, a few hundred million years, Haughton calculated that the Earth was 2.5 billion years old. Being firmly anti-Darwin, however, and unable to conceive of such an age, he later revised this figure to 100 million.[7]

Portrait of Samuel Haughton by Sarah Purser, 1883
TRINITY COLLEGE DUBLIN

College Hall. He underlined the importance of the then current title of King and Queen's College of Physicians in Ireland:

> we were so attracted by the name 'Queen' that we have determined not to avail ourselves of the privilege, but to retain our present title.[5]

Corrigan also drew attention at the time to new legislation which would broaden the entry criteria to allow the College to elect Fellows from any British, Irish or foreign university, and to accept Licentiates who merited this distinction, even without university degrees:

> We shall have power to award without distinction to all those of our profession whose personal conduct and professional merits deserve the fellowship of our College. We shall attain our true position, recognising perfect freedom in education, and our only question henceforth will be, as it ought to be, what a man knows, not where he learned it.[6]

Haughton's Act

The traditional exclusivity of the College was further relaxed by the so-called 'Haughton's Act' of 1867, formally known as the School of Physic Amendment Act. Under this Act, the King's Professors no longer had to be Protestants, and people from all countries, whether or not they had a medical degree, could be appointed. The election of the King's Professors was to be made entirely by the College, and its Fellows no longer had to resign their position to become candidates.

This was a radical move for an institution which had such strong historical Protestant associations, but the College, in effect, was embracing the spirit of the times, and behaving accordingly.

Samuel Haughton

One of the principal architects of the 1867 Act was the Reverend Dr Samuel Haughton, one of the most influential and impressive figures of his time. In 1844 he graduated with an Arts degree from Trinity College, and became a Fellow in the same year. He was deeply religious, and in 1847 he was ordained as a priest in the Church of Ireland. He took his clerical duties seriously, and preached from the pulpit regularly.

Haughton was also a leading scientific figure. From 1851 to 1880 he was Professor of Geology at Trinity, and in 1861 at the age of 41, he also graduated with an MB and an MD and became a Licentiate of the College of Physicians, and later a Fellow there too.

Haughton was responsible for important improvements at Sir Patrick Dun's Hospital, and he helped to extend its provision of services in surgery, obstetrics and gynaecology, and other medical care. He was also an important supporter of reforms in medical education. This nineteenth-century polymath was one of the key figures who backed the admission of women into the medical profession.

Women in Medicine

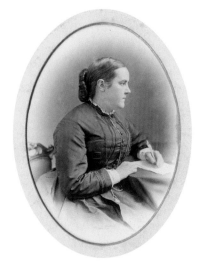

Sophia Jex-Blake, Scotland's first woman doctor, was a leading campaigner for the admission of women into medical schools. She was the founder of two medical schools and the now closed Bruntsfield women's hospital. Jex-Blake fought hard throughout her life for women to have the right to train and practise as doctors.[8]

In the nineteenth century, women had an uphill struggle to make their mark in medicine. The 1858 Medical Act, which had formalised much of contemporary medicine, had rationalised and standardised the level of medical education required from universities.

This worked against the interests of the women who had no access to university education. Those from Britain and Ireland who wanted to pursue a career in medicine had to study abroad in places like Zurich or Berne, where the medical institutions had a more liberal attitude towards women.

However, these European qualifications were not recognised in Britain and Ireland, and a number of females, including the fiery Sophia Jex-Blake, began to campaign for the right of women to register as medical practitioners. Jex-Blake had experienced bitter discrimination from her male fellow students, teachers and members of the public after she and six others were admitted to study medicine at Edinburgh University, from 1869 onwards.

This led to a riot in 1870 which was started by male students objecting to women colleagues in medicine.

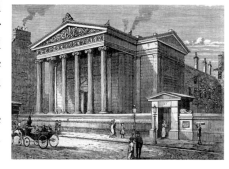

Surgeons' Hall, Edinburgh, now a Museum, where the women studied anatomy, and the scene of the Surgeons' Hall Riot of 1870.

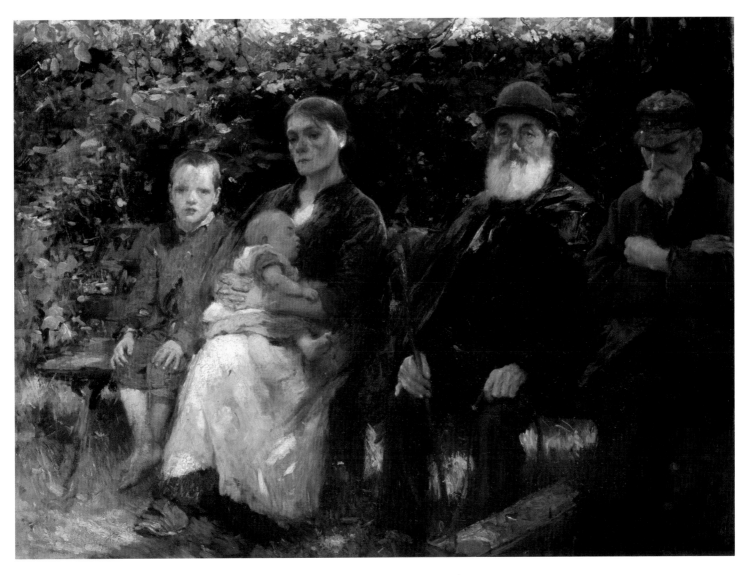

However the so-called 'Edinburgh Seven' continued with their studies until 1873, when they lost a legal case against the University after it decided that they could not continue studying for a medical degree.

However, several leading Parliamentarians at Westminster backed the women's campaign, and this led to the Enabling Act of 1876, which was passed despite strong opposition. This permitted nineteen licensing institutions, if they so wished, to enable women with foreign medical degrees to register as doctors in the British Isles, though they were still not allowed to train there.

Significantly, the Royal College of Physicians of Ireland (then the King and Queen's College of Physicians in Ireland) was the first institution in the British Isles to decide that women with foreign degrees could take the examination for its Licentiates in Medicine. This was seen as a turning point in the campaign.

Other institutions gradually followed suit, but the College had led the way. The reasons for this important development were underlined by Dr Laura Kelly in her book *Irish Women in Medicine, c. 1880s–1920s*.[9] In a comprehensive summary of this complex subject, Dr Kelly emphasised that higher education for women in Ireland had already been taken seriously for a considerable time, and from 1850 onwards women were admitted to classes at the Museum of

In a Dublin Park, Light and Shade, *c*. 1895
Walter Frederick Osborne
NATIONAL GALLERY OF IRELAND

The reality of life for the average family was one of hard work and little comfort. The progress made in the improvement of social conditions by the medical profession, in which female doctors played an important role, helped in the fight against disease caused by poverty and hardship.

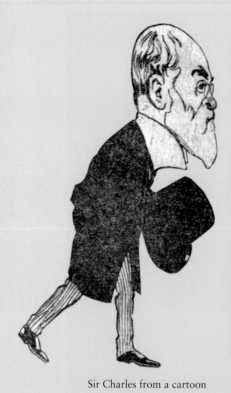

Sir Charles from a cartoon
RCPI

Sir Charles Cameron
1830–1921

Charles Cameron, who became an Honorary Fellow of RCPI in 1898, started work with the apothecaries, Bewley & Evans at the age of 16. He studied chemistry in Germany, and medicine in Dublin. Appointed in 1874 as Dublin's medical officer of health and public analyst for the city, Cameron was responsible for numerous reforms in public health administration. These included housing reform, the closing of dairies and slaughter houses, and the improvement of the water supply and drainage system.[10]

Sir Charles spent nearly six decades fighting to improve the conditions in Dublin's slums, but his reputation in his lifetime was badly damaged by an official report which as Lydia Carroll argues in her biography of Cameron, was driven by political scape-goating.[11] Cameron was President of RCSI in 1885.

Charcoal portrait of Sir Charles Cameron
by Frank Leah, 1921
RCPI

Irish Industry, and also to those of its successor the Royal College of Science, after it was established in 1865.

Dr Kelly also pointed out that the Irish hierarchy had long promoted secondary education for girls, and that this had opened the path for women to a possible career in medicine. It is important to note that as early as the seventeenth century, the College had allowed women to sit for its midwifery licence, and a Mistress Cormack and Mrs Catherine Banford had done so in 1696 and 1732 respectively.[12]

Dr Kelly underlined that the British women who had become medical Licentiates of the College from 1877 had not indicated their intention to practise in Ireland, and therefore they could not be seen as a 'threat' to the existing male Irish medical establishment.[13] She also suggested that some of the leading figures in the Royal College of Physicians, including the Reverend Dr Samuel Haughton, Dr Aquilla Smith and Dr Samuel Gordon had played a crucial role in favouring women Licentiates.

In her book, Dr Kelly speculates that Haughton's religiosity was a factor in his openness to women in medicine:

> It is possible that this religiosity endowed Haughton with the belief that women should be attended by women physicians, and thus encouraged his support of the admission of women to medical schools.
>
> It is likely that Haughton also viewed medicine as a vocation rather than as a profession … a Christian like Haughton might well have felt that a call from God was a real and absolute command that could apply to women as well as men. Medicine and caring for the sick could fall into this category of

vocation and, thus, if a woman wanted to pursue this 'call', she ought to be allowed to do so.[14]

Samuel Gordon

Dr Samuel Gordon was President of the College from 1875–78, at the same time as women were being admitted as Licentiates. Gordon had a wife and nine daughters, and some observers believe that this influenced him favourably towards women in medicine.

This may have been a factor, but then again it might not have played such a large part as some people think. Gordon was a respected physician who would have been well able to make up his own mind about such an important matter.

His obituary in the *British Medical Journal* of 7 May 1898 gives a flavour of the kind of man he was.

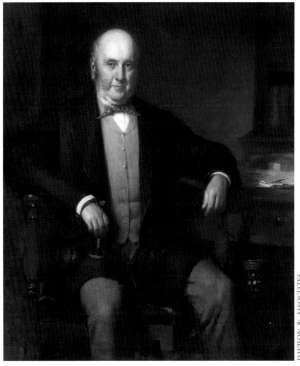

Samuel Gordon, 1816–98
Portrait by Catterson Smith Junior

Dr Samuel Gordon was President of the College from1875–78, during which time it was the first institution in the British Isles to enable women to take the examination for a Licentiate in Medicine. He and his wife had a family of nine daughters.
He was described as 'a sound clinical teacher ... an admirable diagnostician ... and essentially a wise man of great common sense'. [16]
RCPI

> 'Sam Gordon', as his pupils called him with real affection, was a sound clinical teacher. He had not a very showy method of instruction, but what he had to tell was always worth hearing and remembering.
>
> He was an admirable diagnostician, and he gave reasons to his pupils in language simple but forcible, making them follow step by step the facts which led him to a conclusion ... he was essentially a wise man of great common sense, of the most generous instincts, and endowed with a kindliness of nature which secured his popularity everywhere ... there is real and widespread sorrow for the loss of one who held in so large a degree the esteem and affection of all who were privileged to know him.[15]

Even allowing for the fulsomeness which characterised the obituaries of most public and professional figures in Victorian times, there is no doubt that Gordon was highly respected within his profession. Such a man's support for the admission of women to medicine would have carried considerable weight.

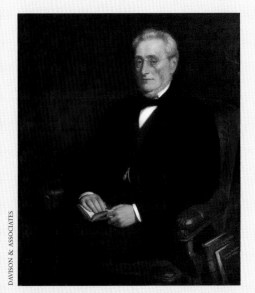

Dr Aquilla Smith, 1806–90

Portrait by S Catterson Smith Junior

Aquilla Smith was a noted physician and antiquarian who was a Licentiate and a Fellow of the College. He was elected Vice-President several times in the nineteenth century. In May 1864 he was appointed King's Professor of Materia Medica and Pharmacy in the School of Physic at Trinity College Dublin. He was one of the supporters of the historic decision by the College of Physicians to award women Licentiates in Medicine. He was an expert in numismatics, and an expert on Tudor and Stewart coinage. His impressive collection of more than 2,500 coins and tokens was purchased by the Royal Irish Academy for its museum.

Sadly, in later years his powers declined, and his virtually inaudible lectures led to student rowdiness in the lecture theatre. A colleague was appointed to finish his course. Aquilla Smith resigned in July 1881, and was succeeded in his post by his third son, Walter.[17]
RCPI

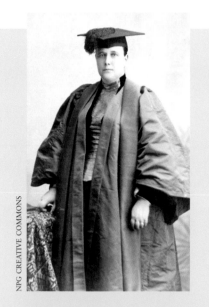

Mary Edith Pechey-Phibson

In 1869 Edith Pechey entered Edinburgh University as one of the first female medical students. As one of the 'Edinburgh seven', she was ousted from the university in 1874 on the grounds that it had been a violation of the by-laws to allow them entry in the first place.

Edith completed her training in Berne, Switzerland and in 1877 was licensed by the College. She established a successful private practice in Birmingham and Leeds and also studied surgery in Vienna.

In 1883 she accepted the position of senior medical officer in Bombay, India, in the first hospital built expressly for women and to be staffed entirely by women. In line with her strong beliefs in women's suffrage, Edith Pechey campaigned for equal pay for her female colleagues. She also worked to abolish child marriage in India and on other social issues. She spent twenty years working in India and was the first woman to be appointed to the Senate of the University of Bombay.[19]

Financial Benefits

Financial considerations may also have played a part in the admission of women as Licentiates of the College, partly because fees were an important source of income. As Dr Kelly suggests in her book:

> In 1874, for example, the total income for the half-year ended 17 October was £801. Of this, £771 came from fees for medical licences.
>
> Similarly for the half-year ended 17 April 1875, the total income was £809, with the sum from fees being £758. By October 1877, it is evident that fees had become an even more important source of revenue for the College; the total revenue for that half-year was £1,201, with the fees totalling £1,048. [18]

First Female Licentiate

The first female Licentiate, and the first woman to be allowed to practise medicine in the British Isles, was Eliza Louisa Walker Dunbar, who was admitted to the College of Physicians in January 1877, shortly after the 1876 Enabling Act became law. She was also granted a licence in midwifery, the first to be given to a woman since those awarded to Catherine Banford in 1732, and Mistress McCormack in 1696, as noted earlier.

The College had in fact already granted permission to Mary Edith Pechey, an English woman and a noted campaigner for women's rights, to sit the examination for the Licentiate, but this permission had been postponed because her degree from Europe was not compliant with College laws. A Committee was eventually asked to decide whether her qualification from the University of Berne was in the list of foreign degrees recognised by the College, and she was eventually granted her Licentiate on 9 May 1877, together with Sophia Jex-Blake and Louisa Atkins. Pechey and Jex-Blake were also granted licences in midwifery. [20]

However, a more liberal attitude to the admission of women in medicine was not shared by all the profession, and a writer in the contemporary *Dublin Medical Press* noted:

> We have already recorded an earnest protest against this laxity with regard to foreign degrees, and we repeat that the license of the Royal College of Physicians must lose a step in public estimation, when it is known that a class of candidates are authorised to write L.K.Q.C.P. after their names, without satisfactory evidence of medical competency. We do not suggest that these ladies would have failed to prove their competency, nor are we able to say whether Swiss degrees are, or are not, reliable evidence of medical knowledge.[21]

Despite this, the College persisted with its policy of admitting women, who had the necessary qualifications as Licentiates, and this policy was gradually adopted by other medical institutions in Ireland. Between 1885 and 1922, a total of 759 women matriculated in Medicine at Irish institutions.[22]

The example set by the College was a significant step forward in terms of the registration of women as doctors in the United Kingdom, and although the Irish institution was in the vanguard of such developments, the others soon caught up.

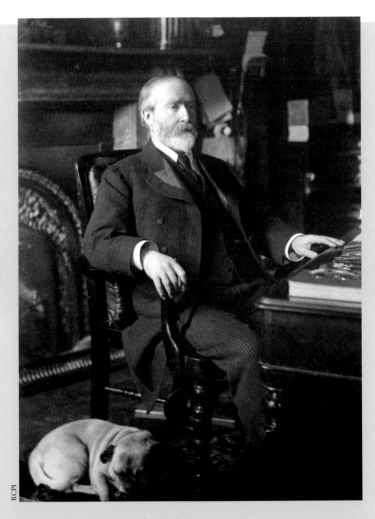

RCPI

Sir Francis Richard Cruise

President of the Royal College of Physicians of Ireland from 1884–86, Cruise was a remarkable man whose name is associated with the first efficient endoscope. This is a medical device with a light attached that is used to look inside a body cavity or organ, which Cruise first described in 1865. He was also one of the first people to use hypnotism as part of medical practice.

He graduated with a medical degree from Trinity in 1858, and two years later he became a member of the Royal College of Surgeons of England. In 1861 he was appointed as an assistant surgeon at the Mater Hospital, and he was elected as a Fellow of the College in 1864. Two years later Cruise and a Mater colleague, Thomas Hayden, wrote about the cholera epidemic of 1866. Sir Francis resigned as a surgeon in 1878, but he served as a physician in the Mater until his death in 1912.

He was a man of many talents, and was a crack shot with a rifle – a skill he had developed in the backwoods of North America, where he had gone to recuperate after a period of excessive work had threatened his health. During one medical social outing, held in the Dublin mountains, he entertained his colleagues by shooting the corks out of champagne bottles from a considerable distance, and without breaking the glass. The feat was all the more accomplished because he had helped to empty the bottles in the first place!

Cruise was a gifted musician who played and composed for the cello. He also founded the Instrumental Club, which played chamber music in public.

Throughout his life he studied the writings of the medieval religious scholar, Thomas a Kempis, and he translated the author's *Imitatio Christi*. The medical historian, Professor John Widdess recalls a poignant portrait of this fascinating man:

> In his latter days he might be seen, driving in a small, tightly-closed brougham to his house in Merrion Square, as Dr John Pollock records 'there is a candle burning within, which serves to illuminate the occupant; a shrunken, aged man, with a white beard, his head bent low over an open book, absorbed by his reading in this doubtful illumination'.
>
> He was known by the Dublin wits as 'Kempis Cruise' because of his religious devotion and scholarship of Kempis. He left his religious books and beautifully-carved crucifix to the Jesuits at Gardiner Street in Dublin.[23]

Cruise was created a Knight of St Gregory by Pope Pius X, and a street in Kempen, Germany was named after him. He had been a pupil of Dominic Corrigan, and they became lifelong friends. Cruise attended Corrigan during his final illness.

Francis Cruise was knighted in 1896, and became Physician-in-Ordinary in Ireland to King Edward VII (1901–10) and to King George V (1910–11). Cruise died in 1912. Representatives of the College complied with his wishes not to attend his funeral, but paid him a handsome tribute at their next meeting.[24]

159

For example between 1877 and 1888, a total of 48 women were admitted as Licentiates of the College in Ireland, compared with only five in the London School of Medicine for Women. However by 1900, the figures were 49 and 93 respectively. [25]

In Ireland, the Queen's Colleges and the Royal College of Surgeons allowed women to take medical qualifications from the 1880s. The Catholic University and TCD opened their doors to women medical students in 1898 and 1904, by which time many British universities, including Bristol, Glasgow and Durham, had done likewise. It should be noted, however, that the University of London was admitting women to its medical degree courses as early as 1878. However the last British universities to admit women medical students in that era were Cambridge in 1916, and Oxford a year later.[26]

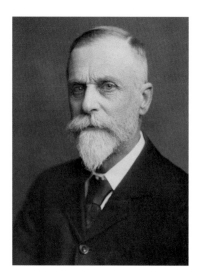

JM Purser
RCPI

First Female Fellow

It took considerably longer for women to be admitted to the College as Fellows. The first nomination, on 3 July 1914, was for Miss Alice Mary Barry of Cork. The College Minutes recorded the findings of a Special Committee set up to consider the matter. Sir John Moore urged that women should not be admitted to the Fellowship and after further discussion, it was decided by fourteen votes to nine, on a resolution proposed by Dr Walter Smith and seconded by Dr JM Purser, that it was 'inexpedient at present that women be admitted to the Fellowship of the College'. [27]

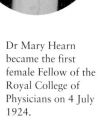

Miss Barry was informed of the decision, and she withdrew her candidature. However on 5 February 1915 the College considered the latest legal opinion on the eligibility of women for the Fellowship. It was decided, by seventeen votes to seven, that 'in the opinion of the College it is desirable that women should be eligible to become candidates for the Fellowship'. The College also asked a Parliamentary Committee to suggest 'such steps as are necessary to place women in the same position as men in the College, and to report to a future meeting of the College'.[28]

Dr Mary Hearn became the first female Fellow of the Royal College of Physicians on 4 July 1924.
RCPI

However, it took almost another decade before the admission of the first female Fellow. This honour went to Mrs Mary Ellice Thorn Hearn, the widow of the Rt Reverend Robert Thomas Hearn, the Bishop of Cork. She had met her future husband when she was studying Medicine at University College Cork, and in compliance with the customs of the times, she discontinued her studies after her marriage.

However, in 1919 she qualified as a doctor from UCC with first-class honours and special distinction in Medicine. She had thereafter a distinguished career in the Victoria Hospital Cork, and in 1924 she became the first female Fellow of the College. There is a well-equipped reading-room in No 6, Kildare Street which has been named in her honour.

Miss Barry of Cork had to wait a little longer. She was elected a Fellow in 1930, during her distinguished service at Peamount Sanitorium in Newcastle, Co Wicklow, from 1929–46.

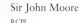

Sir John Moore
RCPI

In *The historiography of women in medicine in Ireland*, Dr Laura Kelly neatly summarises the advances for women in medicine in Ireland for within just over a century:

> By 1898 women made up approximately 0.8 per cent of medical students matriculating at Irish universities. In 2008, 110 years later, 75 per cent of Irish medical students were female, in comparison with 59 per cent of females across the university sector. [29]

Today's female Fellows, Members and Licentiates of the College, and women doctors in general, owe a considerable debt to the early pioneers of women in medicine. These include not only the female campaigners but also the institution of the Royal College of Physicians of Ireland itself, which was some 33 years ahead of the Royal College of Physicians in London whose first female Licentiate in Medicine was not admitted until 1910. [30]

Agreement With Surgeons

Another important development in the late nineteenth century was the agreement between the Royal College of Physicians and the Royal College of Surgeons to hold jointly the qualifying examinations in medicine, surgery and midwifery.

The question of greater cooperation between the two Colleges had been raised many times during the nineteenth century, and there had been several encouraging signs of a possible agreement which ultimately had proved abortive, partly because of differing opinions about the role and status of apothecaries.

Over a decade after the 1858 Medical Act had become law, the surgeons proposed to the physicians that they should consider a conjoint diploma which

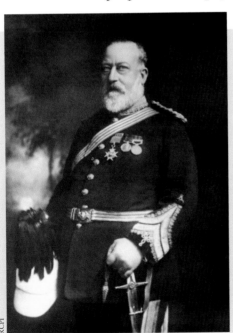

RCPI

Surgeon-General Charles Sibthorpe

Charles Sibthorpe was born in Dublin in 1847. He studied medicine at the Royal College of Surgeons in Ireland, and at the Meath Hospital.

In 1870 he joined the Indian Medical Service as Assistant Surgeon. Following some years of official work in the civilian and military departments, he was appointed Civil Surgeon and Superintendent of the Gaol in Banda, in the Central Provinces (Uttra Pradesh).

In 1875 Sibthorpe was transferred to Madras (now Chennai), and appointed Resident Surgeon to the General Hospital and Professor of Pathology at the Madras Medical College.

He remained at both institutions until 1890, serving successively as Professor of Opthalmology, Anatomy and Surgery. In 1894 he was appointed Surgeon-General with the Government of Madras, a post he held until 1900.

In 1880 he had been elected a Fellow of the Royal College of Physicians of Ireland, and in 1897 he was appointed CB (Companion of the Order of the Bath).

Sibthorpe volunteered for active service with the Indian Medical Service in 1878, and he served with the Peshawar Valley Field Forces in Afghanistan. In 1885 he transferred to active service, this time in Burma, where he was Staff Surgeon to Sir H Prendergast, the Officer-in-Command of the British Forces in Upper Burma.

Sibthorpe retired from the Indian Medical Service in August 1900. He returned to Dublin, where he lived with his sisters until he died in 1906. After their brother's death, the Misses Sibthorpes donated to the College his casebooks which cover most of his time in the Indian Medical Service, as well as a small collection of other documents relating to his time in India. [31]

would qualify students to practise medicine and surgery, but the discussions ended because of financial difficulties which a joint approach might create.

The issue was raised again in 1870 and 1871, and once more in 1876 and 1877, but still no agreement was reached. Six years later the surgeons approached the physicians to re-open negotiations on a conjoint approach, but this attempt ended in failure too because the physicians could not accept the surgeons' proposal to include apothecaries in the scheme.

Nevertheless those in favour of a conjoint examination refused to give up, and this led at last to the establishment of an Irish Conjoint Board, soon after the passing of the Medical Acts Amendment Bill in 1886, which required medical practitioners to hold qualifications in medicine, surgery and midwifery from a university or any combination of two or more medical corporations.

This breakthrough was referred to by Sir John Moore, the Registrar of the College of Physicians, in a speech at the Carmichael School in November 1887. While regretting the disappointment of those who felt disenfranchised by their loss of licensing authority, he stated that:

> The one bright ray in the darkness is that in England, Scotland and Ireland alike, the Colleges of Physicians and Surgeons have been drawn more closely

An Emigrant Ship, Dublin Bay
by Edwin Hayes

The sailing ship at anchor at the mouth of the River Liffey waits for passengers who are migrating across the Atlantic. The painting was completed in 1853, just a few years after the Great Famine. Around this time over a million people left Ireland in order to seek new lives in North America and elsewhere.[32]

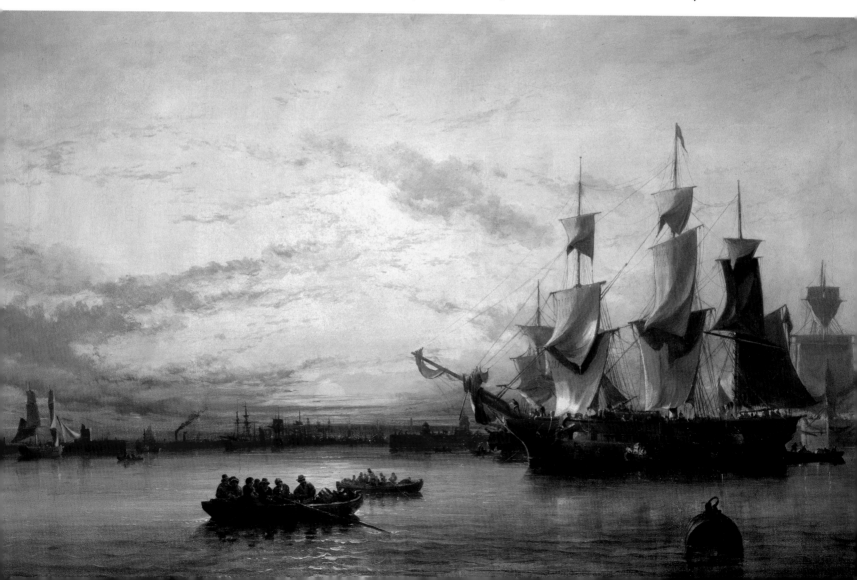

The Land League and Home Rule

The ownership of land, its occupancy and the fate of the poor and dispossessed, as well as wholesale emigration, were some of the major themes of Irish history in the nineteenth century. Under William Gladstone, who declared in December 1868 that his mission was 'to pacify Ireland', the Liberals passed laws which attempted to guarantee fair rents for tenant farmers, and provided protection against unfair evictions. [33]

However Gladstone's Land Act of 1870 only served to increase the violence of what became known as 'the Land War'. His next Land Act of 1881 provided more protection for tenants, but it did not go far enough. Gladstone reluctantly signed the Coercion Acts, which conferred wide powers to arrest dissidents, and although the Land War ended, the discontent remained.

Charles Stewart Parnell, a Protestant who had been educated at Cambridge, became President of the Land League, which refused to accept Gladstone's 1881 Land Act. Parnell concentrated on the political struggle for Home Rule, and with over 80 MPs in his party at Westminster, he was in a strong position to campaign for the measure, with the support of Gladstone.

Gladstone's Liberal party was split by the issue, and Parnell fell from grace over his long affair with Kitty O'Shea, the wife of Captain O'Shea, from whom she was separated. Kitty O'Shea and Parnell had three daughters, one of whom died early.

Charles Stewart Parnell
CREATIVE COMMONS

The relationship became widely-known when Captain O'Shea filed for divorce. Parnell married Kitty but was forced to resign from politics, and died at the age of 45, some years after the Home Rule Bill was defeated. However the issue of Home Rule, and the government of Ireland, continued to cast a dark shadow, particularly in Ulster, in the early years of the twentieth century up to the outbreak of the First World War, and well beyond that.

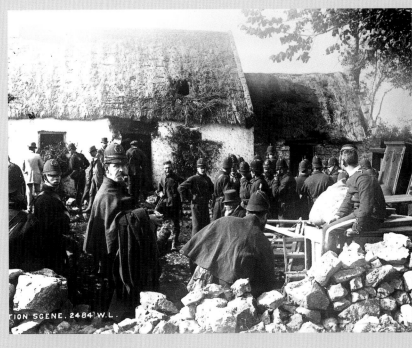

Eviction scene by William Lawrence
NATIONAL LIBRARY OF IRELAND

together, and an *entente cordiale* between Medicine and Surgery has been established.

In proof of this, witness the scene in the Hall of the King and Queen's College of Physicians on Friday, November 11, 1887, when the President and Council of the Royal College of Surgeons of Ireland joined with the President and Fellows of the College of Physicians in a ceremonial for conferring the Diplomas of the two Colleges on the candidates who had been successful at the recent Final Professional Examinations under the Conjoint Scheme. [34]

In 1889 the Irish Conjoint Board was established between the Royal College of Physicians and the Royal College of Surgeons. The Board would award the joint Licentiate of both Colleges, in accordance with the 1886 Act.

The apothecaries had still been left out in the cold, but the two Colleges had at last laid the matter to rest, and had made history together in doing so.

Annie Moore with her Sons. This sculpture stands at the entrance to the port of Cobh as a monument to the many families who emigrated from Ireland.

ALF McCREARY

163

Other Developments

There were other important developments in the final decades of the nineteenth century. In 1879 the College introduced its Membership status, as a progression between Licentiates and Fellows. Three years later, the Royal Academy of Medicine was established, and the College's former Members' Association became the new Academy's Section of Medicine.

One of the most important developments of all in the late nineteenth century was the decision to adopt the new title of the Royal College of Physicians of Ireland. As noted earlier, the physicians had been given the authority under the 1858 Act to do so, but had not taken up the option.

However it seemed a sensible step for the new title to be adopted shortly after the agreement of the Conjoint Scheme with the 'Royal' College of Surgeons, in 1886. There was also the practical point that the new title rolled off the tongue more easily, rather than the somewhat cumbersome 'King and Queen's College of Physicians in Ireland', which the physicians had used for so long, but which was possibly becoming outdated by the late nineteenth century.

New Title

The new title was introduced with the minimum of fuss, and the change was recorded almost matter-of-factly in the Minutes of the period. The last reference to the KQCPI was on 3 October 1890, and the 'Royal College of Physicians of Ireland' was first mentioned in the minutes eleven days later.

It was proposed by the Registrar, seconded by Sir John Banks, and agreed by the College that 'The Letters Patent under the Great Seal of Ireland' granting the title of the 'Royal College of Physicians of Ireland' be 'hereby accepted by

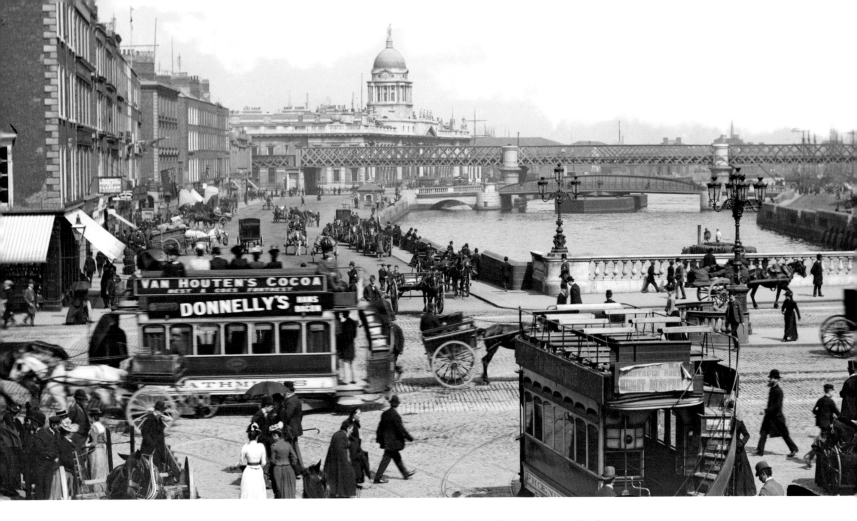

the President and Fellows, and that the College should be affirmed accordingly
to the said Letters Patent'.[35]

The change of title coincided with the adoption of a Supplementary Charter,
which was signed by Queen Victoria in August 1890. It had been a long journey
for the College since the conferring of the first Royal Charter by King Charles
II in 1667, and the second Royal Charter in 1692.

Death of Queen Victoria

Eleven years after the Queen had signed the supplementary Charter for the
Royal College of Physicians, she died, on 22 January 1901, at the age of 82.
Her death marked the end of one of the most eventful reigns by one of the most
remarkable, and until then the longest-serving, sovereign in British history.
Victoria's reign also encompassed significant changes of fortune in the history
of the College. When she ascended the throne in 1837, several outstanding
figures including Graves, Stokes and Corrigan, were busy establishing the
'Golden Age of Irish Medicine'; by the time of her death the College had
become a better-organised, and even more highly respected institution of Irish
medicine.

The death of Queen Victoria marked the end of a very long era. As the people
of Britain and Ireland stood at the cusp of a new millennium and the beginning
of the twentieth century, everyone knew that things would not remain the same.
Sadly, however, they were not to know that they were facing not just rapid
change, but also an historic upheaval of cataclysmic proportions.

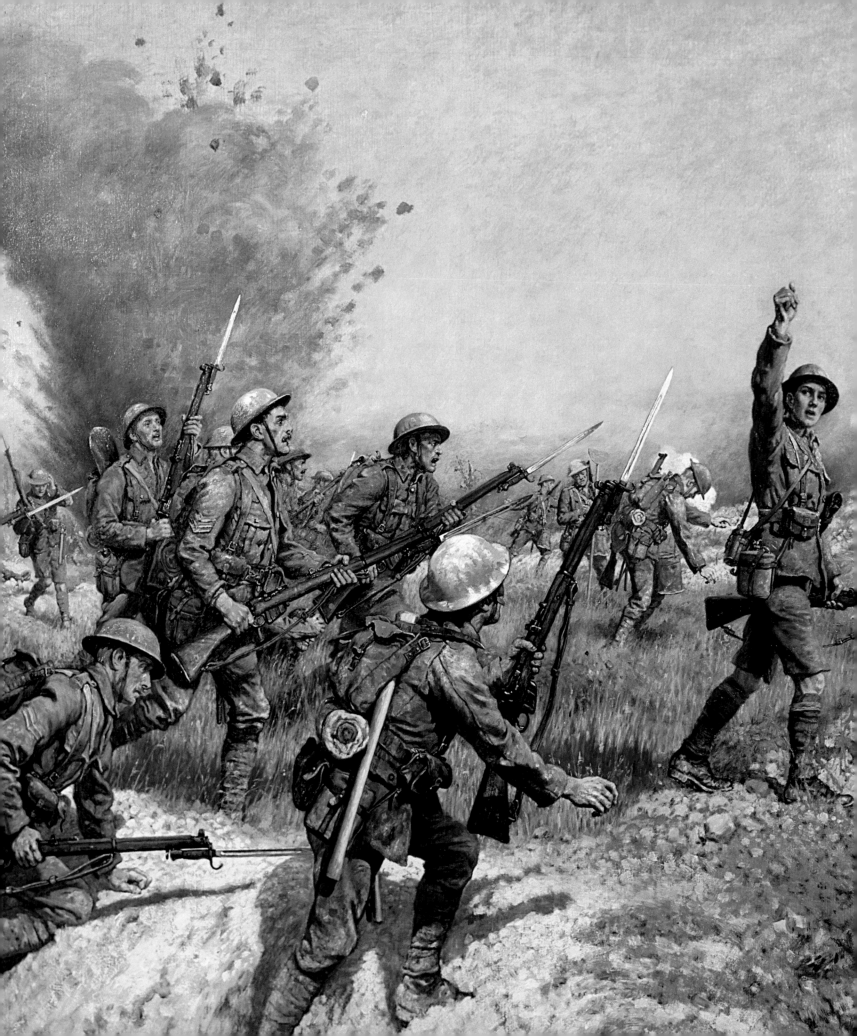

Violence ...
and more violence

The death of Queen Victoria was a watershed.
However, her son, Edward VII, proved to be a much
better King than people had expected.

The Edwardian era had its own style, and the notorious playboy who
had waited for so long for the Throne showed himself to be a shrewd
ruler, with a deft touch in foreign affairs. He also managed to deal
skillfully with the constitutional and other challenges of the new century.

In Ireland the College of Physicians proudly retained its 'Royal' Charter,
as it had done throughout all the changes of Monarchy since the
Restoration of Charles II. As an institution it continued to make an
important contribution to the field of medicine at a time when poverty
and disease were still rife, despite the advances which had been made in
the previous century.

As one medical historian noted in 1901 about the nation's health:

> Affluence was not a word that a student walking the wards of Dublin's
> Meath Hospital would have heard on the lips of his teachers. Its patients
> were drawn from the Liberties and the grim tenements of York Street and
> Kevin Street, ravaged by late stages of tuberculosis, syphilis and cancer.
>
> During the week ending 26 January 1901, hospitals in Dublin admitted
> 17 cases of typhoid fever, 8 of scarlatina, 8 of diphtheria, 2 of typhus. Dublin
> had a higher death rate from typhoid than London, but a lower
> mortality from diphtheria. The annual death rate
> calculated from deaths in Irish urban areas in January
> 1901 was 24.1 per 1000 persons in the population –
> London was 17.9 per 1000.[1]

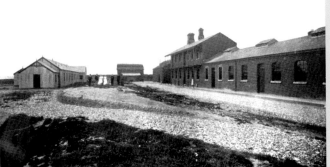

ABOVE: Proclamation of the Easter Rising in
April 1916, and LEFT: *The Battle of the
Somme*, July 1916, painting by JP Beadle
BELFAST CITY COUNCIL

The Easter Proclamation, 1916

DISEASE, DIRT, AND FLIES.

THE GREAT CARRIER OF DISEASE IS DIRT.

The cleaner the person, the clothes and bedding,
the room, and whole dwelling, the less likelihood
there is to become diseased.

DIRT ATTRACTS FLIES, and Fies carry dirt,
and sometimes disease germs, into milk and other
food, producing sometimes disease.

IN HOT WEATHER tainted food causes much
of the illness of infants and young children.
If you desire to guard your children against
disease, keep them, their clothes, and their food
clean.

DESTROY FLIES (the carriers of disease) by
means of cleanliness, which deprives them of food,
and by means of FLY PAPER, which entraps and
kills them.

COVER UP MILK, BUTTER, BREAD, &c., so
that Flies cannot pollute them.   Do not eat RAW
cockles or mussels, as they may contain disease
germs.

CHARLES A. CAMERON,
Medical Superintendent Officer of Health.

PUBLIC HEALTH COMMITTEE,
CASTLE STREET, *August*, 1908.

In 1903 there was an epidemic of smallpox in
Dublin. Some of the people worst affected were
those living in the Church Street – Beresford
area, where the housing conditions were
appalling. The earliest cases were treated in the
Hardwicke Hospital, which housed the smallpox
ward.

Unfortunately, the Hardwicke was situated an
a congested area of the city, close to several other
major institutions. Sir Charles Cameron and the
Dublin Public Health Committee petitioned the
Corporation for a more suitable site for treating
smallpox victims, and eventually some buildings
were acquired near the Pigeon House Fort. The
visiting physician was a Dr Day, the resident
Physician of the Cork Street Hospital.[2]

The Smallpox Hospital, Pigeon House, 1903

DUBLIN CITY LIBRARY AND ARCHIVE

167

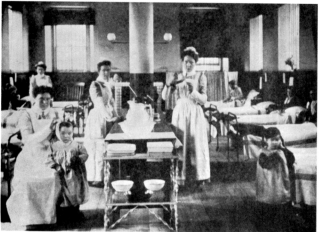

One of the wards in Cork Street Fever Hospital. The hospital coped with all sorts of contagious diseases, including typhus and cholera. Poor sanitary conditions, insufficient nutrition and bad housing all contributed to the continuing spread of contagious disease.[3]

RCPI

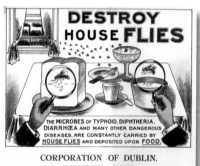

Upheaval

Politically the situation in Ireland deteriorated quickly during the early twentieth century, almost to the point of civil war. By common consent, this was averted only by the outbreak of the disastrous First World War in 1914.

There was added upheaval stemming from the Dublin Lockout of 1913–14, and then the 1916 Easter Rising. Following the end of the Great War, there was further bitter conflict which resulted in Partition, and the establishment of the Irish Free State and of Northern Ireland.

In such circumstances, conducting the normal business of the Royal Colleges in Ireland was a considerable challenge, in a society which was tearing itself apart.

Nevertheless, there was a sense in which this was history repeating itself. The Fraternity of Physicians had after all been established in the aftermath of the violence of the Cromwellian invasion of Ireland, and sustained through the Williamite wars, to emerge at the end of the seventeenth century with not one but two Royal Charters. The development of the College, like that of Ireland itself, had taken place against a background of sustained political uncertainty and violence from the mid-seventeenth century onwards.

However, with characteristic determination, as well as a mixture of vision, magnanimity, muddle, and a certain aplomb, the College carried on, regardless of the state of the world in general, and of Ireland in particular.

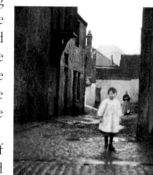

Slum conditions in Tyndall's Alley, off Bridgefoot Street, Dublin

Dublin Lock-Out

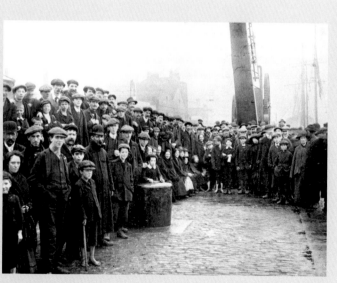

The Dublin lock-out, which lasted from August 1913 to January 1914, was a test of strength between 25,000 workers, led by James Larkin, James Connolly and others, and 400 employers, led by William Martin Murphy, a prominent businessman who had formed the Dublin Employers' Federation in 1912.

The battle was over the workers' right to unionise, but the background to the dispute was the terrible living conditions in the Dublin tenements. In one of the worst incidents, the police charged a union meeting in O'Connell Street on 31 August 1913, and arrested Larkin.

During the ensuing rioting, two people died, and some 200 policemen and many civilians were injured. The workers who had been locked out lost their struggle, and had to return on their employers' terms. However they had shown the importance of their cause, and the bitter memories of the dispute helped shortly afterwards to fuel the flames of the Uprising during Easter Week 1916.

Workers waiting on the docks for the food ships coming from the UK. *Irish Life*, 3 October 1913, NLI

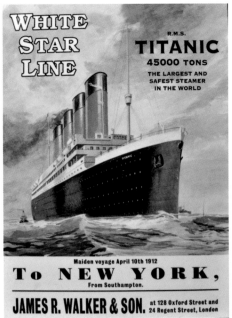

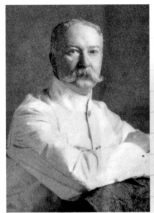

Titanic Loss

The Minutes of most institutions are concerned primarily with their own business. However, there are occasions when a short reference in a Minute to an event of national and international importance underlines the impact of what has taken place, partly because of the stark simplicity of the reference itself.

One example of this is a College Minute of 1912 instructing the Registrar of the College to forward a letter of condolence to the relatives of the late Dr WJN O'Loughlin, a Licentiate, 'who was lost in the wreck of the RMS *Titanic*'.[4]

It was a reminder of the magnitude of the tragedy when the *Titanic* sliced into an iceberg in the calm but icy Atlantic ocean at 11.40 pm on Sunday, 14 April 1912, and sank shortly afterwards, with the loss of 1,513 lives – affecting so many families, on both sides of the Atlantic.

Other Challenges

While the Home Rule issue had reached crisis dimensions in Ireland, with activitists in the North and South involved in gun-running and preparations for a civil war, the Minutes of the College also recorded a perennial problem in its history – a shortage of money. A Minute of December 13, 1913 noted that:

> ... [the] financial state of the College, as reported by the Treasurer, is unsatisfactory, the question [should] be referred to the Economy Committee with a view to suggesting what way the deficit can be wiped out, and how in future the expenses of the College can be reduced.[5]

The expenditure in the previous year had exceeded the College income by £217-17-7, and the Treasurer, HT Bewley asked what steps should be taken to deal with this. The Economy Committee met, and duly recommended a reduction in the salaries of the Registrar and Treasurer, and in the fees of the Examiners.

A reproduction from College Minutes of June 1912, referring to the loss of RCPI Licentiate WJN O'Loughlin, a Senior Surgeon for the White Star Line. He lost his life while on duty with the RMS *Titanic* on her maiden voyage.
RCPI

FAR LEFT: a publicity advertisement for the ship on her way to New York turned out to be overly optimistic.

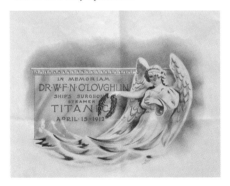

A memorial to Dr O'Loughlin published in the journal, *American Medicine, Vol XVIII*, in May 1912, shortly after the *Titanic* sank.
RCPI

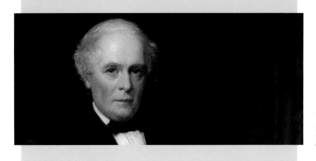

In The Picture

At a special business meeting on 12 March 1912 the College considered a request from the renowned artist, Stephen Catterson Smith RHA, asking that his father's portrait of Sir Dominic Corrigan be transferred temporarily on loan to the National Portrait Gallery.

However, he received a testy refusal which showed how elitist the College could be at times. It was resolved that the President and Fellows could not 'see their way' to lending the portrait to the National Gallery, because it was a presentation to the College 'and is therefore retained by them as a valuable trust'. Nevertheless, in a somewhat sniffy addendum, it welcomed 'members of the public who are interested in art to inspect the portraits in the College'.[7]

Happily, however, the College was more accommodating later on, following a request by Mrs Catterson Smith on notepaper from her prestigious address at 42 Stephen's Green in Dublin. She asked for the loan of 'a portrait of modern size and some drawings by my late father-in-law and by my husband', as contributions to an Irish Art Exhibition to be held in London.

She requested especially the 'small cabinet picture of Sir Dominic Corrigan Bart', which she claimed:

> is, with one exception, the finest specimen of Papa's highly-finished, small portraits, and I should like IT to represent him on the forthcoming public occasion, if the College would be so kind and so public-spirited to lend it for six weeks.

The President and Fellows could not lightly turn down such a tactful request. They stipulated, however, that the painting should be insured for £300, and that 'all risks and expenses' should be undertaken by the Executive Committee of the Exhibition.[8]

Not surprisingly, there was a flanking movement from those who disapproved of these measures, and they put forward an amendment to the proposal, suggesting that the payments to the Registrar and Treasurer should not be cut. However, their rearguard action was to no avail, and the amendment was lost. The College ruled that reductions should apply to all payments made after St Luke's Day in 1912.[5]

The Great War

The immense blunders that led to the Great War of 1914–18 were well summarised by the late distinguished military historian, Sir John Keegan, who described it as a 'tragic and unnecessary' conflict:

> Unnecessary, because the train of events that led to its outbreak might have been broken at any point during the five weeks crisis that preceded the first clash of arms, had prudence or common goodwill found a voice; tragic, because the consequences of the first clash ended the lives of ten million human beings, tortured the emotional lives of millions more, destroyed the benevolent and optimistic nature of the European continent and left, when the guns at last fell silent four years later, a legacy of political rancor and racial hatred so intense that no explanation of the causes of the Second World War can stand without reference to those roots.[6]

It is estimated that some 206,000 Irish recruits enlisted in the British Army during the First World War, and that 3,000 of these – including 400 students – were from the medical profession.

As part of the recruitment drive, representatives of the Armed Forces wrote to the College. The Royal Navy asked the Dean and Registrar, 'if you would be good enough to recommend young qualified practitioners to volunteer for service as Voluntary Surgeons in the Royal Navy, should it be necessary to mobilise the Fleet'. The letter was dated 30 July 1914, two days after Austria-Hungary declared war on Serbia and six days before the United Kingdom declared war on Germany.[9]

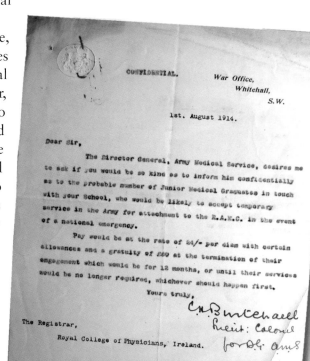

A letter from the War Office at Whitehall, requesting volunteer medical recruits for the Army

RCPI

Sir Andrew Horne
1856–1924

Andrew John Horne was a leading obstetrician who was educated at Clongowes Wood College, Co Kildare, and the Carmichael School of Medicine. He became a Licentiate of the Royal College of Surgeons in 1877, and a year later, a Licentiate of the Royal College of Physicians, of which he became a Member in 1881.

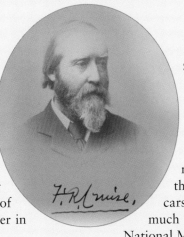

Horne was the founder member and first joint Master of the National Maternity Hospital in Holles Street, Dublin, where he was the *de facto* manager. Though a Catholic himself, he made it plain that the hospital would not be a 'Catholic' institution, but open to students and trainee midwives of all denominations.

He performed the first Caesarian operation there in 1901, but he believed that his colleagues should not be bound by the Catholic Church's attitude of 'Spare the mother, no matter the child'. He taught his students and colleagues to 'operate early, delay is fatal'.

Andrew Horne was also a good administrator, and he and his colleagues helped to expand the maternity hospital to become the largest in Europe.

He was elected a Fellow, Censor, and Vice-President of the Royal College of Physicians, and eventually he became President, from 1908–10. He was knighted in 1913.

James Joyce by Alex Ehrenzweig
CREATIVE COMMONS

Despite his many medical honours, his name is also associated with James Joyce who mentioned him in *Ulysses*. When describing the visit of Bloom to Holles Street, Joyce wrote: 'Of that house A. Horne is lord.' Joyce also refers to him in *Finnegan's Wake* 'Ho, he that hath hornhide!'

Horne apparently never read Joyce, but his son Andrew – who had a distinguished war record – claimed that his father had Joyce thrown out of the maternity hospital in 1904 when, as a student, he was found without permission in one of the wards and had intruded on the privacy of the women patients. Sir Andrew had also objected to a disparaging remark allegedly made by Joyce about the poor 'breeding like rabbits'. Apparently the remark was never made by Joyce, and it misrepresented his outlook.[10]

Andrew Horne senior was a founder member of the Dublin medical dining club, – The Phagocytes – and an accomplished pianist, who played with Sir Francis Cruise in a musical trio. They gave recitals in fashionable Merrion Square where they both lived. These social events were referred to by Dublin wits as 'Cruising round the Horn'. Andrew Horne was a forward thinker, and in 1912 he bought one of the first motor-cars – an 18-horsepower Schneider, in which he had much pleasure in being driven from his home to the National Maternity Hospital, which was only a short distance away.

However there was also a slightly bizarre aspect to some of Horne's behaviour. His wife suffered from diabetes, and as a result her leg was amputated. Her husband apparently had it preserved in formaldehyde, and on her death two years later, he placed it in her coffin.[11]

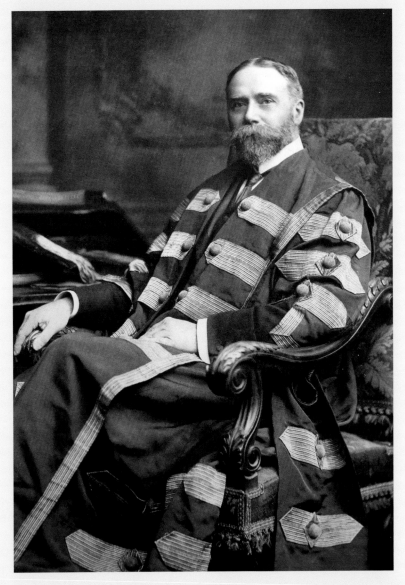

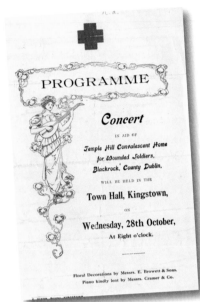

The urgent need for army medical recruits was underlined by another letter to the College on 1 August 1914 from Lieutenant-Colonel CH Burtchaell, an Irish doctor in the Army Medical Service.

He requested that the College would inform him about the probable number of junior medical graduates who might serve in the RAMC on a temporary basis in the event of a national emergency. The College Registrar replied, in a letter three days later, that he was unable to provide the names of any candidates 'at the present time'.

This reluctance to supply names may have been due to the short notice supplied, or because the young doctors were lukewarm about the war effort. However as the conflict continued this attitude was to change to one of strong commitment.

While daunting developments were taking place on the battlefields of Europe, the College was steadily recording, in the early stages of war, the business of the main committee meetings, events and developments which were important in keeping the institution going.

One of the first indications that the European conflagration was beginning to impinge on the normal routine of the College was in a Minute dated 29 September 1914, which proposed that 'owing to the European War in which the British Empire is at present engaged, the College Dinner on St Luke's Day be postponed'.[12]

Help for Belgian Colleagues

In December 1914 the College had to deal with a much more substantial matter. This was a request for help from Professor Jacobs of Brussels on behalf of Belgian pharmacists and medics and their families, who had become destitute because of the havoc created by the war in Europe. Within a month of the invasion of Belgium on 4 August, the country had been entirely taken over by Germany.

Professor Jacobs' appeal was taken up by the College Registrar TPC Kirkpatrick, and CM Benson, Secretary to the Council of the Royal College of Surgeons. A joint meeting of the two Colleges was held in November 1914 and this resulted in the establishment of the Belgian Doctors' and Pharmacists' Relief Fund. A Committee was appointed to collect subscriptions to help the Belgians. The donations would be channelled through the Royal College of Physicians, which received hundreds of responses from the members of the Irish medical profession.

A further attempt to help their stricken European colleagues, the College recommended that the curriculae of four Belgian universities

OPPOSITE: Temple Hill Concert Programme
This concert to raise funds for the Temple Hill Convalescant Home for Soldiers was held on 28 October 1914. Temple Hill is located near Blackrock, and was one of the numerous convalescent homes established in the city. Fundraising for the war effort distracted those with loved ones at the Front from worry, and made those at home feel part of the war effort. This Red Cross Concert was one of many such fundraising events.
DUBLIN CITY LIBRARY AND ARCHIVE

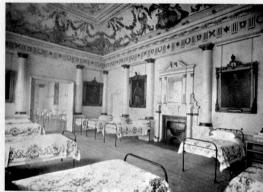

Hospital ward, State Drawing rooms, Dublin Castle

This image is taken from the Souvenir album presented to the Marquis and Marchioness of Aberdeen and Temair, as a farewell gift by members of their staff of 1905–15. During their time the Aberdeens had been very popular with the ordinary people of Dublin, though not so much so with high society, as their approach to the post was too democratic for many. They left Ireland in 1915, having transformed much of Dublin Castle into a Red Cross hospital for wounded soldiers.
DUBLIN CITY LIBRARY AND ARCHIVE

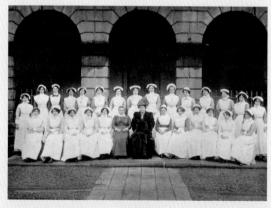

The nurses of the Dublin Castle hospital, gathered around Lady Aberdeen and the Matron Miss AM MacDonnell
DUBLIN CITY LIBRARY AND ARCHIVE

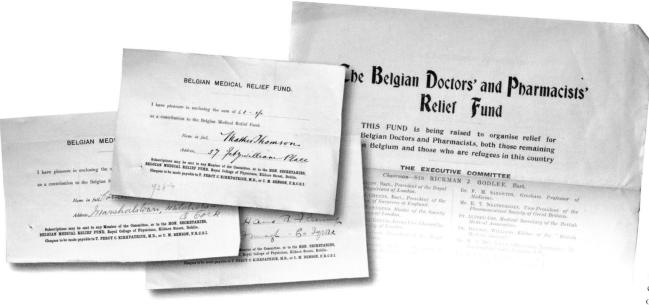

Some of the donation certificates which came in from all over Ireland from doctors and pharmacists, in answer to an appeal for funds to help Belgian colleagues who were in distress and financial difficulties after the outbreak of the Great War.
RCPI

should be recognised on behalf of Belgian students in exile who wished to sit the Conjoint examinations of the two Colleges in Ireland. It was also recommended that Belgian students who could not afford the fees should be excused from paying for the examinations.[13]

Support from a USA colleague

There was also help from America. On January 11 1915 Dr WS Thayer, an Honorary Fellow of the College, wrote from his home in Baltimore, Maryland, and made a contribution to the relief fund. He stated:

> You have no idea how truly our hearts are with you in these troublous days. For myself I feel humiliation that our country is not doing more.
>
> The present Administration is a gentle and timorous one, and we cannot expect much, but the moral sympathies of America are with you all, heart and soul.[14]

Dr Thayer would have to wait for more than two years until the USA entered the war against Germany on 6 April, 1917 – partly because of the unrestricted German submarine warfare which sank many vessels. These included the RMS *Lusitania*, which was controversially torpedoed by a German U-boat off Kinsale in May 1915, causing the deaths of 1,198 passengers and crew. This took place just three months after Dr Thayer's letter was sent to the College in aid of his Belgian Colleagues.

King and Country

Not long before the sinking of the RMS *Lusitania*, the College recorded in its Journal an address which it had presented earlier to Lord Wimborne, the new Lord-Lieutenant, expressing its by now strong support for the war effort:

> At this moment when the forces of our King, drawn from all parts of his Empire, are engaged in a deadly struggle with our common foe for the defence of our homes and liberty, we welcome the opportunity of expressing to you our unwavering attachment to the Empire, and our confidence in the ultimate triumph of the cause for which our people and our allies are fighting.

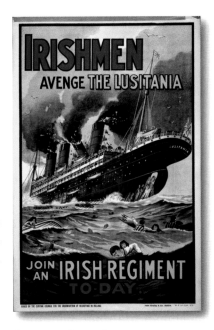

A propaganda recruitment poster following the sinking of the *Lusitania* by a German U-boat, 6 May 1915
CREATIVE COMMONS

The great Irish art collector, Hugh Lane, died on the *Lusitania*. He was the director of the National Gallery in Dublin and bequeathed the Municipal Gallery (the Hugh Lane Gallery), to the city.

173

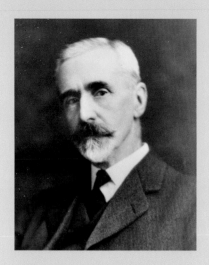

Suffering and Loss

The personal suffering and loss during the Great War was reflected at different times in the Minutes of the College.

Dr Joseph O'Carroll, President of the College from 1916–19, was a consultant to the Military Heart Hospital, and to the Red Cross Hospital in Dublin Castle. Later he became the only consultant physician to the Forces in Ireland, and held the rank of Colonel.

His son, Frank Brendan O'Carroll had been a law student at University College Dublin in 1914, and in September of that year he received a commission in the 6th Battalion the Dublin Fusiliers, which several months later took part in the ill-fated Gallipoli campaign. Young O'Carroll was killed on 10 August, 1915 – only three weeks after his twentieth birthday.

He was one of 36,000 men who died, and his grave is not marked. With thousands of others he is commemorated on the Helles Memorial in Gallipoli.

In memory of his son, Dr O'Carroll endowed a bed in the children's ward of the Richmond Hospital, and commissioned a plaque by Oliver Sheppard for a wall in the building.

After the war Dr O'Carroll was offered an OBE for his services to medicine, but he declined the honour to record his disapproval of British policy in Ireland, during the 'Black and Tans'' activities.

In this great cause, the Fellows, Members and Licentiates of the College are willingly taking their part both at home and abroad, endeavouring, as far as in them lies, to bring help and healing to those who have suffered, and to ward off those attacks of disease which have so often proved the most dangerous enemies of armies in the field.

In lending what aid they can in this the common danger, the President and Fellows feel that they are merely carrying on the great tradition of their College, handed down to them by their predecessors since its foundation by King Charles II.

We desire to assure Your Excellency of our readiness to afford to His Majesty and to his Government our hearty assistance in this time of the Empire's peril, and to express again our loyalty to his Throne.[15]

Military Training

The military authorities took the physicians at their word, and on November 7 1915, the Surgeon-General at the War Office, MWH Russell, wrote thus to Dr Ephraim MacDowell Cosgrave, the President of the College:

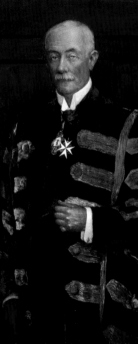

Dr Ephraim MacDowell Cosgrave, President of the College, 1914–16
RCPI

An impression appears to have obtained credence among medical students in their fourth and fifth years that it is unnecessary for them to undertake any military training while engaged in the study of their profession.

This view has doubtless arisen because, owing to the great demand for medical men and the shortage of supply, many who have achieved no military training have been given commissions in the Royal Army Medical Corps.

From the experience of the past year, it has been clearly shown that men who have had previous military training are of infinitely greater value as officers of the Royal Army Medical Corps than those who have no military experience.

Students in their fourth and fifth years have been advised that it is best for them to continue their medical studies in order to qualify for commissions in the Royal Army Medical Corps, but this does not in the least exempt them from using all the means available for obtaining military instruction.

The medical units of the various Officers' Training Corps are organised so that men may obtain this instruction without disturbance of their medical studies, and all senior students, who have not already done so, are strongly urged to become cadets in the medical units of their University's Officers' Training Corps.[16]

Gallantry

There were many examples of the great courage and skill of medical men at the Front, and at a special business meeting of the College on

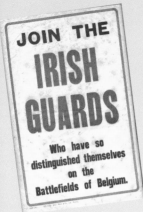

This recruiting poster for the Irish Guards emphasises the heroic part the regiment had played in the early part of the war in Belgium, particularly at the first battle of Ypres.
DUBLIN CITY LIBRARY AND ARCHIVE

Wytschaete Ridge, Belgium, 1916
The Dublin Fusiliers took part in the capture of Wytschaete Ridge, just south of Ypres and of the Messines Ridge ... many Ulstermen of various regiments fought alongside the Dublin Fusiliers in this latter engagement which included the largest underground mine of World War One.[19]
FR BROWNE SJ COLLECTION
DAVISON & ASSOCIATES

10 January 1916, the Registrar was instructed to write to temporary Captain Henry James Burke, serving with the 1st/8th Battalion of the West Yorkshire Regiment, who was awarded a Military Cross, for 'conspicuous gallantry' near Turco farm in France on 8 November 1915.

The Minutes of the College contain a report in *The Lancet* which stated:

> A Sergeant in the front line had his leg crushed by the blowing-in of a dug-out, and Captain Burke found immediate amputation necessary. In order to save time, he carried across the open to get his instruments, while the enemy turned a machine-gun on to him. In spite of their fire, he returned the same way, and coolly performed the operation in the trench while the enemy was shelling it heavily.

The Registrar was instructed to write to Captain Burke to express the College's congratulations on the recognition of his gallantry.[17] The Military Cross was instituted by Royal Warrant on 29 December 1914, and more than 37,000 such medals were issued during the First World War, which gives one some indication of the sheer magnitude of the conflict.[18]

The College also noted at their meeting on 3 March 1916 that the Irish Schools' and Graduates' Association had awarded the Arnott Medal to Captain WFM Loughnan, a graduate of the Royal College of Surgeons in Ireland who was serving in France with the RAMC:

> The Minute recorded that Captain Loughnan went to France with the original expeditionary force, and has shown conspicuous bravery on several occasions. Among other acts, he secured the severed artery of a badly-wounded officer on the battlefield, and under fire, carried him to a place of safety.

The College asked the Registrar to convey its congratulations to Captain Loughnan.[20]

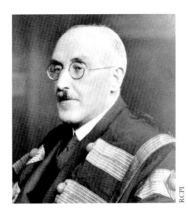

RCPI

Dr William Arthur Winter
President of the RCPI, 1927–30

Dr Winter graduated from Dublin University with an MB in 1892. He became a Licentiate of the College in 1898, and three years later a Fellow. He was appointed as a radiologist in the Royal City of Dublin Hospital, and in 1904 he was appointed as an assistant physician in Dr Steevens' Hospital.

Five years later he was appointed as a full physician at Dr Steevens' Hospital. During the Great War he served in France as a Major with the RAMC, and was stationed at No. 83 General Hospital.

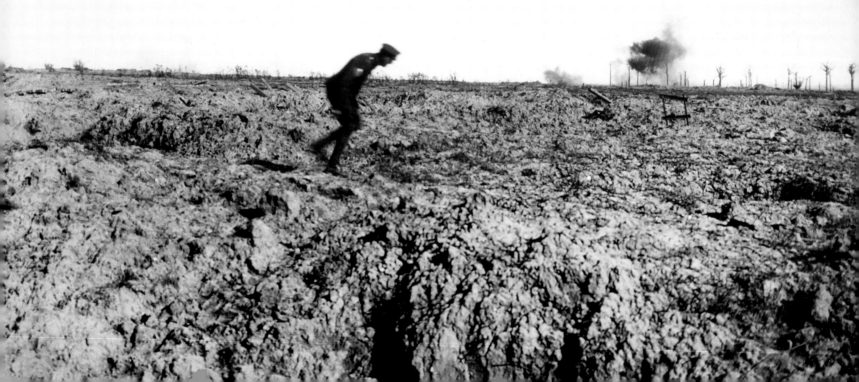

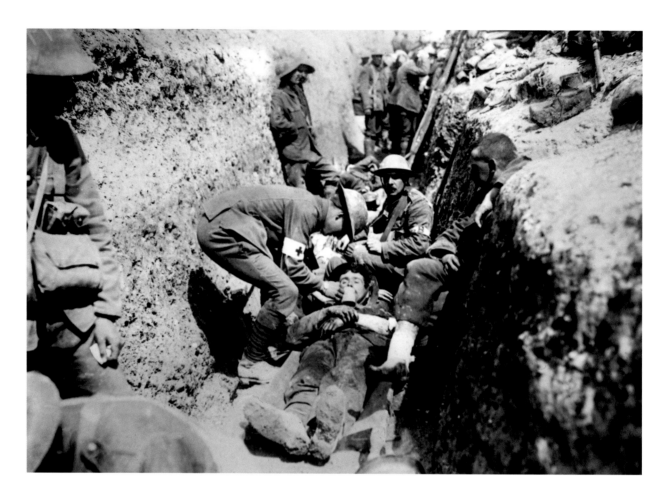

Hell-Fire

The dispassionate language of such a Minute, though no doubt accurate, could not begin to describe the hell of life and death on the battlefields at the Front. This was conveyed most graphically by Erich Maria Remarque, a former soldier in the Kaiser's Army, whose anti-war novel, *All Quiet on the Western Front* remains one of the classics of war literature. In this passage he depicts what it was like for young soldiers as they moved towards the Front:

> The air becomes acrid with the smoke of the guns and the fog. The fumes of powder taste bitter on the tongue. The roar of the guns makes our lorry stagger, the reverberation rolls raging away to the rear, everything quakes. Our faces change imperceptibly. We are not, indeed, in the front-line, but only in the reserves, yet in every face can be read: This is the front, now we are within its embrace … [21]

The conditions at the Front were appalling, with doctors having to operate often without anaesthetics, and with mud and debris everywhere. Many of the unsung heroes were the stretcher-bearers who recovered the dead and injured from no-man's land, often under fire. They carried only the basic supplies of morphine and bandages.[22]

As one historian has pointed out:

> The use of tanks and automated weapons caused new and horrific types of injuries, unimaginable in previous conflicts – and the emergence of wet, cold

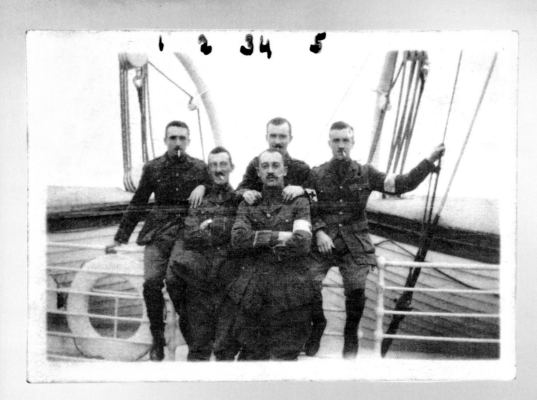

Captain Andrew Horne

The son of Sir Andrew Horne, Andrew Horne junior was a medical student at Trinity when the War started, and he qualified six months early to join the RAMC, and serve in Gallipoli. Horne was one of the last officers to be evacuated from the peninsula, and he later served in Egypt, India and Mesopotamia.

His photo album presents a vivid picture of his war service, and one of his letters to his mother, states that:

> The last thing I saw of Helles was our ships pumping shells into our hospital, and the Turks shelling the W-beach, still thinking there were troops there. Nobody can believe we had such a time and came through it alive, but here we are.[23]

ABOVE: The last five officers to leave Gallipoli aboard HMS Letitia, 11 January, 1916.
BACK ROW FROM LEFT: Captain Horne (Irish); Captain Angus (Scottish); Lieutenant Allison (Canadian); Captain Rees Thomas (Welsh) and Lieutenant Leeson (Canadian).
BELOW: A Turkish shell landing in Suvla Bay with (inset) a photograph of Captian Andrew Horne.

Photographs are from Horne's war album
NATIONAL MUSEUM OF IRELAND

After the war, Andrew Horne was Assistant Master at the National Maternity Hospital from 1924–6. He shared his father's broadmindedness about religion and culture, and withdrew his candidature for the Mastership of the Hospital in 1931 when the Roman Catholic Archbishop of Dublin, Edward J Byrne opposed his appointment because he was a Trinity College graduate.[24]

Care of returning sick and wounded

The majority of hospital ships arriving in Ireland docked in Dublin and contained an average of 400 soldiers. From 1914 to 1918, approximately 70 institutions located throughout Ireland provided facilities for the treatment of 16,000 returning sick and wounded. These included auxiliary wards and hospitals and a number of specialist institutions established by RAMC Command (Ireland) for the treatment of specific diseases. In 1915, for example, the War Office appointed Lieutenant-Colonel William Dawson, Inspector of Lunatic Asylums in Ireland, as RAMC (Ireland) specialist in nerve diseases. On 16 June 1916, Dawson took charge of the Richmond War Hospital, located in Dublin's Grangegorman Asylum. The Hospital catered for 32 soldiers suffering from mental disorders. From the date of opening till its closing on 23 December 1919, the Richmond War Hospital treated 362 patients, of which two-thirds were discharged to friends or ordinary military hospitals, two returned to duty and 31 sent directly to civil asylums. While the institution was helpful in the RAMC's attempts to provide treatment for mental cases, it was undeniably small. Therefore, in October 1916, the War Office requested Dawson to facilitate them by placing an asylum with 500 beds at the disposal of the RAMC. Similar arrangements had been managed successfully in Britain. In Ireland the vastly overcrowded asylums made this an unlikely prospect. Yet, in April 1917, the War Office acquired Belfast's Civil Lunatic Asylum and incorporated it as part of the Belfast War Hospital. The hospital received Irish men suffering from mental illness during active service and also treated men, not of Irish birth, who belonged to Irish regiments. The first military cases arrived on 15 May 1917. Staff consisted of men who had enlisted in the RAMC for the duration of the war and who had previous experience working in asylums.[27]

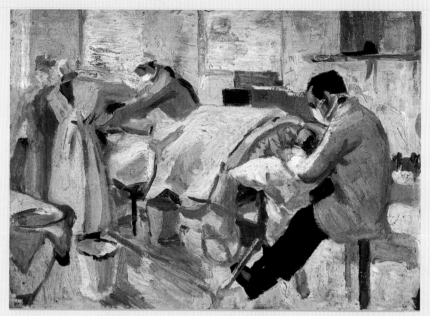

An operating theatre in a hospital ship
Oil painting by Godfrey Jervis Gordon (Jan Gordon)
WELLCOME LIBRARY, LONDON

and squalid trench warfare brought with it untold discomfort and suffering. These were four long years of torture and pain, with excruciating human losses.

From conditions such as trench foot, mustard gas poisoning, hideous facial injuries and shell shock, to illness such as tonsillitis, or life-threatening Spanish flu, even in-growing toenails and lice … few men escaped unscathed.[25]

Sir Patrick Dun's Hospital and the Great War

The staff of Sir Patrick Dun's Hospital played an important role in the War, and supplied no fewer than 80 trained nurses, who served in the Army or Navy from 1914–18.

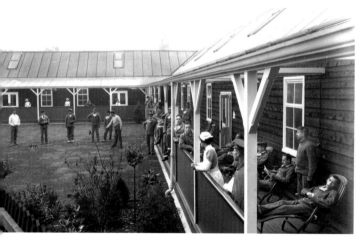

A temporary UVF hospital was set up at Queen's University Belfast in 1915. In this photograph, as a means of relaxation, men play quoits in the hospital grounds.
PUBLIC RECORD OFFICE NI

Some 400 or more former students of the Hospital served in the RAMC and in the Naval and Air Medical Services. In the Hospital the Iveagh and Wicklow Wards were set aside for sick and wounded soldiers, where up to 30 beds were maintained.

In 1920 a brass Memorial Tablet, set in an oak frame, was unveiled in the Hospital, with the names of 30 people who had died in the conflict. A Memorial bed in the Hospital was endowed by others who had served in the War.[26]

Dr Robbie Smyth

Robbie Smyth, seated here in the middle of the second row, was an outstanding rugby player. He won two Irish caps in 1904, and he played for Sir Patrick Dun's Hospital in the Dublin Hospitals' Rugby Cup between 1900–1905. The Dublin Hospitals' Cup is thought to be the longest-standing rugby competition in the world.
In January 1881, a group of surgeons and physicians had met in Dublin to discuss the establishment of a rugby competition between teams from the Dublin hospitals. One of those who supported the idea was the surgeon, William Thornley Stoker, whose brother Bram Stoker was the author of the Gothic novel, *Dracula*.
RCPI

One of those who died was Dr Robertson Stewart Smyth. Smyth was a house-surgeon for a year at St Patrick Dun's Hospital in 1905, and then joined the RAMC.

He was posted to India, and on the outbreak of the First World War, he served in France. He was promoted to the rank of Major, and was Mentioned in Dispatches by the British Commander, Lord French 'for his gallant and distinguished action in the field'.

In December 1915, Major Smyth was twice gassed by enemy action. The next year, while recuperating in London, he resigned from the Army. He died in April 1916, at the age of 36. His remains were taken to his native Banbridge in Co. Down, where he was buried.

He had been a typically well-rounded young doctor who had played for Dun's in the Dublin Hospitals' Rugby Cup from 1900–05. During this time his team won the trophy five times, and Robbie Smyth played for Ireland twice in 1904. In an obituary in *The Lancet*, an unnamed friend wrote:

> … [his] loveable disposition and engaging personality gained him many friends. His death will be deeply regretted by all who knew him, and he will always be held in affectionate remembrance by the friends he made in his all too short life.[28]

Dr George Sigerson
1836–1925

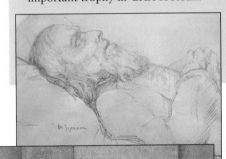

The drawing below by Estelle Solomons of the deathbed scene of Dr George Sigerson is part of the RCPI Archive. Sigerson, who was born in Strabane, was a well-known Irish physician, scientist, politician, academic, writer and poet.

He was a major figure in the late nineteenth century Irish Literary Revival, and also an influential member of the GAA. He donated his salary as a UCD Professor to help establish the Sigerson Cup, which was first competed for in 1911, in a Gaelic football competition for third-level students. The inaugural winners were UCD, and the Sigerson Cup remains an important trophy in GAA football.

RCPI

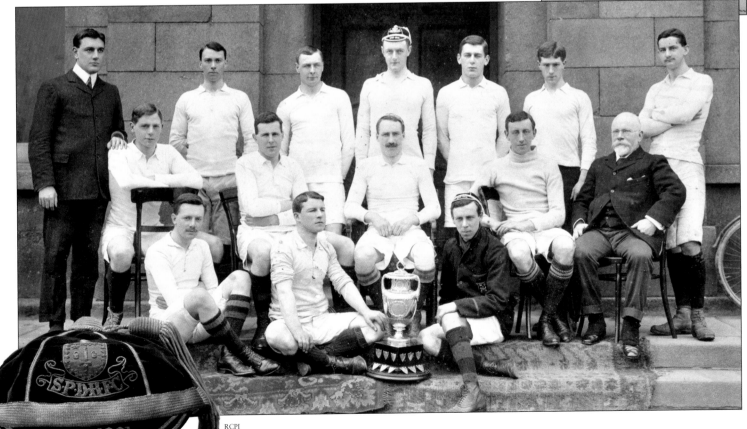

RCPI

179

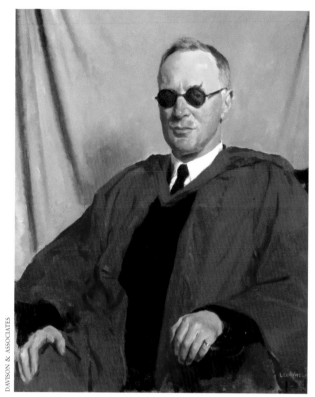

Thomas Gillman Moorhead, who had a distinguished War record and who was also a leading member of the Irish medical profession. He lost the sight of both eyes following an accident, but with immense courage continued his career. He was President of the College from 1930–33.

Portrait by Leo Whelan

Thomas Gillman Moorhead

One of the most noteworthy medical figures of the period was Thomas Gillman Moorhead, a physician at Sir Patrick Dun's Hospital, and later Chairman of the Board of Governors. He served with the Royal Army Medical Corps, attached to the Royal Dublin Fusiliers during the First World War. Moorhead later survived a serious peacetime injury, and managed to continue with his notable medical career.

Thomas Gillman Moorhead was born in Benburb, Co Tyrone on 15 October 1878. His middle name was the maiden name of his mother, Amelia Davis Gillman. He grew up in Bray, where his father Dr William Robert Moorhead was a family doctor. His two brothers were also doctors.

TG Moorhead read Medicine at Trinity College Dublin where he won many prizes, and he graduated in 1901. He was awarded an MD the next year, and became a member of the College in 1905. A year later he was elected a Fellow.

He became a respected teacher in medicine and allied subjects, and his classes at the Royal City of Dublin Hospital and at Sir Patrick Dun's Hospital were popular.

Following the outbreak of the First World War, many casualties were treated at Dun's Hospital, as noted earlier, and at other voluntary hospitals in Dublin. Moorhead was a physician at Dun's Hospital, and played a full part in this work. However in 1915 when many of the veterans of the ill-judged Gallipoli campaign were badly affected by illness, he joined the RAMC and served in Alexandria, which was the main military base for Gallipoli, where troops of the 10th Irish Division were heavily involved. Some 21,000 British and Irish soldiers, and nearly 11,500 from Australia and New Zealand perished in this disastrous blood-bath for the Allies, after which Winston Churchill (who bore most of the political responsibility for the failure) was forced to resign as First Lord of the Admiralty.[29]

By 31 December 1915, the majority of the troops had been evacuated from Gallipoli, and four major hospitals for British and Anzac troops, as well as two for Indian troops, and an Egyptian Government hospital were set up in Alexandria.

TG Moorhead, who had the rank of honorary Captain and later became an honorary Lieutenant-Colonel, worked in the largest general hospital, which had some 2,500 patients.

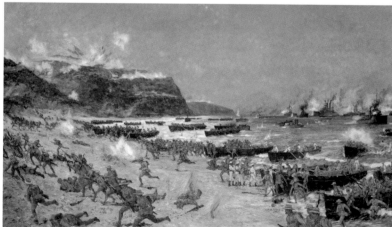

Gallipoli landings by Charles Edward Dixon
The Landing of Anzac, April 25, 1915
WAR ART ARCHIVES, NEW ZEALAND GOVERNMENT

He had a staff of forty medical officers, all of whom lived in tents. Moorhead's commanding officer was a Colonel Healy, a Dubliner, and the matron was an Irish nurse who had trained at St Vincent's in Dublin. Moorhead and his colleagues had to deal with many challenges, including a jaundice-like epidemic which was diagnosed as a form of hepatitis.[30]

In 1916, while on leave in Dublin, Moorhead was elected to the Chair of Medicine at the Royal College of Surgeons, and on November 1 he gave the inaugural lecture of the College's Biological Society. In the presence of a distinguished audience, including the Lord-Lieutenant, the Church of Ireland Archbishop of Dublin and the Surgeon-General, he outlined some of the challenges he had faced in Alexandria.

He said that an Army in the field had two foes, 'bacilli and bullets, and of these in most campaigns the former was by far the most dangerous'. In Gallipoli the tropical heat of the summer and the abundance of flies made conditions especially trying, 'but it was appalling to think that over 96,000 cases of medical illness occurred, a total that was probably in some measure responsible for the failure of the campaign'.

A copy of a serious, yet also a jocular and friendly letter, of 12 January 1916, from the outstanding bacteriologist and immunologist, Sir Almroth Wright to a colleague concerning a new anti-gangrene vaccination for inoculating troops at the Front. Wright, who later became an Honorary Fellow of the College, worked with his colleagues at an Army general hospital at Boulogne during the Great War. He was knighted in 1906.
RCPI

Professor Moorhead was thanked for his talk by the Lord-Lieutenant, Lord Wimborne, and the meeting closed 'with the playing of the National Anthem' – an interesting comment on that part of Dublin society of 1916, just a few months after the Easter Rising. So, too, was the sympathy expressed at the meeting to a Past President of the College, Sir Robert Woods, and Lady Woods, whose son had been killed in action.[31]

Later Career

Following his return from the War, Moorhead's medical career continued to flourish. In 1925 he was appointed Regius Professor of Physic at Trinity College Dublin. In the same year he made extensive visits to medical institutions in the USA and Canada, but the following year he suffered a calamitous accident when travelling in London to attend a meeting of the British Medical Association. While at Euston Station he tripped and fell badly, and, when his head hit the platform, became totally blind from a bilateral retinal detachment.

Moorhead however was a man of great courage who refused to allow this to end his medical career. With the help of professional clinical colleagues he continued to undertake consultations, and he was well-respected as the Chair of many committees.

His friends used to accompany him on Saturday afternoon walks, he played bridge with Braille cards, and he continued his interest in fishing, and even

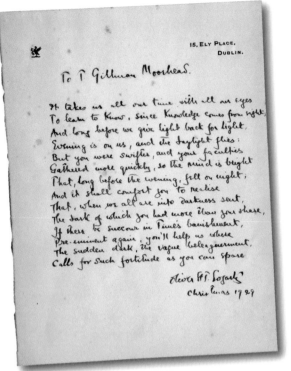

A poem written in 1929 by Oliver St John Gogarty, paying tribute to the courage of his friend TG Moorhead in coping with his total blindness after an accident three years earlier.
RCPI

mountaineering. He also remained a regular theatre-goer and held weekly dinner parties at the Royal Irish Yacht Club in Dun Laoghaire.

TG Moorhead won the admiration of his many colleagues and friends, including the noted doctor, athlete, politician, author, poet and wit, Oliver St John Gogarty. He wrote *As I was Going Down Sackville Street*, which was regarded as 'probably the best as well as the most entertaining book he wrote'.[32] Gogarty, incidentally was also the inspiration for Buck Mulligan in James Joyce's *Ulysses*.

During Christmas 1929, three years after Moorhead's accident, Gogarty wrote a short sonnet, praising the Professor's talents and also his fortitude:

> It takes us all our time with all our eyes
> To learn to know, since knowledge comes from sight;
> And long before we give back light for light,
> Evening is on us, and the daylight flies;
> But you were swifter, and your faculties
> Gathered more quickly …

After Professor Moorhead's death, his widow presented this poem to the College.[33] Moorhead's first wife had died in 1935, and three years later he married Sheila, daughter of the author Stephen Gwynn.

In his last remaining years Thomas Gillman Moorhead suffered great pain. He died on 3 August 1960. In his rich, adventurous and varied life he had been not only an outstanding representative of the College, but also an outstanding human being.

The Easter Rising 1916

Many accounts have been written about the Easter Rising, from many different perspectives, and doubtless much more will be written about this watershed period in Anglo-Irish history for years to come.

On Monday 16 April some 1,600 members of the Irish Volunteers and the Irish Citizen Army seized strategic roads and buildings in Dublin, and temporarily took control of the city. From the steps of the General Post Office, which had been overtaken by the rebels, Patrick Pearse proclaimed the new Irish Republic.

The rebellion was doomed to failure in the face of the vastly superior fire-power of the British, and within a week the rebels had surrendered. Initially the Rising had been greeted with a mixture of surprise, bewilderment, indifference and hostility by the general public, but the strong reaction by the Army, the mass of casualties and the Government's execution by firing-squad

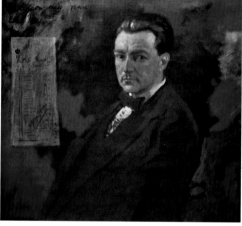

A portrait of Oliver St John Gogarty, the well-known Dublin doctor, author, politician and wit, which was painted by William Orpen in 1911. They had dined in style at the Café Royal in London, and apparently Orpen had paid the hefty bill. As a reminder to Gogarty, the artist included a copy of the receipt in the left-hand background to the portrait!
RCSI

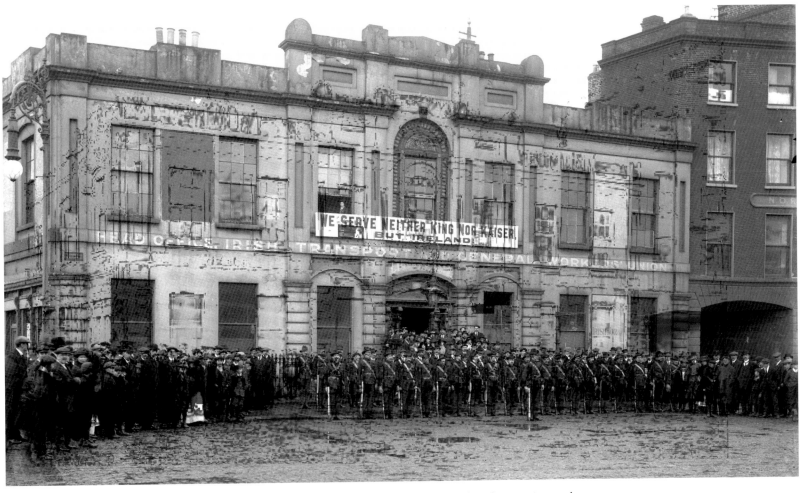

In 1914 the Irish Citizen Army lined up under the banner 'We Serve Neither King nor Kaiser', outside Liberty Hall, making their allegiance clear.

KEOGH PHOTOGRAPHIC COLLECTION
NATIONAL LIBRARY OF IRELAND

of the ringleaders, helped to swing public opinion firmly against the Establishment, and the British cause and connection was lost.

After six days of hostilities, 132 soldiers and policemen were killed, and 397 were wounded. However there were greater casualties among civilians, including 318 dead and 2,217 wounded. Only about 64 rebels died, as well as the 15 executed ring leaders.[34]

European context

While the focus of this chapter is to try to determine how the events of Easter Rising in Dublin affected the Irish medical profession, rather than to cover the associated political and military developments. It is worth considering one observation by the historian Edward Madigan, which helps to place the events of April 1916 in context.

> The Rising – an undeniably foundational, nation-making event – would not have occurred and cannot be fully understood outside the context of the First World War.
>
> The nationalist rebellion that erupted in Dublin in April 1916 was as much an event of the World War as the sinking of the *Lusitania* in 1915, or the Arab revolt in which TE Lawrence was involved. It was comparatively small in scale, and took place on the periphery of the industrialised killing on the western and eastern fronts, but it was nonetheless part of the chain of violent episodes that made up the global conflict.

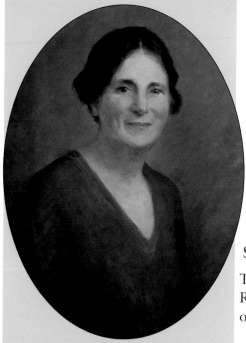

Dr Kathleen Lynn
1874–1955

The daughter of a Church of Ireland clergyman, Kathleen graduated in 1899 from the Catholic University Medical School in Cecilia Street, Dublin.

She was a well-known suffragist and an active Irish nationalist, who played a significant role in the Easter Rising. She worked in the soup kitchens during the Dublin lock-out, and was Chief Medical Officer to the Irish Citizen Army during the insurgency. She looked after the wounded from her base in the City Hall, and her car was used for carrying guns, and also as a sleeping place for Countess Markievicz.

Kathleen Lynn was imprisoned in Kilmainham, but was released on the intervention of the Lord Mayor of Dublin, Laurence O'Neill, because her medical services were needed during the Spanish flu pandemic from 1918–20.

She worked constantly for the poor, and is best known for her pioneering work in establishing St Ultan's Hospital for Infants in Dublin. She died in 1955 and she was given a full military funeral. Her diaries, and a portrait, are held in the College.[37]

Portrait by Lily Williams

DAVISON & ASSOCIATES

Unless we place them in the context of a World War in which the British state was deeply invested, we cannot properly comprehend the British response to the Rising, the subsequent rise in republicanism, the success of the Sinn Fein party in 1918, the First Dáil, Partition and the War of Independence.

These events, these phenomena, gave birth to modern Ireland, and they were all either part of, or inextricably linked to, the First World War.[35]

Sir Patrick Dun's and the Easter Rising

The Dublin hospitals played an important part in treating casualties of the Rising, and none more so than Sir Patrick Dun's Hospital, which was close to one of the main areas of the fighting.

On the Monday and Tuesday of Easter Week 1916, several dead and wounded were taken in. From then onwards, the situation deteriorated rapidly, as TG Moorhead recorded in his history of Sir Patrick Dun's Hospital:

> ... it was on Wednesday, April 25, that the real time of strain and anxiety began, during the Battle of Mount Street Bridge.
>
> Sisters, Nurses, and Resident Students went to the Bridge to carry in the wounded, and were for four and a half hours under heavy and continuous fire. Eighty wounded soldiers and three civilians were brought into the Home that day, and as many as possible of these were conveyed through the narrow passage crossing Love Lane to the Hospital.
>
> Up to Sunday, the 29th, the strain continued most acutely; on the afternoon of that day, one of the Irish leaders came to the Hospital and said that he wished to be taken to British Headquarters, as he wished to surrender. From that time onwards, conditions slowly and gradually returned to normal.

After the Rising had ended, the British Commander-in-Chief Sir John Maxwell sent a letter of thanks to the Hospital Board, and the Governors also thanked the hospital staff, including, 'Dr Watson, by whose exertions the Hospital was provided with food, and a very serious situation averted'.

During the period of disturbance, Dr Watson motored on several occasions, and at great personal risk, to Wicklow, and brought back large supplies of potatoes, eggs, meat, bread and other food, including gifts from many friends of the Hospital, resident in County Wicklow.[36]

Many female medical staff were Suffragists and Nationalists, belonging to Cumann na mBan – the Women's Council – which played an important role in both the 1916 Rising and the subsequent War of Independence.

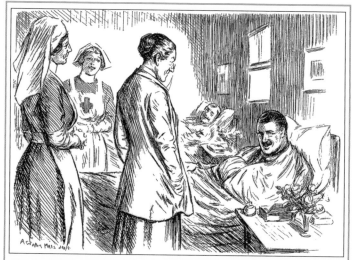

Eminent Woman Surgeon, who is also an ardent Suffragist (to wounded Guardsman).
"Do you know your face is singularly familiar to me. I've been trying to remember where we have met before."
Guardsman. "Well, Mum, bygones be bygones. I *was* a police constable."
PUNCH, AUGUST 1915

John Lumsden

John Lumsden was born in Drogheda in 1869 and was educated in Dublin and Taunton. He received his MB in 1894, and his MD degree in 1895. He was a senior visiting physician on the staff of Mercer's Hospital in Dublin and in 1902 was the Principal Medical Officer to the Commissioners of Irish Lights. However, it was his role as Medical Officer (and later Chief Medical Officer) at the Guinness Brewery that proved a turning point for him.

The Guinness family had a tradition of philanthropy and therefore Lumsden's work for Guinness focussed on the well-being of the employees, many of whom lived in appalling conditions in the slums and tenements of inner-city Dublin.

Lumsden encountered a high rate of tuberculosis amongst the employees and realised that overcrowding was probably a factor. In 1900 he was given the approval of the Guinness board to spend two months inspecting the homes of each employee, in order to ensure that they lived in proper housing, and to look for ways to prevent or to treat the disease. He also studied the diets of employees and established cookery classes for the wives of employees. Finally, he helped to set up the first Guinness sports club.

Dr Lumsden was also asked to provide first-aid classes for employees at the Guinness Brewery: these were so popular that they later evolved into the first registered division of the St John Ambulance Brigade of Ireland. This was founded by Dr Lumsden in 1903, and became the first Commissioner, a post he held until his death.

Dr John Lumsden
GUINNESS STOREHOUSE

Within days of the outbreak of War in 1914 Lumsden helped 70 of the men who had trained in the St John Ambulance Brigade to report to the Royal Naval Base at Chatham. He also enabled the Brigade to set up three auxiliary hospitals at Temple Hill, Blackrock, Monkstown and Mountjoy Square, in order to cope with the wounded who arrived on hospital ships at Dun Laoghaire and Cork. Dr Lumsden was a Major in the RAMC from 1917–18.

During the Easter Rising of 1916 he became a familiar figure as he dashed around carrying a white flag and his medical kit, to tend to the wounded on both sides. For these acts and his formation of the St John Ambulance Society, he was knighted by King George V.[41]

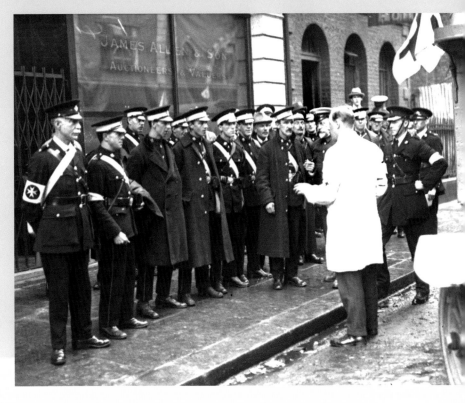

St John's Ambulance Brigade inspection, just after the 1916 Easter Rising.

CASHMAN COLLECTION
RTÉ STILLS LIBRARY

Dr Ella Webb

Dr Ella Webb, who became a member of the St John Ambulance Brigade of Ireland in 1914, was educated at Alexandra School, Dublin, Queen's College, London, and at Göttingen in Germany.

She graduated in 1904 and was married in 1907 to George R. Webb, a Fellow of Trinity College Dublin (FTCD).[38] They moved into Hatch Street in Dublin and, as well as raising her family and running a private practice, Ella also held a free-dispensary in Kevin Street.[39]

Dr Webb was appointed as an anaesthetist to the Adelaide Hospital in 1918 (the first woman member of the medical staff) and became MD in 1925.[42]

Dr Ella Webb
RCPI

Dr Webb studied mortality among children in Dublin under one year old, which was abnormally high in 1915,[39] and carried out pioneering work in preventative medicine with children. She became famous for prescribing a teaspoonful of Guinness for infants recovering from gastroenteritis.[38] She was also the founder of the Children's Sunshine Home in Stillorgan, Dublin in the early 1920s which was originally a convalescent home for children suffering from rickets.[40]

She was made a Lady of Grace of the Order of St John of Jerusalem and was awarded the MBE in 1918 for her medical work during the Easter Rising. She was also a member of the Joint Committee of the British Red Cross Society.[41]

Surrender of Countess Markievicz
outside the College of Surgeons

K Ford, based on a painting in the
Royal College of Surgeons in
Ireland

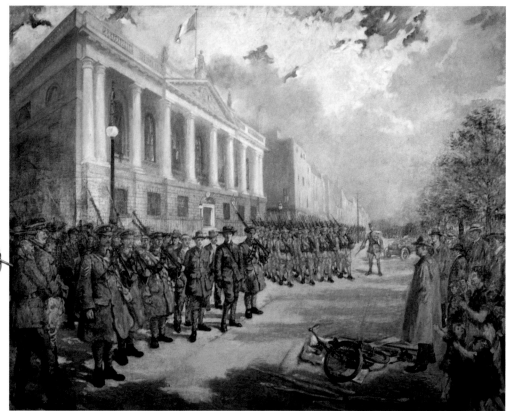

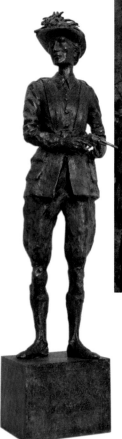

Statuette of Countess Markievicz
RCSI

Countess Markievicz was a colourful
figure in Irish society, and a prominent
figure in the 1916 Easter Rising. She was
one of the commanders of the insurgents
who occupied the Royal College of
Surgeons building on St Stephen's Green.
She was sentenced to death, but this was
commuted to penal servitude for life. In
1917 she was released during an amnesty.
She was a strong supporter of Éamon de
Valera, and was imprisoned several times
for her political activities. She died in July
1927 in Dublin, in the presence of
de Valera, and also of her Polish husband,
the Count Casimir Markievicz, who had
travelled from Warsaw to be with her.[44]

Other leading doctors were caught up in the events of Easter Week 1916, as recorded by Professor JB Lyons:

Dr Kathleen Lynn, later a co-founder of St Ultan's Hospital for Infants, organised a casualty station in the City Hall. Richard Hayes, Dispensary Medical Officer for Lusk, Co. Dublin, was at North Cross, but relinquished his command to Thomas Ashe in order to tend the wounded on both sides.

Dr AD (Louis) Courtney, a house-surgeon in St Vincent's in 1916, recalled how, soon after noon on Easter Monday, a number of casualties were brought in to the Emergency Room.

Two were already dead, killed by stray bullets; another was shot in the shoulder. Next day a number of wounded Volunteers were admitted, and St Vincent's took overflow cases from Sir Patrick Dun's Hospital. Canon Walters, the parish priest from Haddington Road, was also admitted, but died from abdominal wounds sustained while going on a sick call.[43]

The Royal Colleges and the Easter Rising

The Royal College of Surgeons was occupied during the Easter Week of 1916 by insurgents under the command of an officer named Michael Mallin and Countess Markievicz.

On Easter Monday morning the Countess and two other rebels had entered the College at gunpoint, and they were later joined by others who took shelter against the prevailing gunfire sweeping St Stephen's Green.

More than 100 people ended up in the College including some professional nurses. Living conditions were difficult, with mattresses strewn on the floor, barricades erected from books in the Library, and space beneath the Chemistry lecture theatre fitted out as a makeshift mortuary.

The occupants of the College, which was isolated from the other areas of conflict, were under constant bombardment, and they suffered greatly from hunger and fatigue.

After nearly a week of occupation, and following Pearse's unconditional surrender, the insurgents left the Royal College of Surgeons, and gave themselves up to the British Army's Captain de Courcy Wheeler.

From 30 April to 27 May, the College was occupied by 400 soldiers of the 5th Lincolnshire Regiment, with twelve officers commanded by a Colonel Walter. Each officer was subsequently presented with a silver cigarette case by the grateful College.

The following April, the Royal College of Surgeons was granted its claim of £764 for damage to the building. Compared to other buildings in Dublin, however, the damage was relatively light. There remained several bullet-marks, and some portraits, including that of Abraham Colles, were perforated.

A painting of Queen Victoria by Catterson-Smith the elder was cut out of its frame, allegedly by Countess Markievicz. In fact it had been taken by one of the insurgents, a boy who had cut it up to make leggings. By doing so he incurred the wrath of his commander, Mallin, who 'reprimanded him severely and boxed his ears'.[45]

In comparison to these stirring events at the Royal College of Surgeons building on St Stephen's Green, the home of the Royal College of Physicians in nearby Kildare Street was relatively unscathed, but the events of that day were mentioned at a later monthly business meeting of the College, on 2 June 1916.

The remains of Liberty Hall in Dublin, after the Easter Rising in 1916, during which 132 soldiers and policemen were killed, and nearly 400 were wounded. The casualties among civilians were much higher, totalling 318 dead and 2,217 wounded.

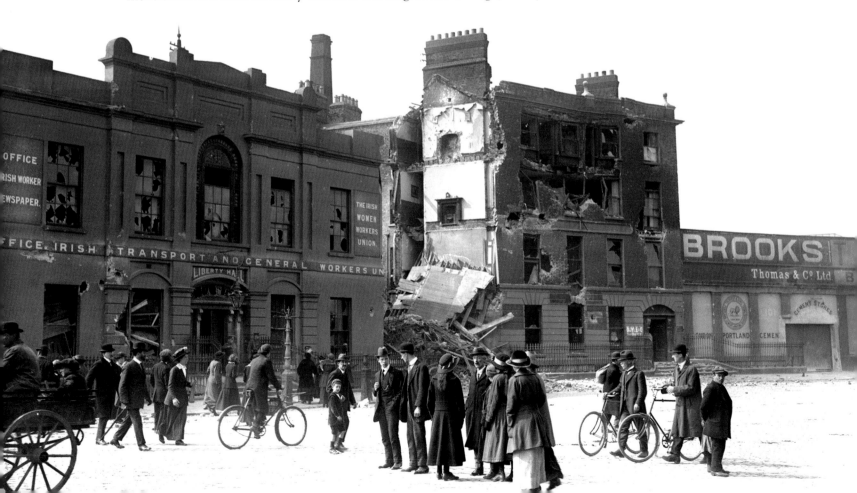

It was noted that during the recent Rising in Dublin, some damage had been done to the Royal College of Surgeons while in the hands of the insurgents, and Minutes state:

> It was proposed by Dr Kirkpatrick, seconded by Dr Montgomery, and resolved that the President and Fellows of the Royal College of Physicians of Ireland have heard with regret of the damage done to the Royal College of Surgeons during the recent Rebellion.
>
> The President and Fellows trust that if necessary the President and Fellows of the Royal College of Surgeons will avail themselves of the hospitality of this College.[46]

This short but significant reference masks much of the turmoil of the times, but the brevity and the almost matter-of-fact tone contains an assurance of solidarity among professional medical colleagues, and a certain stoicism in facing up to the stern challenges of those days of conflict.

Significant contribution

There was also a message dated 7 June 1918 from the College to the new Lord-Lieutenant Lord French. It was almost a replica of a previous letter from the College to the previous Lord-Lieutenant several years earlier.

However this time there was an important addendum. The College also emphasised to the Lord-Lieutenant that:

> … a considerable number of the Fellows and Members of the College are serving with His Majesty's forces, and of those who have obtained the License of the College since the outbreak of war, some ninety per cent have entered the Navy or Military Service.[47]

This demonstrated not only the significant contribution of the College to the war effort, but also the fact that even up to a few months before the war ended, that support remained firm.

Farewell

One of the most poignant messages of all was contained in a formal address from the College in Dublin to the College of Physicians in London, shortly after the Great War ended on 11 November 1918.

Dated December 1918, it expressed congratulations to the London College on the 400th anniversary of its foundation, but added:

> The great trial through which the world has been passing during the past four years and a quarter has, we feel, cast a cloud over this notable occasion, just as it has brought sorrow and suffering into so many of your homes and your lives.
>
> This trial has however proved the worth of your College, as it has proved also the worth of so many of her sons. Your Linacre, your Harvey and your

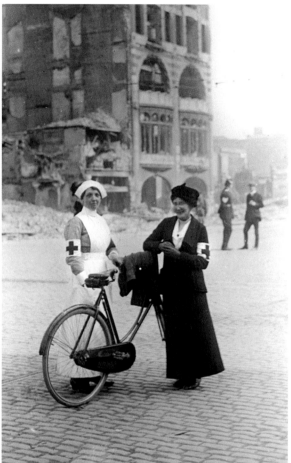

Two nurses beside the Dublin Bread Company, a restaurant on the lower east side of Sackville Street. It was occupied by the rebels from, 24–26 April, 1916.

Sydenham have in the past won renown throughout the civilised world by their achievements.

Today every citizen of our worldwide empire owes to your College a debt of gratitude for health and healing brought by you to their gallant sailors and soldiers stricken in the cause of freedom.

We in Ireland rejoice in having the names of not a few of the illustrious sons of your College, including your learned President, inscribed on our Roll of Honorary Fellows.

As the clouds of war pass away, and the sun of peace is again about to warm the hearts of men, our prayer is that, with that peace may come for your College a future as bright as its past has been glorious.

May your College continue as of old to send forth those whose learning and skill will illuminate the dark places where lurk disease or death.

We glory with you in your great history, we rejoice with you in your present joy, and we hope with you, as we trust in you, for the future.

Farewell.

The Registrar was instructed to send an 'engrossed' [sic] copy to the Royal College in London.[48]

The tone of the message, by today's standards, seems effusive and perhaps overblown. However, it was a document of its times, and reading between the lines of the formal language, there is a sense of the suffering and the hurt of the previous four years, as well as a hope – which unfortunately was in vain – for better times ahead.

The final, and perhaps unusual, 'Farewell' was not just a form of Collegiate solidarity and professional regard, but also the drawing of a line under all that had taken place. It was not only a salutation, but perhaps also an epitaph for a civilization that had disappeared for ever.

The Royal College of Physicians of London

Although the Irish physicians sent a gracious letter to their English colleagues on their historic anniversary, the London College did not manage to hold a celebration of their Quater-Centenary in 1918, due to the prolongation of the Great War.

On St Luke's Day, 18 October 1918, the London College held its annual Harveian Lecture, in honour of William Harvey, its outstanding former Fellow, and afterwards the President, Norman Moore explained to the large audience why no official celebration of the 400th anniversary was planned. His remarks were recorded in the Minutes of the College and also in a subsequent edition of the *British Medical Journal*:

> This day may be regarded as the four hundredth anniversary of the Foundation of our College, and the original Letters Patent, which founded it, are placed on the table before me. They are dated September 23, 1518, the tenth year of King Henry VIII.
>
> We should like to have celebrated the four hundredth anniversary of this event with a brilliancy suited to it, but the times in which we are living forbid

Thomas Sydenham
RCPI

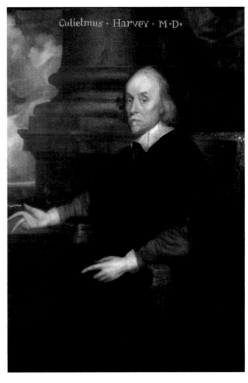

Culielmus · Harvey · M·D·

William Harvey, 1578–1657, discoverer of the circulation of blood, donated his own library and collections to the Royal College of Physicians, London, in 1656 creating the *Musaeum Harveianum* – possibly the earliest named 'museum' in England.

Portrait in the Royal College of Physicians, London
ALF McCREARY

189

it. Our sons have gone out to meet our enemies in the gate, and many of them will never return. We venerate their actions and their memory, and their absence might not alone have prevented some appropriate celebration, but when we reflected on what a war in which we were engaged, more or less every one of us, in defence of our liberties and of those of Europe, and indeed of all mankind, we feel that we could not at present take part in this happy kind of ceremonial suitable to times of peace.[49]

However the President went on to mention that there had been a celebration elsewhere on 23 September 1918, which marked the 400th anniversary of the very day of the founding of the College.

This had taken place at the Front in France, where sixteen Fellows of the Royal College in London had held a very special dinner. The dinner, and its aftermath, was described thus in a 1972 history of the College by one of its Fellows, Dr AM Cooke:

… they met in Boulogne and celebrated the occasion with a seven-course dinner and appropriate wines … Unhappily the harmony of the occasion was disturbed by enemy action, and the party was compelled to break up earlier than intended. The diners had prepared an illuminated Latin Address composed by Major Jex-Blake, which was delivered to the College after the Harveian oration on St Luke's Day by one of their number, Major Michael Foster.

The President presented Major Foster with two silver coins as mementoes of the occasion: a denarius of Caligula, who had associations with Boulogne, and a drachma from Larissa, where Hippocrates is believed to have practised.[50]

The letter from the Fellows of the London College gave a graphic account of life on the Front, and also recorded the raw feelings of senior medical officers serving with the British troops. The English translation from the original Latin was reproduced in the *British Medical Journal*. After conveying their greetings to the College, the Fellows, who included two Major-Generals and several Colonels and Lieutenant-Colonels, stated:

The fourth year of the war, which all agree was begun by German madness, is now done; we fighting men see, alas!, what kind of new regiment of fevers has descended on Earth, as if set free from Pandora's Box, and how many diseases, lice and flies, and noxious vapours have brought: and in how great a catastrophe shall the savage foe of our race, and of the whole human race, who has put ruthless war to its foulest uses, be thoroughly beaten down. But the chances have now been for some time favourable, our arms flourish, and will flourish yet more; justice at length will prevail.[51]

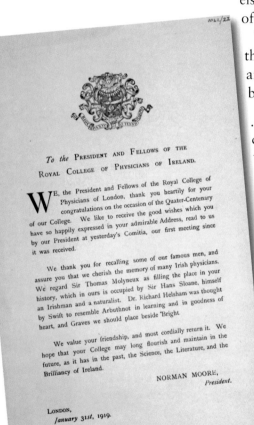

31 January 1919, the President and Fellows of the Royal College in London wrote a letter to the President and Fellows of the Royal College in Dublin, thanking them for their earlier conveyance of good wishes.
ROYAL COLLEGE OF PHYSICIANS, LONDON

The Great War Ends

The message from the Fellows proved prophetic, and within only a few weeks, the Great War had ended. Just over two months later, on 31 January 1919, the

President and Fellows of the Royal College in London wrote a handsomely-produced letter to the President and Fellows of the College in Dublin thanking them for their earlier conveyance of good wishes. A copy of the letter was also placed in the Annals of the London College:

> We thank you for recalling some of our famous men, and we assure you that we cherish the memory of many Irish physicians. We regard Sir Thomas Molyneaux as filling the place in your history, which in ours is occupied by Sir Hans Sloane, himself an Irishman and a naturalist. Dr Richard Helsham was thought by Swift to resemble Arbuthnot, 'in learning and in goodness of heart', and Graves we should place beside Bright.
>
> We value your friendship, and most cordially return it. We hope that your College may long flourish and maintain in the future, as it has done in the past, the science, the literature, and the brilliancy of Ireland.[52]

Despite the horrors of the Great War and the continuing violence in Ireland, which was so threatening to Anglo-Irish relations, the warm exchange of letters from the Presidents and Fellows of the Colleges of Physicians in Dublin and London underlined the close professional relationship of the two bodies which had existed throughout the long years of their histories in times of war and peace, and which would continue to exist as the United Kingdom and Ireland faced into a most uncertain political future in the twentieth century.

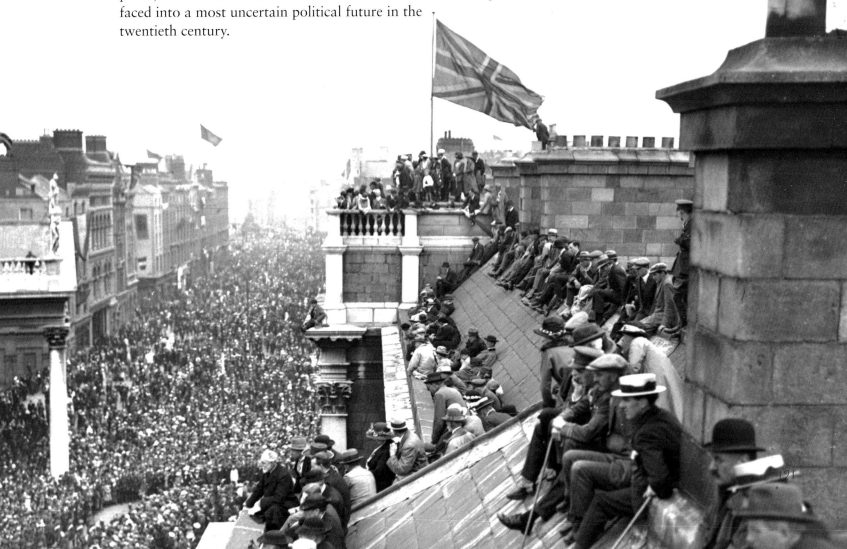

Irish Regiments march through Dublin's centre for the August 1919 Victory Day parade. Spectators sit on Trinity rooftop under the Union Jack.

Into the Unknown

As the Great War ended on 11 November 1918 the nations of Europe tried to come to terms with the enormity of what had happened. In Ireland, however, there was still much unfinished business.

The violence continued, and civil war stalked the land until the partition of the island brought an uneasy peace. The formation of an Irish Free State and the establishment of a Northern Ireland administration was an example of *realpolitik* which arguably alienated as many people as it satisfied.

However, those on both sides of the border had to adapt to the radically new situation as best they could. They were not to know about the immense degree of trouble and suffering that still lay ahead, both in Ireland and on an international scale.

As well as all of this, there were the ravages of the Spanish flu pandemic of 1918–20, which caused the deaths of millions worldwide, and of at least 26,000 people in Ireland – almost as many as those Irishmen who had died during the Great War. A reference in the College Minutes of 5 March 1920 warned that 'an epidemic of the disease may occur again during the present year, and people should be prepared beforehand in case it does so'.[1]

It was against this sombre background that the College of Physicians moved into the future, in a world which was to prove vastly different from anything that the institution had known during its long and colourful history.

Past and Present

The political view in London of post-War Ireland was summarised eloquently by Winston Churchill, when he stated:

> Great empires have been overturned. The whole map of Europe has been changed. The position of countries has been violently altered. The modes of thought of men, the whole outlook on affairs, the grouping of parties, all have encountered violent and tremendous changes in the deluge of the world.
>
> But as the deluge subsides and the waters fall short, we see the dreary steeples of Fermanagh and Tyrone emerging once again. The integrity of their quarrel is one of the few institutions that has been unaltered in the cataclysm that has swept the world.[2]

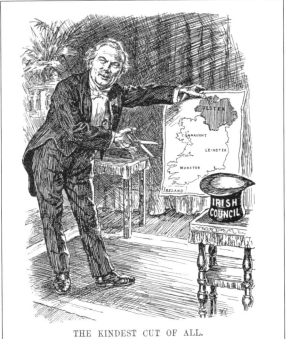

THE KINDEST CUT OF ALL.

Sadly, Churchill's disparaging political comments about these beautiful northern counties could still apply, but his words could have equally referred to the 'dreary' steeples of Dublin or Cork, or other parts of the island at that time.

Just as the outbreak of the Great War in 1914 had averted civil war in Ireland, the end of the conflict provided further space and time for the violent quest for Irish independence.

The Government of Ireland Act of 1920, which made provision for the establishment of Northern Ireland, was bitterly rejected by the powerful Sinn Féin Party and other nationalists.

Nevertheless King George V bravely travelled to a troubled Belfast in 1921, and on 22 June he opened the new Northern Ireland Parliament in the City Hall. The King had last set foot in Ireland during a visit to Dublin in 1912, and the events of the intervening period of the Great War, and the violent struggle for Irish independence, had troubled him deeply.

In his address to the Unionists and their wives in Belfast's City Hall, he made a heartfelt plea.

> I appeal to all Irishmen to pause, to forgive and forget, to stretch out the hand of forbearance and conciliation, and to join in making for the land which they love a new era of peace, contentment and goodwill.

His well-meaning words seem particularly sad today, given all that has happened since then. King George V and Queen Mary returned to London, but the Irish War of Independence continued, with brutality from all quarters.

However some months later a truce was established, and the Anglo-Irish Treaty of 6 December 1921 created an Irish Free State with dominion status. Ominously, it was

The Welsh Wizard (Lloyd George). 'I now proceed to cut this map into two parts and place them in the hat. After a suitable interval they will be found to have come together of their own accord – [aside] – at least let's hope so; I've never done this trick before.' A cartoon from *Punch*, 10 March 1920, which underlined the complexity of Partition and Lloyd George's tentative hope that it might provide a British answer to an Irish problem
LINEN HALL LIBRARY

William Conor was commissioned to paint a pictorial record of the Opening of the First Northern Ireland Parliament by George V on 22 June 1921 in the Council Chamber of Belfast City Hall. His superb painting was criticised by some unionists because it made the King look smaller than the Queen – which was in fact the case – and because of his portrayal of some of the ladies' hats.
NORTHERN IRELAND ASSEMBLY

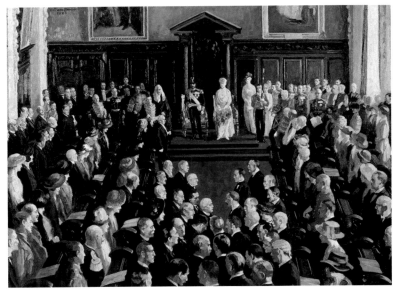

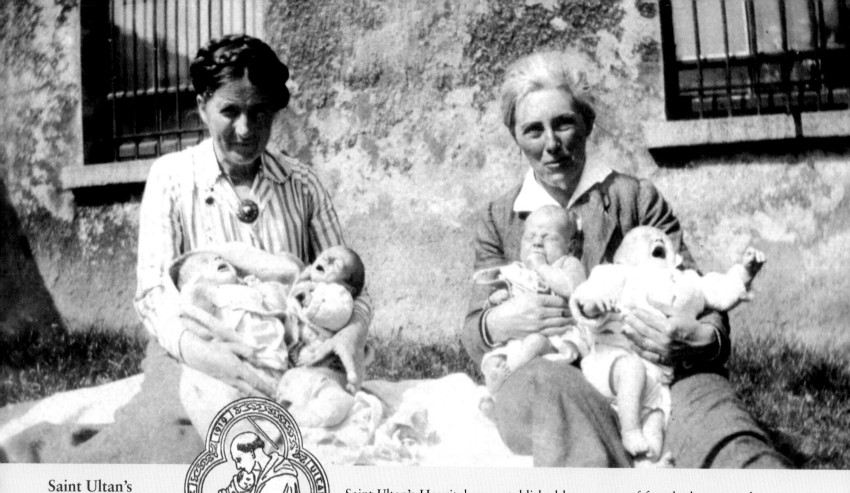

Saint Ultan's Hospital, 1919–84

The name of the hospital came from the seventh century Saint Ultan of Ardbraccan, Bishop of Meath, who had looked after local children during an outbreak of yellow plague.

Saint Ultan's Hospital was established by a group of female doctors and activists, who were deeply concerned at the high level of infant mortality in Dublin, and the rise of infant syphilis in the wake of the First World War.

A central figure was Dr Kathleen Lynn. A Committee, Cóiste Cosanta na hÉireann, was founded in May 1918 to set up the hospital, and the members worked hard to raise funds and find a suitable site. It opened, at 37 Charlemont Street on Ascension Day, Thursday, 29 May 1919.[3]

In 1926 Dr Margaret Enright was appointed Bacteriologist. She had been an assistant bacteriologist at UCC, and conducted research on the microbes found on babies' comforters. This research was important, since the biggest killer of infants in St Ultan's was gastroenteritis, an infectious disease. In 1926 it was the cause of 21 of the 48 deaths in the hospital.[4]

Saint Ultan's was also at the forefront of the fight against tuberculosis in Ireland. Dr Dorothy Stopford Price had pioneered the introduction of the BCG vaccine to Ireland, and proved its effectiveness at Saint Ultan's. The hospital, continued to grow, with the opening of the Dr Kathleen Lynn Surgical Ward in 1965, the result of the Memorial Committee's fundraising. However, by the 1980s, plans for the restructuring of hospital provision in Dublin were threatening Saint Ultan's, and it was closed in 1984. A fund was established to deal with the assets of the former hospital, with the money going to other Irish hospitals, and the hospital's administrative papers to the Royal College of Physicians of Ireland.[3]

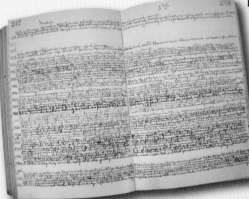

MAIN PHOTOGRAPH: Kathleen Lynn (left) with babies Mairyrad, Muhr and Ursula. Beside her, Madeleine Ffrench-Mullen holds Séan and Harry.
ABOVE, pages from Kathleen Lynn's tightly-written diary from May 1916–55.

194   RCPI

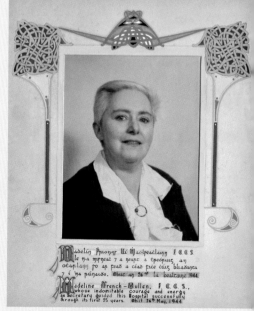

Madeleine Ffrench-Mullen
RCPI

passed in the Dail by a majority of only one vote: further trouble lay ahead.

The resultant Civil War between those for or against the Treaty was fought with the utmost savagery. It ended in April 1923, with well over 1,000 people killed. The Boundary Commission began its work in 1924, and the next year, the Partition of Ireland was ratified.

Partition, however, remains a live issue, and the future of the island depends on the degree to which democratic governments can overcome violence to find a political solution acceptable to all.

Great War Veterans

Meanwhile, the doctors who had returned to Ireland from the Great War did their best to adapt to the new order after 1918. Some like Thomas Gillman Moorhead, moved from the trauma of the Gallipoli conflict to a Professorship at Trinity and to a distinguished medical career.

Sadly, however, a number of doctors did not come back. The names of many of these lived on, but only in the memories of their friends and families, and also on the war memorials in churches and on cenotaphs throughout the land – including the memorial in Sir Patrick Dun's Hospital which has been mentioned already.

The College gave its support to such commemorations, before an unfortunate amnesia about the Great War overcame the politicians and the people of the Irish Free State. On 4 June 1919, however the President and Fellows declared themselves willing to support a proposal to establish a war memorial for the RAMC.[5]

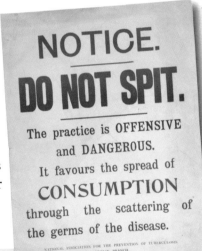

The Irish Peace Delegates.

The Irish peace delegates. the five Anglo-Irish Treaty signatories, 1921. From left to right: Eamonn Duggan, Michael Collins, Arthur Griffith (centre) Robert Barton and George Gavin Duffy. The Treaty gave Ireland dominion home rule status in the British Empire. Southern Ireland was to be called 'the Free State'. It was signed on 6 December 1921. Instead of bringing peace, however, it led to the outbreak of civil war.

RTÉ STILLS LIBRARY, CASHMAN COLLECTION

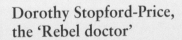

NOTICE.
DO NOT SPIT.

The practice is OFFENSIVE and DANGEROUS. It favours the spread of

CONSUMPTION

through the scattering of the germs of the disease.

NATIONAL ASSOCIATION FOR THE PREVENTION OF TUBERCULOSIS DUBLIN BRANCH.

Dorothy Stopford-Price, the 'Rebel doctor'

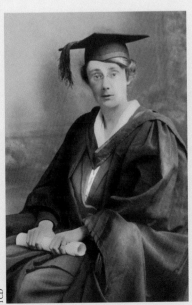

After graduation at Trinity, Stopford-Price worked as a dispensary doctor in West Cork. There she combined visits to the 'ladies of the county' with first-aid classes to the IRA, and treatment for those wounded during the War of Independence, and later, for the anti-Treaty side during the Civil War. She was also a medical officer for the local RIC Barracks.[6]

In 1921 Dorothy Stopford-Price started on the work which would lead to the eradication of TB in Ireland. At a time when the medical profession in Ireland looked to the UK for guidance, Price taught herself German so she could access the latest scientific

Photograph of Dorothy Stopford, graduating as a Bachelor of Medicine, Trinity College Dublin. 1921.

knowledge coming out of Germany, where many of the leaders in the field were researching. Stopford-Price's work also placed her in opposition to one of the strongest powers in Ireland at that time – the Catholic Church, and especially the Catholic Archbishop of Dublin, John Charles McQuaid.

She had come to know Kathleen Lynn during her time as a medical student in Dublin, and went to work in 1923 as a house surgeon at Saint Ultan's hospital. In 1949 Saint Ultan's opened a dedicated BCG Centre, and when in the same year, the National BCG Committee was established by Noel Browne, Minister for Health, it was based at Saint Ultan's, with Stopford-Price as its Chair.[7]

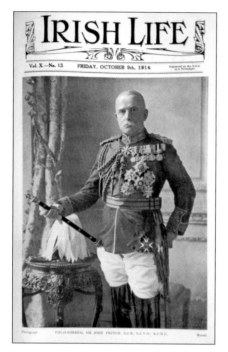

IRISH LIFE

Vol. X.—No. 13. FRIDAY, OCTOBER 9th, 1914.

FIELD-MARSHAL SIR JOHN FRENCH, G.C.B., G.C.V.O., K.C.M.G.

Lord French

The Lord-Lieutenant was the son of a
retired naval officer whose ancestors
originally came from Ireland.
A physically attractive man whom
women found irresistible, he was not
however good with money. He spent
lavishly on horses, women and risky
investments, running up debts, and then
turning to others, especially his sister
Charlotte Despard, suffragist and
pacifist, for relief.

Danger and Uncertainty

As an institution the College also did its best to move forward, but this was a
time of continued danger and uncertainty. Few references were made to the
conflict as such, but reading between the lines of the Minutes, there is more
than a whiff of gunpowder and a strong indication of the political trauma of
those times.

On 2 January 1920 the College sent a message to the Lord-Lieutenant Lord
French recording, 'heartfelt congratulations on your marvellous escape from
the dastardly attack on your life, made this afternoon'. Lord French duly
replied, expressing his thanks for the College's concern.[8] The continued dangers
of living and working in such a conflict were underlined by a Minute of
4 March 1921 concerning an Order issued to the Secretaries of Dublin
Hospitals, which resolved that:

> The Irish Medical Association be informed that the College is of the opinion
> that the Order of the Competent Medical Authority with regard to wounded
> persons in Hospitals is in contravention of the recognised obligation of
> medical men to observe the confidence of the patients.[9]

The College determined, but only by 10 voted to 6, that representations should
be made to the military Commander, General N Macready to inform him that
the latest Order was 'contrary to the general ethical practice of the profession'.

Five days later, however, the College received a polite but firm reply written
by Macready, who stated:

> While I quite realise that such Orders may not be in direct conformity with
> the ethical practice of the Medical Profession, the conditions in this country
> are such that it is impossible to conform to normal rules and practices.

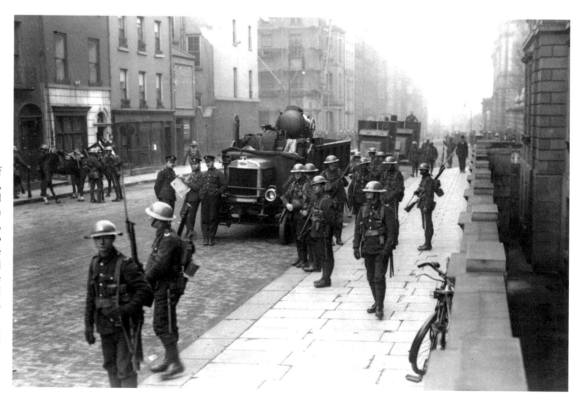

During the War of
Independence,
armoured cars and
British soldiers search
Kildare Street, Dublin,
on 1 January, 1921. To
the right is the
National Museum and
further along, the
pillars of the Royal
College of Physicians
can be seen.

196

Kevin Gerard Barry
1902–20

Kevin Barry, a medical student at University College Dublin, was an activist with the Irish Volunteers and was sentenced to death by court-martial for the murder of three soldiers in 1920. Despite pleas for clemency, he was hanged in Mountjoy Prison, Dublin on 1 November. It is said that 'his conduct in custody was marked by cheerfulness and fortitude'.[14]

Barry became a Republican martyr, who is still remembered in many ballads and verses, and he is one of the best-known students in the history of Irish medicine.

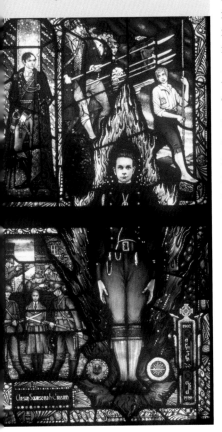

The Kevin Barry Memorial stained glass window by Richard King, in the University College Dublin (UCD) Lecture Theatre, Earlsford Terrace, Dublin.
RTÉ STILLS LIBRARY

You may be interested to learn that from documents which have fallen into my possession, belonging to the organisation which is currently disturbing this country, there is clear evidence that the Orders in regard to notifying certain particulars about the patients have to a considerable degree hampered the extremists in their efforts to hide persons who have been wounded while attempting to carry out murder and outrage.

This being the case, I fear that it is impossible for me to modify the Orders already given, and I can only hope that the medical profession, along with other well-disposed persons of this country, will bring pressure to bear on those who are responsible for the present disturbed state of Ireland, and on whose shoulders must fall the responsibility for Orders and regulations which are necessary to curb their activities.[10]

More Disturbances

The continued disturbances added to the burdens of members of the medical profession. On 23 March, the President and Fellows of the College wrote to the Post-Master General to oppose increased charges of services and told him that, 'medical practice in or near Dublin is greatly hampered, and life endangered, by the insufficiency of the Telephone service and the delays in the Postal service'.[11]

In the midst of the prevailing uncertainty, the College was at pains to declare its loyalty to the ruling Establishment. In June 1921, it presented an Address of Welcome to the new Lord-Lieutenant Lord Fitzalan, in which it reminded him that since 1654, 'the President and fellows have done what they could to watch over the health of the people of Ireland, and to further the education of medical men'.[12]

The noble Lord replied in a like manner, and he expressed his assurance that:

A great tradition will be by you fitly maintained and strengthened. You are trustees for the public health of Ireland, and in the pursuit of the profession, remote from differences of class or politics or creed, you are enabled to make an unchallengable contribution towards the welfare and happiness of your country.[13]

The violence continued, and more doctors were directly affected. A Minute of 7 July 1922 recorded that the President and Fellows of the College:

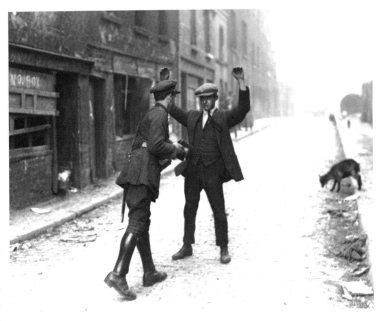

An Irish Free State soldier is pictured here holding a gun as he searches a suspected Republican in Mary's Lane during the Civil War. Republicans were against the Anglo-Irish Treaty and were called 'Irregulars' by the Provisional Government.
RTÉ STILLS LIBRARY, CASHMAN COLLECTION

Dr Colman Saunders, a medical student at UCD, recalled the perils of moving around Dublin's streets: 'Science subjects were studied in Earlsfort Terrace, Zoology at 86 St Stephen's Green, and medical subjects in Cecilia Street'.

The Black and Tans were most hated but Saunders recalled that they were more scared of disease than any bullet: '... we soon learned if we were picked up after curfew and thrown into a lorry, to say we were students from Cork Street Fever Hospital, on which we were immediately kicked out onto the street'.

197

... sympathised with their friend and colleague Dr Alexander Nixon Montgomery on the occasion of the disaster which has deprived him of his home in Upper Sackville Street, Dublin, it having been destroyed by fire in the unfortunate disorder of the past ten days.[15]

At a College business meeting of 9 March,1923 those present considered a Motion:

... that this College deprecates individual violence as a mode of political conversion; that it offers its sympathy to those members of the medical profession who have been subjected to such violence, and protests strongly against vocational reprisals, such as have recently been carried out against a group of medical men in Dublin.

It was resolved that 'copies of this resolution be sent to members of the Ministry, to the Dublin daily newspapers, and that the *BMJ*, *The Lancet* and the medical press be circulated'. However the motion was lost 9–4 on a show of hands, and nothing was sent to the media or the medical press.[16]

New Order

Following the upheaval since 1916, it became clear that the old order was changing, and that the Irish Free State was to be the new centre of power.

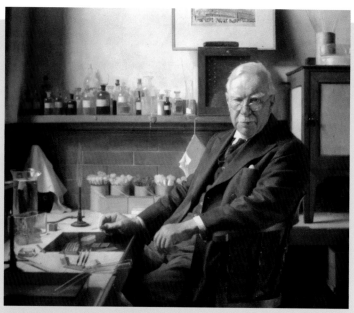

Sir Almwroth Wright

The College placed much importance on its professional links with the outside world, and several well-known medical figures became Honorary Fellows. They included Sir Almroth Wright, who was elected unanimously on New Year's Day in 1932.

Wright was an outstanding immunologist and bacteriologist, and also a dedicated medical researcher who campaigned strongly for proper support for important medical research programmes.

Sir Almroth Wright by Sir Gerald Kelly, PRA
Exhibited at the Royal Academy in 1934 and now in the
Wright-Fleming Institute.

Born in Yorkshire in 1861, he was the second son of an Irish Anglican cleric, who spent some time as the rector of St Mary's in Belfast. Almroth Wright was educated at the Royal Belfast Academical Institution and at Trinity College Dublin, where he studied Arts and Medicine.

He could have followed a career in literature but he chose medicine. He carried out important research in bacteriology and he was active in studying the wound infections among troops in the Great War. When he left the Army Medical Service, Almroth Wright developed a world-class department at St Mary's Hospital in Paddington. He became a friend of George Bernard Shaw who, with some poetic licence, depicted him as Sir Colenso Ridgeon in his play *The Doctor's Dilemma*.

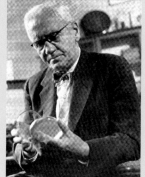

Sir Alexander Fleming

Sir Almroth Wright retired in 1946 at the age of 85. He was succeeded at the London Institute of Pathology, which he had done so much to establish, by his colleague Sir Alexander Fleming, the discoverer of penicillin.[17]

The College of Physicians, just like John Stearne in the mid-seventeenth century, had to be aware where that power was focused, and on 9 March 1923, the President and Fellows wrote to Tim Healy to congratulate him on his appointment as Governor-General of the new Irish Free State:

> During the 269 years of its existence, our College has seen many changes in the country, but throughout this long period its policy has been ever to promote the study of medicine, and to foster all true efforts for the improvement of the health of the people. Our trust is that in the future we shall be permitted to continue in the pursuit of these aims, and we place freely at the disposal of the Government our services of advice in the remoulding of both medical education and public health administration, which must of necessity follow on the constitution of the new State.
>
> To His Gracious Majesty whom you represent, to the Government of which you are the head and to yourself, we offer our loyal and dutiful service.[18]

The new Governor-General Tim Healy replied in kind and stated:

> You can, I am sure, always rely on the co-operation of the Irish Free State Government in your efforts for medical education and sanitary reform.
>
> On behalf His Majesty and the Government, I express my gratitude for your assurance of the same loyal and dutiful service which has distinguished your College in the past.[19]

It took several years to complete the necessary legislative details to bind the College into the new State. In 1926 the Royal College of Physicians of Ireland (Adaptation of Charter) Order was passed to make the RCPI Charter valid under the laws of the Free State, with the 'Royal' title intact, despite the revolutionary and republican mindset of the Ireland of those days.

Indeed, that awareness of the Royal title has remained an important dimension of the RCPI's identity, and over a decade after its title was confirmed as part of the Free State's legislation, the College sent a message of congratulations to King George VI on his accession to the British Throne, expressing 'the sincere hope' that he and the Queen, 'will have a long, a prosperous and a happy reign'.[20]

In family terms it proved to be happy for the Royal Family but as the terrible events of the reign unfolded, the irony of that sincere greeting from the College to the Windsors in 1937 became all the more apparent, and poignant.

Dr Charles Dickson MC
1886–1978

Charles Dickson, a former Fellow and Registrar of the College, won an MC for gallantry in the First World War, and was a well-known doctor, administrator, historian and author.

He was born in Dromore, Co Down, on 20 January 1886, and educated at the Royal Belfast Academical Institution and Queen's University, where he developed an interest in the Gaelic language. He graduated in 1908 with first-class honours in medicine.

Three years later he was awarded an MD, and later worked as a medical officer in the civil service, with the National Health Insurance commissioners.

He was an RAMC officer from 1915–19, and served at the Battle of the Somme. In August 1917 he won the Military Cross for gallantry in restoring a field-dressing station under heavy enemy bombardment by high explosives and gas shells. Tragically, in the same month, his brother was killed in action.

Following the Partition of Ireland, Dickson – who by that stage was a fluent Irish speaker – lived in Dublin. He was Chief Medical Officer in the Irish civil service from 1923 until his retirement in 1954, at the age of 68.

He was Secretary of the Royal Academy of Medicine from 1954, and editor from 1962–70 of the *Irish Journal of Medical Science*, to which he contributed many informed and neatly crafted articles. In 1966, fifty years after the Somme, he revisted the battlefield with an RTÉ crew to reflect on the courage of doctors and others in clearing up the carnage.

In his later years he lived in the Killiney area, and he died on New Year's Day 1978.[21]

Portrait by Thomas Ryan
RCPI

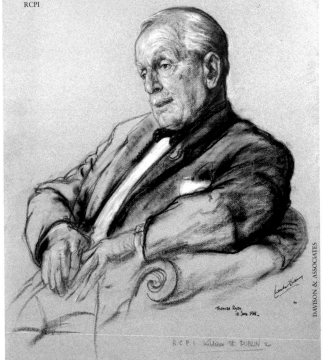

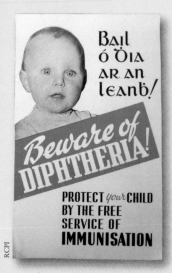

The campaign against diphtheria in Cork Street Fever Hospital 1934–1952

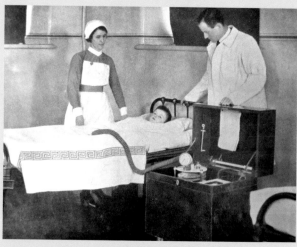

Post Diphtheric Paralysis being treated with the Bragg-Paul Pulsator, Cork Street Fever Hospital, 1935

In 1934, Dr CJ McSweeney became Medical Superintendent of Cork Street Fever Hospital, Dublin, a position he retained until his death in 1953. A progressive physician, who was a strong proponent of preventative measures and the use of therapeutic aids, McSweeney devoted much time in his first decade in Cork Street to the fight against diphtheria of the 'gravis' type, which had claimed the lives of thousands of children, especially those under 10 years of age.

Diphtheria accounted for a large proportion of admissions to the hospital. Dr McSweeney noted in 1934 that the 'gravis' type of diphtheria prevailing in Dublin was much more virulent that that occurring in many other areas in Ireland and the UK, and case mortality was therefore higher.

Although the number of patient admissions remained high during these years, the introduction of a mass immunisation scheme by Dublin Corporation in 1940 resulted in a progressive decline in mortality rates.

Dr McSweeney regularly wrote about the need for a mass diphtheria immunisation programme, and claimed that these deaths were 'all preventable and in an enlightened community would not occur'. The remedy was the 'immunisation of all children as soon as they attain their first birthday, followed by re-inoculation, if found necessary, before they begin school life'.[22]

McSweeney's wish became a reality in 1940, when the Government introduced a diphtheria immunisation scheme in Dublin in connection with wartime evacuation for children organised by the Department of Defence. However, the scheme was not compulsory for all children.

In 1947 admissions of patients suffering from diphtheria in Cork Street declined greatly, down to 179 from 431 the year before. In the 1953 Medical Report there is no mention of diphtheria at all.

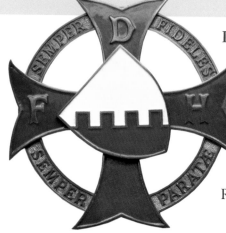

In the Doldrums

Unfortunately, the College did little to enhance its national reputation in the following decades, compared to the achievements of previous years.

The Presidents and Fellows continued their regular meetings, and dealt with routine business, but their failure to grasp the opportunities, albeit challenging, of the new era characterised one of the less impressive periods of the College story.

This was succinctly described by the late Dr John Feely, a former College Registrar:

ABOVE: Dublin Fever Hospital Crest

RIGHT: Dublin Fever Hospital china

> With undergraduate medical education firmly established and regulated, and much of the teaching passing to the Royal College of Surgeons in Ireland, the College (of Physicians) entered a tranquil period.
>
> Living in its Victorian past as 'a Dublin-based medical club' of some 100 Fellows, the College missed the opportunity of playing an important role in the emerging independent Ireland of the first half of the twentieth century.[23]

The reasons for this period of relative hibernation were complex, and remain a matter of conjecture. However this has to be seen against a

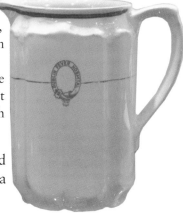

background of post-partition Ireland where a deep fissure now existed in the political and social life of the two jurisdictions on the island.

Both the Free State and Northern Ireland had to find their way in completely new territory, and there were few, if any, experiences from the past to help guide them on their arduous journey.

The post-partition period in the Free State was a time of economic challenge, and continued political machinations. The dominant figures were Eamon de Valera, and the Roman Catholic Archbishop of Dublin Dr John Charles McQuaid, who between them built a theocratic state in which the Protestant population, and the hitherto largely Church of Ireland College of Physicians, had to find a different role.

The Taoiseach and later President, Eamon de Valera was a particularly powerful figure. One writer noted that:

> To part of his own people he was a hero of 1916, the last of the commandants to surrender, the one leader to survive the national struggle, who never flinched in his purpose, the one man of his time with a pre-eminent claim to govern the Irish people.
>
> To another part, he was a danger to the state, a politician of tricks and turns, who was capable of disastrously wrong decisions, to whose actions most of the misfortunes of the country since 1921 were attributed, and, that most dangerous of power-seekers, a man with an invincible sense of his own righteousness.
>
> …Yet this much even his detractors must concede: he possessed an unshakeable courage and resolution, his patriotism was unalloyed and passionate, and in the flat years of post-revolutionary politics, he was the only figure in Irish public life with magic to his name.[24]

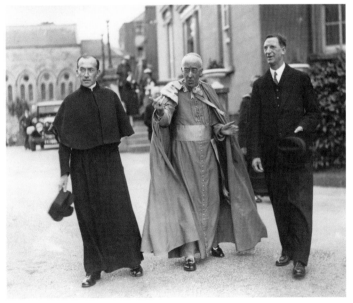

Eamon de Valera, with Archbishop John Charles McQuaid and the Papal Nuncio Paschal Robinson, during the historic Eucharistic Congress, which was held in Dublin in 1932.
UCD ARCHIVE/IRISH TIMES

However that alleged 'magic' was also diminished in the eyes of many, when de Valera, in retaliation for the British imposition of heavy import duties on Free State agricultural products, put in place high taxes on British goods. During the resultant economic war, which ended in 1938, the Irish economy, particularly its agricultural sector, suffered severely.

He also established a new Constitution in 1937, in which the Free State, became known as Éire, and which gave a special position to the Catholic Church.

Archbishop McQuaid needed no prompting to further his vision of a Catholic state, and one of his comments, in 1944, gave an indication of the mood of the times:

> No Catholic may enter the Protestant University of Trinity College without the previous permission of the ordinary of the Diocese. Any Catholic who disobeys this law is guilty of moral sin, and while he persists in disobedience, is unworthy to receive the sacraments.[25]

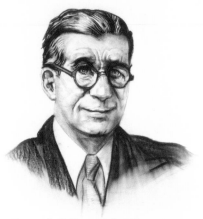

Joseph Warwick Bigger
1891–1951
Portrait by Sean Keating

Joseph Warwick Bigger, who was elected a Fellow of the College of Physicians in 1922, developed a special interest in pathology and bacteriology.

He published a series of papers on antibacterial substances. His discovery of the 'phenomenon of persistence', a name given to the fact that a small proportion of a population of bacterial cells always survives when treated with a lethal concentration of an antibiotic, arguably his most important contribution to science. He built a strong international reputation for the study of bacteriology in TCD by producing the first textbook on the subject suitable for medical students. His Handbook of Bacteriology was first published in 1925. He diagnosed his own leukemia, while studying a film of his blood in a laboratory. He died on August 17, 1951.

RCPI
DAVISON & ASSOCIATES

A bronze statue and plaque commemorating General Richard Mulcahy at Collins Barracks, Dublin. His motto was 'Let us be brave then, and let us work'.

It would be unwise to attribute the insularity, economic depression and Catholic narrowness of post-partition Ireland solely to de Valera and McQuaid; as modern historians are noting, the causes of the Irish malaise were much more complicated.

However the broad sweep of political, ecclesiastical and social life in Ireland from Partition until after the Second World War may partly explain why the College, with its historically 'Anglican' background, found it so difficult to avoid adopting a bunker mentality.

Jonathan Bailey, a former Secretary of the College, and an Anglican, said:

> We were not without Catholic friends in the Fifties and Sixties, but I believe that the Protestant community was defensive and insular. However I think that the Government handled it rather well, because it was not prepared to lose that section of Irish society where the preponderance of the business life had been in Protestant hands. It took many more years to open out Irish business to produce a more reflective mix of the two main traditions of the country.
>
> In such an atmosphere within Ireland in the years following Partition, the College of Physicians in a way 'hunkered down'. I don't think that its people they quite knew where they belonged.[26]

Professor Risteard Mulcahy, the distinguished cardiologist and a Fellow of the College of Physicians, is the son of General Richard Mulcahy, a leading protagonist in the Irish Civil War. He believes that the 'quiet period' of the College was due to the general political background of the times:

> When the Treaty was signed, the Irish undertook that there would never be any pressure on the Protestants, and that they would be fairly treated. In my opinion this is what happened, and they were more than fairly treated.
>
> However I think that some of the leading Protestants had gone underground after 1916, and even before that. The gaining of Catholic emancipation meant inevitably that eventually the Catholics would take over. It took some time for them to become some of the leading figures of society, and it also took time for the merging of the relatively small Protestant minority. There was a great deal of political change, and there may have been a loss of confidence among the Protestant professionals.[27]

General Richard Mulcahy

Mulcahy was a leading military figure in the Irish struggle for independence. Professor Risteard Mulcahy, his son, now in his early nineties, retains warm and vivid memories of his father.

> He was totally devoted to the country, and he had no personal ambitions of any sort. He was a man of great ability and education, and he was a wonderful Irish speaker.
>
> Someone asked me recently who was my great hero, and I said that of course my father was my hero. He was an amazing man. He

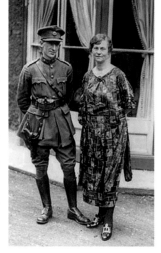

General Richard Mulcahy and his wife Josephine (or Min). Following the death of Michael Collins on 22 August 1922, Mulcahy was catapulted into the role of National Army Commander-in-Chief.

was head of the Army for six years during the war of Independence and the Civil War, and when he was pushed out in 1924, he remained in politics for the rest of his life and became a Minister on several occasions – in Education, Local Government and Public Health.

There were only two things I could do. One was to join the Army or go to university, so I was pushed into medicine. My father was curious in his way that, although he had been head of the Army during the whole revolutionary period, I don't think he wanted his children to go into the Army. I think he was proud of my ability in medicine.[27]

Routine Business

With hindsight it is easy to be critical of the College in post-partition Ireland because of its low public profile. However it could also be argued that the Presidents and Fellows in the post-partition years deserved credit, at the very least, for keeping the institution going, at a time when they had enough on their hands otherwise maintaining a health service in a new and relatively impoverished State.

Some of the business recorded in the College Minutes was decidedly routine, with lists of successful examination candidates, and all too frequent accounts of the passing of aged colleagues who had made distinguished contributions to medicine and to the RCPI itself.

These included Sir Andrew Horne, who died on 5 September 1924. Three weeks later the President and Fellows at a College meeting paid tribute to him as one of its 'most esteemed ex-Presidents', whom they described as 'a gentleman of innate courtesy and urbanity of manner, and who filled the Presidential Chair some years ago with dignity and impartiality'.[28]

There were also some strictly 'housekeeping' matters, such as rewiring the College in 1932 at an estimated £210, and the purchase of a Hoover cleaner at £31 8s 0d, a costly acquisition in the currency of that time.

The College also received some special gifts. These included a gold watch which had belonged to Sir Henry Marsh, presented in 1932,[29] and also, a plaster model of the marble bust of the distinguished Royal College of London physician, Thomas Sydenham. This was presented to the Irish College in 1936 by Dr Mary Hearn, the first female Fellow of the College.

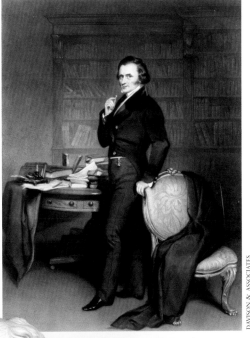

Sir Henry Marsh and his pocket watch presented to the College in 1932.

RCPI

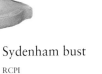

Sydenham bust

RCPI

Second World War

The attitude to the Second World War was very different in Ireland to that at the time of the Great War. While Northern Ireland was directly involved through its links with the rest of the United Kingdom, the Free State – or more properly, Éire – remained aloof because of Éamon de Valera's policy of neutrality.

However it was a particular kind of neutrality. German aircrew who crash-landed in Éire were interned, but their British counterparts were either allowed to fly away in their repaired planes, or quietly sent across the border to Northern Ireland. Some 70,000 Irish people joined the British forces, and they won nearly 800 decorations, including seven VCs. Around 200,000 Irish citizens worked in British factories throughout the war, and equally significantly, food exports from Éire to the UK were vitally important.[30]

This period was referred to in Éire, with massive understatement, as 'the Emergency' but it was partly an Irish solution to an English and European problem.

It is certain that the Germans knew what was going on. The bombing of Dublin by the Luftwaffe may have been an 'accident', or something more sinister. Whatever the motive, 34 people died, 90 were injured and some 300 houses were destroyed, when Dublin's North Strand was bombed on 31 May 1941.[31]

Many Irish doctors and other medical staff joined the British Forces during the Second World War, including those from the North where conscription was not enforced.

The College of Physicians during the Second World War

Despite such trauma, there was scarcely any mention of the Second World War in the College Minutes, and it was as if this titanic struggle was taking place on a different planet. It is perhaps not difficult to understand, however, why the College made so little reference to the War which, strictly speaking, was not 'their' war. For example, on 28 September 1939, just after the War broke out, the Minutes record merely that the St Luke's Day Dinner was postponed, that the College was purchasing a ventilator fan for the Middle Hall, that the College would accept an estimate for fixing blinds, and that a new carpet should be bought for the Reading Room.

However some of the comments made during the course of the conflict give an indication that something of significance was taking place outside the country. On 2 February, 1940 there was a College business meeting which considered a request for help from the staff of the Jagiellonian University in Krakow, and it was decided that if the letter seeking assistance was genuine, it would be forwarded to the Minister for Foreign Affairs.[32]

On 7 June 1940 the College considered a letter from Lady Talbot de Malahide and the Secretary of the Irish Red Cross concerning relief for Polish professors interned in Germany.[33]

Numbers 29 to 32 North Strand Road, Dublin, as they appeared on 4 June 1941 following the air raid of 31 May. This photograph was one of a series commissioned by Dublin Corporation for use as evidence in the assessment of insurance claims.

DUBLIN CITY LIBRARY AND ARCHIVE

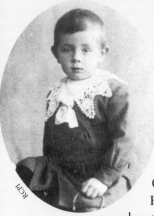

RCPI

Major-General Francis Joseph O'Meara
1900–67

Many Irish doctors served with the British Forces during the Second World War, including Major-General Francis Joseph O'Meara. He served in the Royal Army Medical Corps, and his extensive personal papers and photographs were given to the College by his family.

He was born in 1900 in Co. Cork and was educated at Clongowes Wood College and Trinity College Dublin. He joined the Officer's Training Corps in 1918, but left to study Medicine.

He received his MB from Trinity in 1923 and served initially with the RAMC in Egypt and India. At the start of the Second World War he set up an Ambulance Corps at a casualty station in France.

In June 1940 he was captured, and spent the next four years in different prison camps. His papers include a report on two German doctors in the camps, and about their treatment of British captives. He mentions a man who was an informer for the Germans, and who also tried to unsettle the British detainees.

O'Meara's writings also give a flavour of the underlying tensions the male POW camps including:

> … [an] association and understanding between men, quite independently of nationality, with prison records for civil crime. … a further complication was, of course, the behaviour of homosexuals.[34]

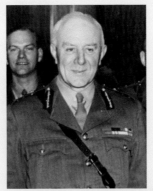

RCPI

He gives graphic details of the treatment of different nationalities:

> On capture the Eastern European was starved for 14 days. He was then too weak to give trouble or escape. By that time he had arrived at a POW Cage, and was given a diet of 600 calories a day, composed of bread, cabbage and swede turnips.
>
> If he was alive at the end of 6 months, he was taken … for slave labour. If he had died, his body had been thrown one morning into a trench … and covered with earth in unconsecrated ground, probably in a wood. His death was probably due to TB of the lungs or intestines, diarrhoea or typhus.[35]

The extremely cold winters resulted in many deaths:

> In October a senior German medical orderly used to ask a senior POW doctor how many graves he would require before the end of winter. The information obtained was passed quietly to the grave-digger at one of the three cemeteries in the nearby town or village – Lutheran, Roman Catholic or Jewish.[36]

O'Meara also described the attitude of the German High Command. In 1940, French prisoners were to be conciliated and treated well. The British were to be ill-treated, and given limited food and water. There was a review every few months.

As the war progressed, the attitude of the Germans changed:

> After the November 1942 occupation of North Africa, instructions were issued to ill-treat the French, and to improve the treatment of the British. By August 1943, the instructions were to conciliate and improve the conditions of the British in every way that local conditions permitted.
>
> The Russians suffered great hardship under these calculated, callous instructions.[37]

O'Meara's repatriation took place in May 1944, by train via Karlsruhe, Metz and Marseilles, and then in a 30-hour journey in a hospital ship to Barcelona, where the Spanish Red Cross attended to him.

He then sailed in a Swedish vessel by way of Algiers and the west coast of Ireland, and into Belfast Lough, where he passed through 'an invasion fleet and its assembled escort'. After a civic reception in Belfast, he set off for Liverpool, and passed through another 'invasion fleet' on the Mersey. He was then given a month's leave, and continued with his Army career.[38]

After the War, O'Meara remained a career soldier, and went back to Germany as a consultant physician to the British Army of the Rhine, from 1945–50. He eventually became the Director of Services, Western Command. He died in Hertfordshire in 1967.[39]

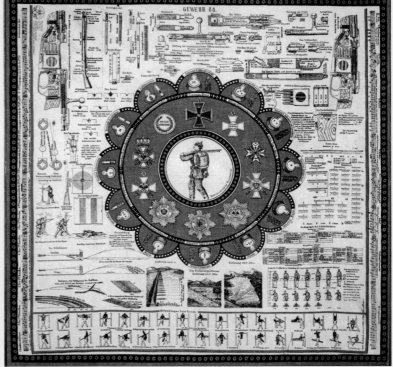

RCPI

In recognition of his outstanding service with the Royal Army Medical Corps during the Second World War and his work with prisoners of war, O'Meara was presented with a handsome memorial. It is inscribed 'For Valour, Nobility and Humanity', and has the imprimatur of the RAMC and Trinity College Dublin.

Dr Bethel AH Solomons
1885–1965

Dr Bethel Solomons was the first Jewish President of the College of Physicians, from 1946–49, and the first Jewish Master of the Rotunda. He was a distinguished consultant in obstetrics and gynaecology, and gained a reputation as a progressive doctor who was deeply concerned for the welfare of his patients.

Solomons was also an outstanding sportsman, and a larger than life character. He represented Ireland at rugby, and won ten international caps from 1908–10. Later he became an Ireland team selector and a vice-president of the Irish Rugby Football Union. He was also well-known as a colourful figure in Dublin literary and social circles, and had an interesting personal life. He produced a lively autobiography, *One Doctor in His Time*, published in 1956.

In 1914 he was appointed as a gynaecologist to Mercer's Hospital, and became a Fellow of the College of Physicians in the same year.

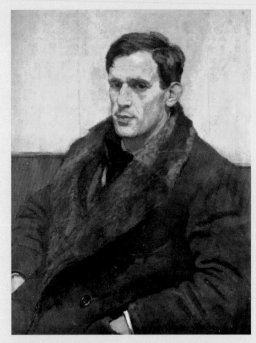

Portrait of Bethel Solomons by his sister Estella

As Master of the Rotunda Solomons gained a high reputation as an innovative doctor, and, like one of his medical predecessors, Sir Andrew Horne, he achieved literary fame through a mention in James Joyce's *Finnegan's Wake:* 'in my bethel of Solyman's, I accouched my rotundaties'.

He was also hard-headed about finance, and as Master of the Rotunda he convinced the Board, including several Protestant clerics, to accept funding from the Irish Hospitals' Sweepstake.

Solomons was a member of the Jewish Representative Council, and a founder and the first-President of the Liberal Synagogue in Dublin. With a medical colleague, he established a dispensary for Jewish women. The Bethel Solomons medal is awarded each year to an outstanding midwifery student at the Rotunda.[40]

Solomons presented a College flag to the College on 1 July 1927, and over 21 years later – on St Luke's Day 1948 – he marked his retirement as President with the gift of a ciborium in silver gilt, which features a statuette of St Luke on the pedestal. The silversmiths who crafted the Solomons' ciborium were Messrs Alwright and Marshall of Dublin. Alwright said later that he had had difficulty in sourcing a suitable visual depiction of St Luke, but had eventually found one in the *Book of Kells*, in the Trinity College Library.[41]

The stem of the ciborium shows the figure of St Luke, with his traditional symbol of an ox at his feet. The dish is decorated with a band of Celtic design copied from the *Book of Kells*, and the lid topped with a finial in the shape of a hand. The earliest record of St Luke's being celebrated by the College dates back to 1676.

RCPI

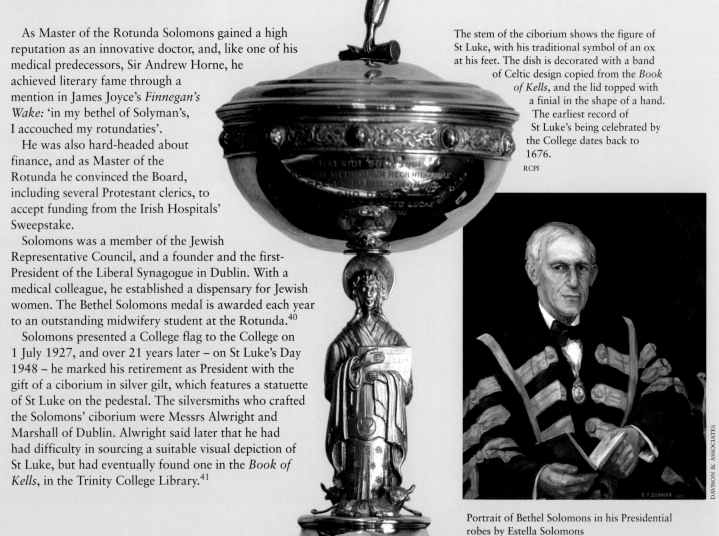

Portrait of Bethel Solomons in his Presidential robes by Estella Solomons

RCPI

DAVISON & ASSOCIATES

206

On 2 May 1941 a business meeting tabled a letter from a Dr MacSorley, thanking the College for its sympathy on his recent experience during 'an air raid on his house in Belfast'. Though no details were included, this almost certainly referred to the night-time attacks on Belfast by the Luftwaffe on the nights of April 7–8 and 15–16 April, with widespread deaths, injuries and destruction of property.

At one stage during these attacks the situation was so bad that Éamon de Valera, in response to a 4.35 am telegraph call from Belfast, authorised the urgent dispatch of fire-engines from Dublin, Dun Laoghaire, Drogheda and Dundalk to help out in the North – another illustration of the unique nature of Éire's 'neutrality', as well as the sense of kinship on the island.[42]

Two days after those who attended the College business meeting on 2 May in Dublin had noted Dr MacSorley's letter about the damage to his house in the Blitz, there was another major attack on Belfast. The Luftwaffe dropped nearly 90,000 incendiaries and some 291 tonnes of high explosives on the city in just over three hours, mostly on the harbour complex, though 191 civilians in nearby areas were killed. It was estimated that nearly 1,000 people died during the combined air raids in Northern Ireland.[43]

Near the end of the War, the College Minutes acknowledged the continued suffering of the conflict, when it was noted on 6 April, 1945 that a Dr Spencer Sheill had lost his son, Captain Gordon Spencer Sheill MC, an officer in the RAMC, who had died 'in Germany'.

In the years that followed, the shadow of war lurked within the lines of the Minutes. On 7 May 1948, the College considered a request for a room in No 6 Kildare Street on behalf of an Irish Association 'to arrange for the dispatch of help for the children of devastated Europe'.[44]

Post-War Period

Following the end of the Second World War, it seems clear that the state of Ireland had not improved significantly since the early days following Partition. One historian has written of:

> an ideology, a conscious turning-away from the world of vulgar modernity represented by the old imperial master, 'pagan England'.
>
> The astonishing deference shown to church leaders, the willing acceptance of censorship, the embracing of wartime neutrality; the GAA's ban on its players playing *or even attending* scheduled 'foreign games': all proceeded from a common sensibility.
>
> At its root was a determination to discover uniquely Irish answers, to insist on the autonomy of the Irish mind. It was a nice idea, but it had nothing to do with economic or sociological reality, and it nearly wrecked the country.[45]

Low Profile

During this period, the College continued to keep a relatively low public profile

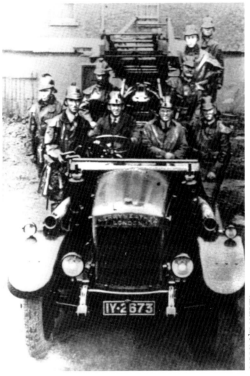

PADDY O'FLAHERTY

Dundalk firemen who voluntarily came to Belfast's aid during the blitz on the city in the Second World War.
F Clarke, E Norton, C St George (engineer), John McEneaney, Brannigan, N Murphy, Patrick Rooney, Kevin Corry, and M Murphy.
In total, seventy men and thirteen fire engines were assembled and dispatched from Dublin, Dundalk, Drogheda and Dún Laoghaire.[46]

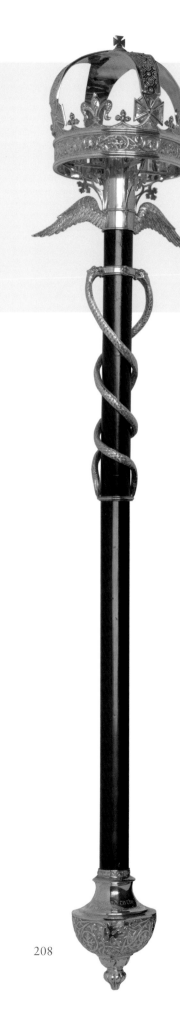

Dr William Geoffrey Harvey
President of the RCPI, 1943–46

Dr Harvey, who was elected as a Fellow of the Royal College of Physicians in 1908, served in France during the Great War, and worked as a physician and anaesthetist at the Urgency Cases Hospital in Revigny. In his later career, he was a dermatologist and physician at the Adelaide Hospital in Dublin.

On 21 March 1947, Dr Harvey presented a Caduceus to the College. It takes the form of two silver serpents entwined around an ebony staff, which had a silver crown. The Caduceus was made in Dublin by Messrs Alwright and Marshall, of Fade Street.[48]

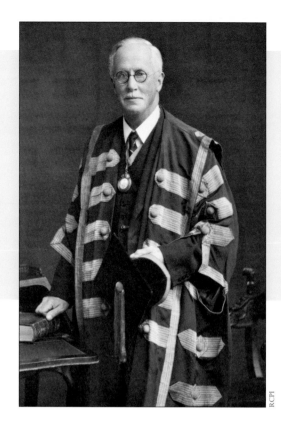

as a medical institution, though some of its leading figures were worthy of note – and several of these presented the RCPI with beautiful pieces of silver.

On 21 March 1947 Dr William Geoffrey Harvey, who had been President from 1943–46, gave the College a Caduceus, which is still used on official occasions.

Dr Harvey, who was a brilliant student at Trinity College, was elected a Fellow in 1908. He was also a veteran of the Great War, and served as a physician and anaesthetist at the Urgent Cases Hospital in Revigny. In his later career, he was a physician and dermatologist at the Adelaide Hospital in Dublin. He died in 1958.[47]

Dr Thomas Percy Claude Kirkpatrick, 1869–1954

Dr TPC Kirkpatrick was one of the most significant figures in the history of the College, of which he was Registrar from 1910–54. He was also General Secretary of the Royal Academy of Medicine for roughly the same period.

A noted physician, bibliophile and medical historian, he was known to his many colleagues affectionately as 'Percy' or 'Kirk'.

He was educated at Foyle College in Derry, and then took a First in History at Trinity College before graduating in Medicine at TCD in 1895. He became a Member of the College in 1903, and a year later he was elected a Fellow. Some 38 years later, he was elected as a Honorary Fellow of the Royal College of Physicians of London.

Kirkpatrick was an anaesthetist at Dr Steevens' Hospital, and later became an honorary visiting physician there. He took a special interest in venereal diseases, and to encourage his patients – many of whom were prostitutes – to seek treatment. He held special clinics for women early in the mornings to help preserve their anonymity.

Prolific

Dr Kirkpatrick was a prolific author on medical subjects and on medical institutions, including the TCD Medical School (1912), the Rotunda Hospital (1913) and Dr Steevens' Hospital (1924). He also wrote about, *inter alia* Sir William Petty, Edward Hill, Oliver Goldsmith and Abraham Colles.

Kirkpatrick was an outstanding bibliophile and collector of information about Irish doctors, and the 'Kirkpatrick Index' in the College is regarded as an invaluable source for many researchers, including biographers. Over 4,000 of his collection of medical books and pamphlets were bequeathed to the College. The remainder of his considerable non-medical collection, including a first edition of *Ulysses*, was auctioned by Sothebys.

Dr Kirkpatrick was a confirmed bachelor, who lived with his sister Sybil at 11 Fitzwilliam Place in Dublin. He was a clubbable man, who was fond of billiards and conversation with his friends.

He was also held in great esteem by his medical colleagues. Following his death on 9 July 1954, the President of the College Dr Edward Freeman described him as 'an affable, loyal and devoted official' who had obtained a position 'which afforded him opportunity to expand his keen interest in books, in affairs and in people':

Thomas Percy Claude Kirkpatrick, 1869–1954, anaesthetist, historian and bibliophile, Registrar of the Royal College of Physicians, 1910–54.

Portrait by Leo Whelan
RCPI

> No-one who has seen him in any setting where people were happy, will forget his beautiful smile slowly spreading across his face as he looked around the scene; just as few of the Fellows who asked him a possibly foolish question at a College meeting could bear him any ill-will for the caustic and witty reply, if the same smile accompanied it.
>
> We have all admired the courage with which he overcame the physical disabilities of the last few years, and all of us who could do so regard him, and have been proud and privileged that such a man was our friend.[49]

Dr Kirkpatrick had been appointed Registrar on St Luke's Day 1910, and in his term of office he had helped to guide the College through some of the most momentous events in its history, including two World Wars, and Partition in Ireland. He was a distinguished and highly-regarded figure from the past, who somehow had survived intact well into the first half of the twentieth century.

In many senses, his ilk, and his particular longevity in high medical office, would never be seen again. The death of Thomas Percy Claude Kirkpatrick was the end of an era, but also the beginning of the end of a long chapter in the history of the College. Nothing would, or could, be quite the same again, though it would take a few more years for RCPI to emerge properly into the fullness of the modern age.

DAVISON & ASSOCIATES

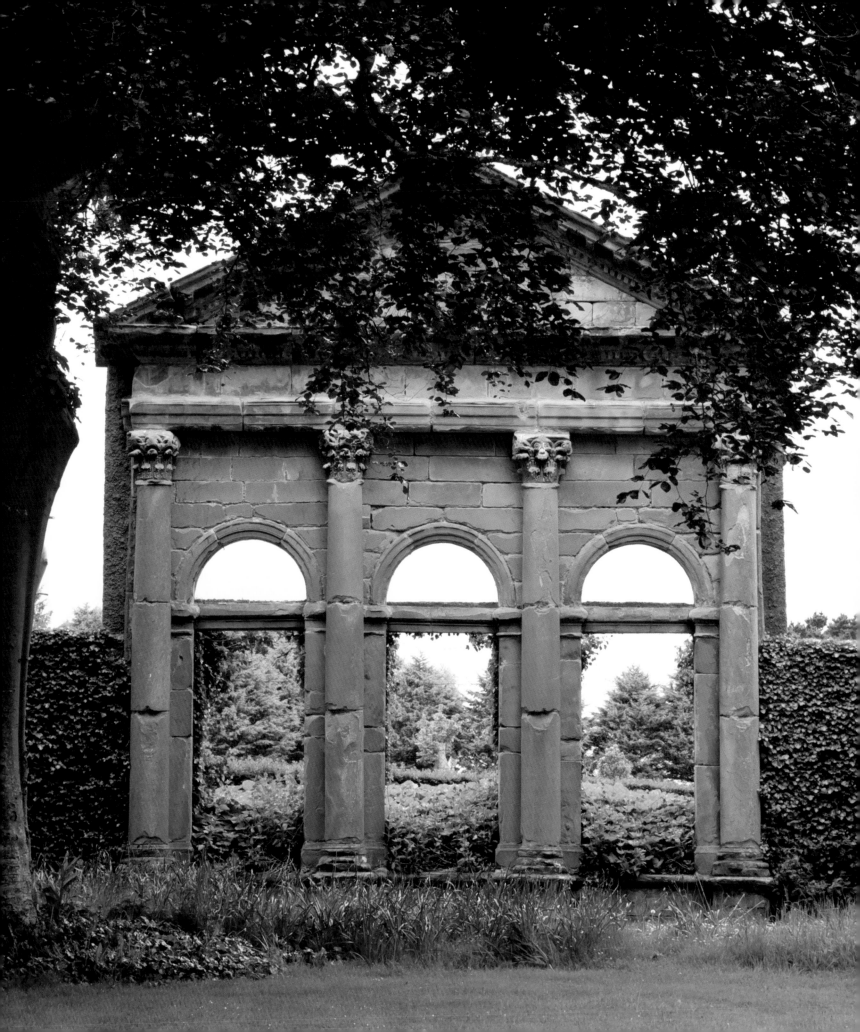

Brave New World

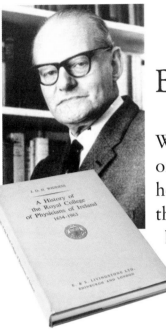

When Professor John Widdess completed his history of the Royal College of Physicians in the 1960s, he had covered the story from its establishment in the mid-seventeenth century until 1961. The book had been commissioned in July 1954, at which time the Library Committee had agreed that the College would provide a subsidy of up to a total of £450 for a print run of 1000 copies.[1]

Professor John Widdess
EOIN T O'BRIEN

Professor Widdess, one of the foremost medical historians of his time, had the luxury of spending roughly a decade in researching and writing the book – a period which would scarcely be feasible in today's world.

Nevertheless he is due considerable credit for undertaking the challenging task, and subsequent authors of the College's story are in his debt for his research and insights. Even though the book was ready for printing in 1963, it took another four years for the publishers to send revised estimates, and the College accepted a tender of 2,000 copies for sale at 40 shillings each.

It was published in 1967, just in time for the College's Tercentenary celebrations. In the final chapters Professor Widdess made little mention of the later story of the College, but as has been noted previously, these were relatively dormant years.

A symbol of change – the original sandstone façade from the upper storey of 6 Kildare Street, now stands in the garden at Woodbrook House south of Dublin. Sir Henry Cochrane, owner of Woodbrook House leased the basement and floor over the basement at No 6 Kildare Street for his company Cantrell & Cochrane.[2] The factory was originally located on the corner of Kildare Street and Nassau Street with another in Belfast.
DAVID COCHRANE
BOBBY STUDIO

However he did underline the important point that in 1961 an agreement between the College of Physicians, Trinity College and Sir Patrick Dun's Hospital had effectively wound up Dun's Trust. The amount raised from the sale of the Trust funds and property was just over £25,000, and the College of Physicians' share was £11,619. Some 56 years earlier, the final Dun's estates in Co Waterford had been sold under the 1903 Land Purchase Act. From the middle of the twentieth century, therefore, the long and often complex, but also beneficial, connection between Sir Patrick Dun and the College of Physicians began to recede into history.

Professor Widdess died in 1982.

Postscript

In 1967, a former College President Dr Edward T Freeman wrote a short postscript to the Widdess book. He sounded a distinctly upbeat note, stating that:

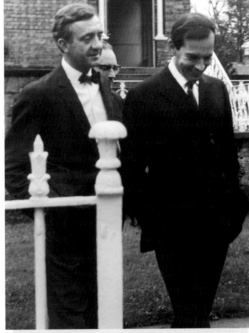

Dr Christiaan Barnard (right) is photographed with Professor Risteárd Mulcahy, the internationally renowned cardiologist and health campaigner, c. 1971.
PRIVATE COLLECTION

During 1967, the year in which Professor Widdess' history of the College of Physicians was published, several particularly significant medical milestones were reached. On 1 December that year Dr Barnard and a team including his brother Marius, performed the first successful human heart transplant, at Groote Schuur Hospital in Cape Town, South Africa, on Louis Washkansky, who survived for eighteen days before dying of pneumonia.[3]

211

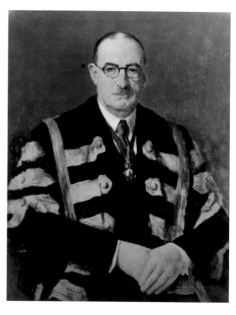

The roll of living Fellows now stands at 155, and contains the names of graduates of all the Universities and Medical Schools of the Country, as well as several from the emerging nations of the Far East and Africa.[5]

Freeman noted the earlier establishment of the Conjoint Board and co-operation with the Royal College of Surgeons. He also mentioned that, from 1959, the College of Physicians had instituted its Dublin Diploma in Obstetrics.

His postscript further emphasised that during the two previous decades an increasing number of overseas students, particularly from Asia and Africa, were coming to Dublin for training at the College, and that there was an increase in overseas doctors sitting the examinations for Membership. He concluded his message with these words:

> ... an immense opportunity presents itself to help people in their need for western medical training, and to extend the influence of Irish medicine far beyond the confines of this country and into regions undreamt of by Stearne, by Dun or by Corrigan.[5]

This was a bold vision of a 'brave new world' for Irish medicine but the big challenge was to make it a reality. In the next few decades there were concerted efforts by senior medical and other staff to move the College further out of the doldrums, to turn it into an institution upholding the highest possible clinical standards and also enable it to acquire a significant role in helping to determine the country's healthcare policy as a whole.

Dr Edward T Freeman was President of the College of Physicians from 1952–55, and the first Catholic in the post since 1925. He wrote a short postscript to the Widdess' history in 1967 and took an upbeat view about the future of the College, which was slowly emerging from its 'long sleep' of previous decades.
MATER HOSPITAL DUBLIN

Buildings

One of the first priorities, however, was to refurbish the antiquated building at No 6 Kildare Street, and to make it fit for purpose. The basement at one time had been used a sugar store by the soft drinks firm, Cantrell & Cochrane, because of its exceptionally dry atmosphere, but the business of the College was sharing medical expertise, not sugar.

Some of the stories about the accommodation in No 6 during those days were Dickensian. Dr Alan Grant, the first Northerner to become President, 1977–79, recalls his early visits to the College from Belfast, with the first of these in 1947:

> At that time the trams trundled to Nelson's Pillar, and horse-drawn carts were still to be seen in the city, while a horde of push bicycles filled the streets at rush hour.[6]

Dr Grant took the clinical examination for Membership, which was held at Dun's and Steevens' Hospitals. He recalled:

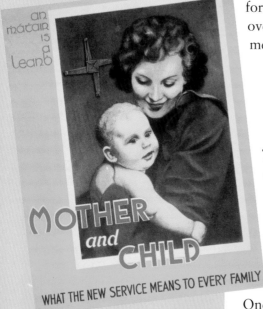

This is a copy of a booklet produced for the proposed Mother and Child Scheme, 1951. The Minister for Health, Dr Noel Browne, resigned after his attempt to bring in free maternity care was rejected. The Scheme was never implemented, in the face of resistance from the medical lobby and the Catholic Church.

Noel Browne was described by a biographer as a man who, 'could retreat from challenges and confrontations into an interior monologue which was so intense that it all but blotted out the world outside. And all of this evoked an understandable and occasionally regretful intolerance among many of those who might have been his allies, of his wayward, headstrong, often self-contradictory and self-indulgent but sometimes prophetic voice'.[4]

212

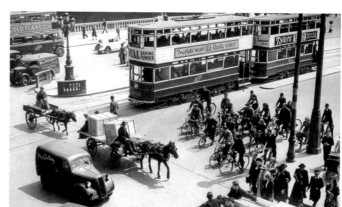

Dublin traffic c. 1947
CREATIVE COMMONS

It was a fair and searching clinical examination conducted at a leisurely pace. A civilised contrast to the frenetic and dehumanised occasions in London.[7]

Grant's next memorable visit was in 1954, when he was admitted as the only Fellow that year. He recalled:

> The ceremony took place in the College Hall where the President, Dr Freeman, and about six senior Fellows sat at a large table. There were no carpets. The walls were a dull mustard colour, with brown surrounds. The windows were grimy, and the dull light showed flaking paint and cobwebs. It was cold. The velvet gowns of the Fellows, which added a sombre dignity to the scene, were practical and warm.[8]

After the meeting, the requisite fee was paid to the Registrar, Dr Charles Dickson, in the Library:

> This large room was heated by a small smoky fire. Dr Dickson sat behind a table piled with papers and books, and talked of the native County Down which he had left so many years ago, and to which I returned forthwith. There was no time to examine the tattered ancient volumes lining the walls. Financial stringency was obvious. The Registrar, frail and devoted, did his best to cope. It is almost impossible for us to visualise such an atmosphere where time stood still, and we had a relic of another Ireland and another age.[9]

Dr David Mitchell, a former Treasurer (1975–85) and a former President (1969–72), also described the atmosphere in the College around 1970. The reception area was at that time:

> ... a dark store-room full of an assembly of books and journals, and of no permanent value or future use. Calendars of minor foreign academic bodies and other ephemeral publications cluttered its shelves and floor, which they sometimes shared with Miss Gardiner's bicycle. This room was cleared out, redecorated and made into an office for the Treasurer and his secretary. The previous Treasurer, Dr Bewley, had felt no need for an office in the post.[10]

Miss Gardiner, the Secretary, was a legendary figure.

> She had kept the accounts, as well as all other documentation. When the examination entries increased to an extent that made separate accounting necessary, a part-time secretary was engaged.[11]

The limited phone service at the College was improved from the single telephone in the Library by installing an extra outside line, and by placing a public phone box in the Front Hall.

A Cold House

The lasting impression for most people, however, was the sheer coldness of the building, which Dr Mitchell described as follows:

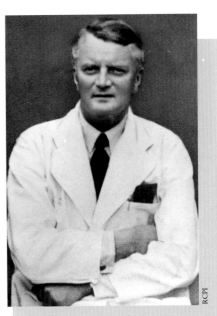

Dr Christopher Joseph McSweeney, Medical Superintendent of Cork Street Fever Hospital (1934–1953) and a prominent physician in the fight against poliomyelitis in Ireland.[12]

In the mid-twentieth century poliomyelitis was feared throughout society; it affected mainly children and left an indelible impression upon individuals and communities alike. Immunisation programmes against tuberculosis, diphtheria and poliomyelitis had greatly reduced the incidences of these illnesses by the 1970s and 80s.[13]

In the 1960s many countries, including Ireland, were beginning to realise that they were facing new health problems requiring different solutions. Infectious disease was being conquered but demographic trends and the growing proportion of old people were leading to a greater prevalence of chronic disease, and mortality from cancer of the lung and coronary thrombosis was increasing.[14]

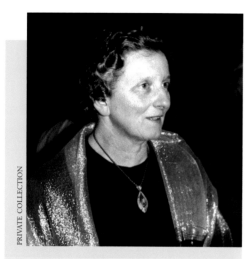

Gladys Gardiner

'Miss Gardiner', as she was known to everyone, was a person who took the unexpected in her stride. In 1969 some 180 places had been set for the St Luke's Day Dinner, which was thought to be a record attendance. Six people arrived unexpectedly, and declared themselves willing to pay cash for their dinner. Miss Gardiner very wisely took their money first, and then went across the street to Power's Hotel, complete with a large basket on her arm. The hotel must have known her well, because she had no trouble in borrowing sufficient extra plates (the College and the caterers had no spares). The extra six unexpected diners were accommodated without fuss, and the College was richer for the experience, in more ways than one.

In her later years, Miss Gardiner had failing health, but even then and during her final illness she continued to help the College in many different ways. She died in February 1991. Dr David Mitchell, who had worked with her closely and had known her well, paid this heartfelt tribute

Her absolute discretion, combined with her special sense of humour, and an ability to appreciate and remember the ludicrous or the absurd, made a unique contribution.[17]

214

The small, smoky fire in the grate at the south end of the Library was all Dr Kirkpatrick needed, and no-one else was considered. Miss Gardiner, whose desk was beside his ... always had a large cardboard box under her desk, in which her feet kept warm. The elegant stove in the College Hall was usually lit not long before meetings, and seemed to heat the back of the President's chair exclusively.[15]

One of the characters of those years was indeed Miss Gladys Gardiner, who was officially the College Clerk but who was also one of those individuals whose inside knowledge and experience makes them almost indispensible for the daily running of an institution. For thirty years she ran the College almost single-handedly. As Dr Mitchell recalls:

She was devoted to the College ... and she had a remarkable knowledge of the things that do not go into Minutes or official records. She had a remarkable memory, not only of personalities and events, but of her very personal filing methods.

She always remembered in which book she had stored an unexpected cheque, or in which part of which drawer a vital document had been secured. The College seemed to be her life.[16]

Improvements

It was clear that something had to be done about the inside of a building where the long-suffering Miss Gardiner had to keep her feet warm by placing them in a cardboard box heated by a hot water bottle. However, there were needs even more urgent than this, because experts warned the College that the ornate façade of No 6 Kildare Street was crumbling and that falling masonry might one day injure passers-by.

In January 1963, the College decided to restore the entire front of the building in Portland stone. Part of the old Victorian façade, which dated from

Early memories – Professor John Murphy

The rather 'olde-worlde' ambiance of No 6 was confirmed by Professor John Murphy, who recalls the atmosphere of the College during his student days:

As a third-year medical student with UCD, I needed to borrow a book which was in the RCPI library. With some trepidation I came down to No. 6 Kildare Street. There were no lights on, and when I knocked on the locked door, Mr Carney, the College Porter let me in.

The place was extremely dingy. The library, which today is very elegant, was then chaotic. There were books on the shelves, books on the floor, and on the fireplace. There was a senior gentlemen, Dr Dickson, to whom I was not introduced, and a charming lady of hard-to-determine years. She was dressed in a fairly severe tweed suit, with her feet in a cardboard box. This was Miss Gardiner, and she was very nice to me.

I have no idea how she found the journal I wanted, and when I asked for a place where I could transcribe, she offered to let me borrow it. When I offered to supply my name and address, she said, 'Don't bother, you've got an honest face. Return it when you are finished with it.' So I duly returned it.[17]

Professor Murphy's next involvement with No 6 was when he sat the MRCP examination in Obstetrics and Gynaecology:

I was the only one sitting in that discipline. The invigilator was a kind lady who brought me coffee and scones and made the thing as cheery as possible. Later on, those who had qualified for membership received a handshake and a parchment, and that was it.[18]

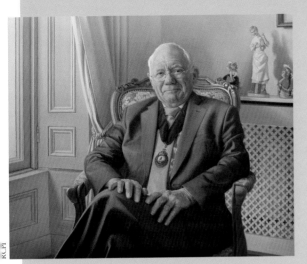
Portrait by Alexander Carey Clarke

Professor John Murphy

Professor John Murphy was a leading figure in the College who was President in the year 2006–7 before spending nearly five years as Professor of Obstetrics and Gynaecology at the Royal College of Surgeons in Ireland in Bahrain. John Murphy was a stalwart of the College who served in several important roles, including Library Committee (1985–2006), Council Member (1988–2014), Vice-President (1994), Dun's Librarian (1995–7), and Treasurer (1998–2006). On his return from Bahrain, he continued to work for the College for two days a week developing projects concerned with simulation in Obstetrics and Gynaecology. Professor Murphy said: 'In my professional lifetime, the College has developed from being a small, exclusive body into a dynamic and thriving medical institution, which is deeply involved with education, training and setting standards. I have enjoyed my time with the College and it was a great privilege to have been associated with so many colleagues, who were so generous with their time and expertise.'[18]

Corrigan's time, was moved to Woodbrook House as 'a charming gloriette', facing the garden front: its three arched windows framing the sea.[19]

The cost of replacing the front of No 6 was £18,500 and – as in previous times – the College was short of money. It was decided to invite the Fellows, Members and Licentiates to take out debentures, which the College had done when the building was being erected in the 1860s.

This time, however, 'The emotional appeal was less cogent, and perhaps twentieth-century Fellows were less generous'. But in 1965 a 'mysterious' Special Committee was set up to provide advice 'in the event of certain monies being displaced at the disposal of the College', and, 'rumour connected the Committee's advice with the Honorary Fellowship that was awarded to the Earl of Iveagh in 1968'.[20]

By early 1967 the building funds raised, including debentures, came to only £11,000, but the Fellows and Members rejected 'out of hand' a proposal that they should subscribe annually until the full amount was raised. Mitchell noted sharply, 'At this date the idea of the Fellows

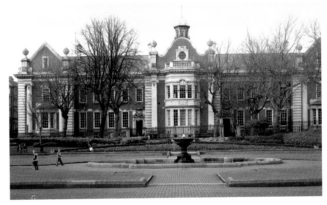

The Iveagh Play Centre, Bull Alley
RICHARD WATSON

ABOVE: The Guinness family have been benefactors of health and social housing over the decades. Lord Iveagh, Edward Cecil Guinness, replaced the infamous Dublin slums at Bull Alley with the Iveagh Play Centre in 1915. The children were taught a wide range of practical subjects with the added bonus of cocoa and a bun. There were annual Christmas parties. In the mid-1960s new inner-city housing development led to a demand for a vocational school. The Iveagh Trust finally closed the Centre in 1977 when the Vocational Educational Committee purchased the building – which now houses the Liberties Vocational School.[21]

Ballymun tower blocks, designed by English architect Arthur Swift, and completed in 1967.
NATIONAL PHOTOGRAPHIC ARCHIVE

While the College was improving the conditions of both its exterior and interior, many social housing plans were also being developed. Ballymun Housing Estate was built to cope with the Dublin housing crisis in the 1960s, as slum dwellings were demolished. Places in one of the seven 15-storey tower blocks were highly coveted at the time, but eventually the estate created its own problems as the promised urban development never happened.[22] The towers were also criticised as having an anti-social layout.

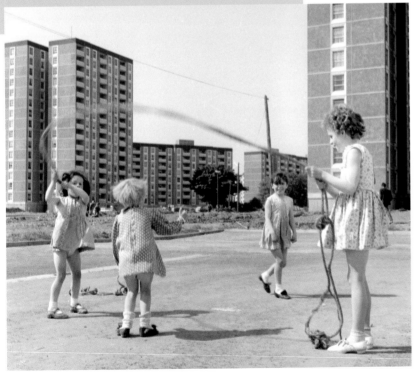

215

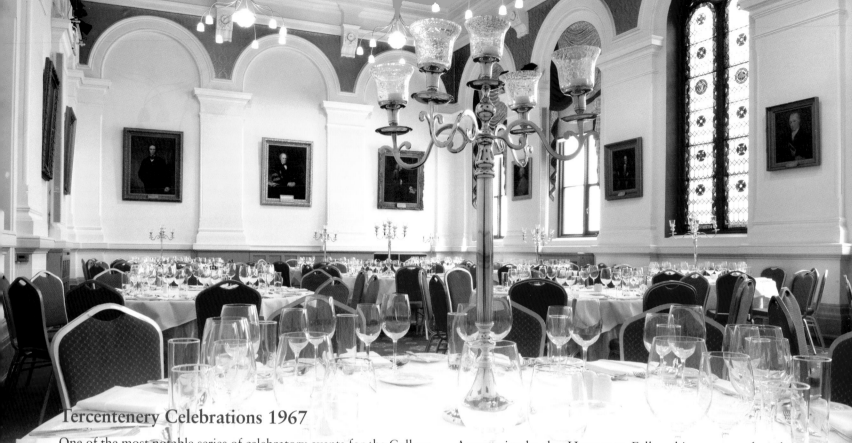

DERMOTT DUNBAR

Tercentenery Celebrations 1967

One of the most notable series of celebratory events for the College took place in 1967 when it celebrated the Tercentenary of the grant of the Royal Charter by King Charles II in 1667.

President Éamon de Valera entertained the Fellows and their guests at his official residence, Áras an Uachtaráin, on 15 May, and the next day he was made an Honorary Fellow. He also attended a Tercentenary Dinner, which was attended by the Presidents and senior representatives of the Royal Colleges of Physicians of London, Edinburgh, Glasgow, Australia, Canada and South Africa, as well as the President of the American College of Physicians.

The citation for the President was delivered by Registrar Dr Charles Dickson, that doughty Ulsterman and long-serving College stalwart who had won an MC in the Great War and was a fluent Gaelic speaker from his early days, and throughout his long career when he settled in Dublin after the Partition of Ireland.

Appropriately the Honorary Fellowship was conferred on President de Valera in Gaelic and then in English.

The Irish President thanked the College, signed the Roll of Honorary Fellows, and a Toast was proposed by the President of the London College, Sir Max Rosenheim.

In reply, the President of the College, Dr Alan Thompson warned eloquently and passionately about the increasing specialisation within medicine which he likened to 'an internal brain drain'. Warming to his theme, he said:

> In many a hospital today we may find a small rump of disgruntled general physicians, too old and too disillusioned to call themselves by any other name, banished to the draughty wards of some building long condemned as unfit for specialist habitation; a disconsolate band of Elijahs waiting for the ravens to bring them droppings from the tables of the specialists – some waif or stray, perhaps, some displaced person who has unaccountably escaped the attentions of the cardoloigist, the neurologist, the rheumatologist, the endocrinologist, the gastroenterologist, or some other personification of the one-track mind.[23]

It was magnificent rhetoric. Even by 1967, however, it was already a voice from the past. Within the next decades a whole series of specialist institutes and faculties would be set up, and important structural changes within the College, and relating to its way of dealing with its members and Fellows, pointed towards a positive and outward-looking blueprint for the future.

As one medical historian noted: 'Following years of stagnation and depression, the Irish economy expanded in the 1960s. An air of optimism swept through the education and health services.[24]

The College cast off the last vestiges of its former exclusivity, and medical excellence became its main touchstone for achievement.

RCPI/ IRISH PRESS

President Éamon de Valera was made an Honorary Fellow of the College on St Luke's Day 1967, as part of the historic Tercentenary celebrations.

paying an annual subscription to the College was unacceptable.'[25] The costs kept rising and the final bill amounted to almost £20,000. However a special Tercentenary appeal shifted all but 81 of the debentures, and the rebuilding of the façade was completed. It was not until 1978, however, that all the debentures were repaid, except for one which was due to a Fellow who could not be traced.[26]

A number of other significant additions and alterations were accomplished, including the building of a new platform in the College Hall to make it suitable for the increasing number of lectures and other well-attended meetings which required a proper auditorium. This also led to subtle, but symbolically important, changes in the seating arrangements for College dinners.

On the lower level, the Winter Hall, which had been opened in 1940 as an adjunct to the Library and which had not properly fulfilled its purpose, was altered extensively in 1972 and let temporarily to the Medical Registration Council.

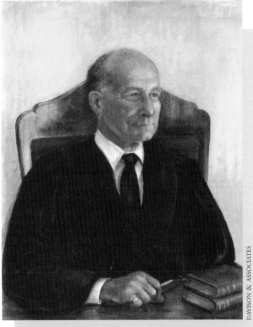

Portrait by Y Cumming Bruce
RCPI

Robert Collis
1900–75

Robert Collis, MRCPI, was an outstanding paediatrician. After spending time in Dublin he vowed to help eradicate the terrible slum conditions in the city. He set up the National Cerebral Palsy Clinic and sought out a patient he had seen at a children's Christmas party – that child was the renowned Christy Brown, who wrote with his foot, and was encouraged by the literary Collis. His autobiography *My Left Foot* became a bestseller and was made into a successful film.

Christy Brown wrote a Foreword to Collis's autobiography, *To be a Pilgrim*, published posthumously after a riding accident. He noted that Collis had 'led a many rainbowed life in so many spheres: physician, paediatrician, child psychologist, writer, playwright – a life so varied and diffuse as to be almost impossible to pin down between the covers of any book, and like many another rare thing, the things that go unsaid are as valid and meaningful as those that are said so beautifully'.[27]

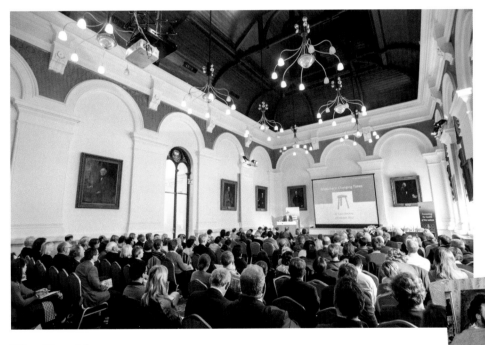

RIGHT: A recent 'masterclass' in Corrigan Hall
RCPI

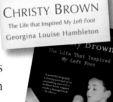

The Troubles

The outbreak of the Troubles was a major catastrophe, which imprisoned the North in a political, social and community straitjacket for nearly four decades from the late 1960s. Its effects also spilled over to other parts of Ireland and the United Kingdom.

Physicians from the North had always played an important role in the life of the College and in medicine in Ireland, these included James Macartney from Armagh in the nineteenth century, and Ulstermen such as Professor TG Moorhead and Dr Dickson in the twentieth century.

217

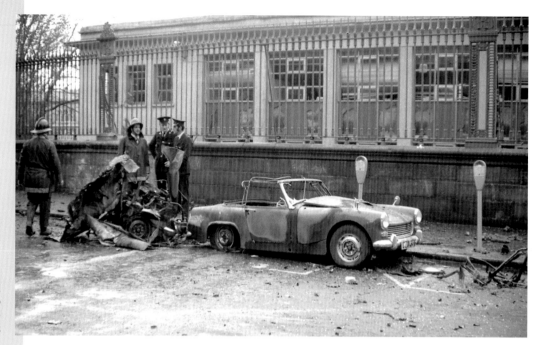

Trinity College Dublin Medical
Faculty, following the car bomb
on Nassau Street in 1974
DUBLIN CITY LIBRARY AND ARCHIVE

Bomb Damage

By the early 1970s, the Troubles in Northern Ireland had been raging for several years, and although the major loss of life as well as the damage and destruction had been confined largely to the North and the border counties, the violence also spilled over into the Irish Republic.

Several bombs in Dublin during this time killed and injured a number of people, and one of these exploded near No. 6 Kildare Street, shattering antique glass in the College Hall. The empty frames were filled by plywood sheets, and three years later they were replaced by modern glass, which tried to match the originals as nearly as possible.

Around the same time, the College building was rewired for £13,000 and insured for £235,000. After the bomb, the College took a malicious damage claim against the Dublin Corporation, but it was never paid.[28]

The College's first Ulster-based President, from 1977–80, was Dr Alan Grant from the City Hospital in Belfast. He outlined graphically some of his logistical problems in travelling from the North:

> Travel to Dublin was disturbed by such euphemisms as 'suspect devices' near the Border. The train journey could be interrupted by a ride in a rickety bus from Goraghwood to Dundalk, adding an hour to the journey. On occasion, the train was fired on in South Armagh.
>
> Going by car, a 'diversion' might mean a tour along flooded rough tracks. To return to the North late at night could be an interesting experience. Diverted to Dundalk on a pitch-black night, I got lost up some side road, only to be roused to full consciousness by two gentlemen with Armalite rifles. What does one do? Stop and claim to know 'the Boss' or put the boot down and swerve up some even more forsaken track? The latter course was followed, and in due course the Guards were met. In such a state of the country, we appreciated the President and a faithful few coming to Belfast for a College dinner in 1969. It gave us a feeling of belonging, which still exists.[29]

The dinner Grant refers to here was described colourfully by Dr David Mitchell in his interim history of the College as, 'an inauspicious start'. He added:

> For the first time, British troops had suddenly appeared on the streets, as had the 'barricades', put up by the local residents against terrorism. The general atmosphere of tension and fear did not make for the success of a dinner of a college from 'Éire'.[30]

The Dublin group included the redoubtable Registrar, Dr Charles Dickson, then aged 84, who had been born, brought up and educated in the North, where he had attended Royal Belfast Academical Institution and Queen's University.

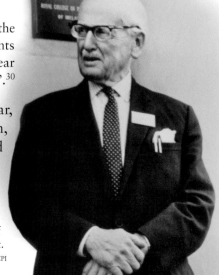

Dr Charles Dickson, who was awarded a Military Cross
in the Great War, retained his dignified military bearing
even in his mid-80s. In 1969 he returned to his native
Ulster as part of a group attending a College of
Physicians' dinner in troubled Belfast.
RCPI

The Corrigan Club

The Corrigan Club was established as a means of bringing together physicians from Northern Ireland and the Republic to discuss matters of mutual medical interest, but also to encourage closer personal links between colleagues from north and south of the Border.

The idea originated after a meeting of the Association of Physicians in Cardiff in 1959, and was mooted by Dr Ivo Drury, who became President of the College in 1986, and Dr Desmond AD Montgomery, a leading endocrinologist at the Royal Victoria Hospital in Belfast. Ivo Drury later outlined the details of the decision:

> We had a chat on our train journey and, when saying goodbye, I said it was a pity that we only met at meetings in England. The idea stayed with me, and on my return home, I reflected on the absurdity of the position, whereby physicians in Dublin and Belfast hardly knew one another. (Corrigan Club booklet)

Dr Drury then wrote to 'Dad' Montgomery:

> ... too many people were blowing up bridges, and that I felt that I would like to try building a bridge if he would help me at the other end. He was delighted, and we agreed that he, in Belfast, and I, in Dublin, would discuss with some colleagues the idea of a Physicians' Club.[31]

On 11 March 1960 the first meeting was held at the Mater Hospital in Dublin, and, as Dr Drury noted:

> ... the Northern members graciously suggested that the Club should be named after Dominic Corrigan.

The list of 32 Founder Members includes many of the outstanding physicians of the time, including the cardiologist, Professor Frank Pantridge from the Royal Victoria Hospital in Belfast, who developed the world's first mobile defibrillator. This led to the invention of mobile coronary care units which has saved countless lives worldwide.

Pantridge was a remarkable character, who served with the RAMC during the Second World War and won a Military Cross during the fall of Singapore when he became a Japanese prisoner-of-war. He was badly treated and served much of his captivity as a slave labourer on the Burma railway. As a result he developed an illness which was with him for the rest of his life.

The Corrigan Club met annually, and varied the venue of its meetings to different parts of the island, including Dublin, Belfast, Derry, Galway, Craigavon, Cork, Maynooth, Newcastle and Dundonald.

Professor Desmond Montgomery, 'Dad', Consultant Physician in charge of the metabolic unit at the Royal Victoria Hospital, Belfast, 1958–79
ROYAL VICTORIA HOSPITAL

The Club was regarded by physicians as an important point of contact, particularly during the Troubles when people from the Republic were extremely wary of coming to the war-torn North.

Professor Brian Keogh from Dublin and Dr Stanley Roberts from Belfast were later Presidents of the College, and they formed close ties due to the Corrigan Club as well as the RCPI. Dr Keogh said:

> When the Corrigan Club met in Dublin, Stanley and his wife stayed with us, and my wife and I stayed with them when the Club met in Belfast. We've remained good friends for many years.

The Corrigan Club still meets, though the current age profile is somewhat higher than in earlier days. Yet undoubtedly it played an important role in bringing together physicians from all parts of the Ireland, particularly during the long period when the Troubles made this particularly difficult.

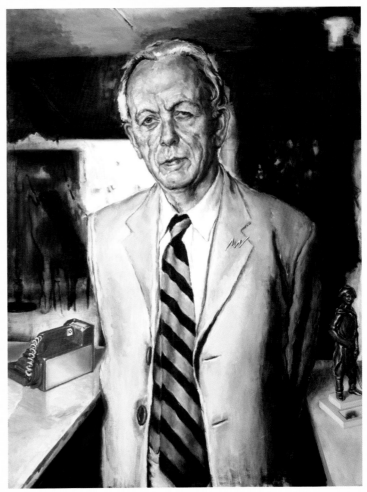

Dr Frank Pantridge. The defibrillator is shown to his right in this painting by Martin Wedge

Dr David Mitchell
1909–95

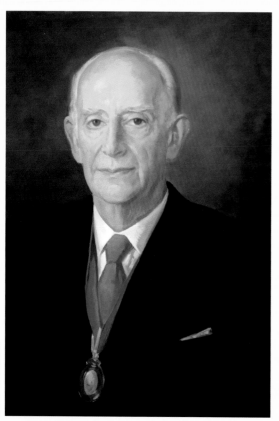

Portrait by David Hone
RCPI

One of the most important figures in the history of the College was Dr David Mitchell, who was widely recognised as 'one of the main movers in the bid to restore the stature of Irish medicine in the second half of the twentieth century'.[32]

Mitchell was an outstanding scholar and medical author, and a distinguished physician who spent most of his career at the Adelaide Hospital. He won many professional honours and accolades, including the Fellowships of the American, London and Edinburgh Colleges of Physicians.

He was elected a Fellow of the RCPI in 1938 and was President from 1969–71.
A senior colleague, Dr Alan Grant, described him thus:

> He had a vision of the College actively promoting, and being the major influence, in medicine and its sub-specialities, first in the Republic, and in the long term, in the whole island. No longer would the College remain an exclusive Dublin medical club.

It was a great Presidency by any standards. The nadir of our fortunes had passed, and the momentum of progress continued after David Mitchell had completed his term. It might be noted, however, that he made sure it did, as he became Treasurer and unofficial keeper of the College conscience. Little that went on in the College escaped his observation.[33]

One of Mitchell's biographers also noted that as President of the RCPI:

> … his wisdom and firmness were regularly employed to resolve conflicting interests, most notably when he introduced a new membership examination to replace one in existence since 1880, but also in his efforts to harmonise postgraduate medical training in Ireland …
>
> His reserved manner masked considerable kindness and generosity. In his professional life he valued learning, integrity, and self-discipline, and expected these qualities from others. He could be outspoken, but the honest and innate pursuit of excellence that motivated him was respected by all with whom he dealt.[34]

Food For Thought

The renaissance of the College after what a former President Professor Brian Keogh referred to as 'the Long Sleep', meant a renewal among other things, of social activity.

The first annual 'June Dinner' was held in 1968, and became a regular feature in the College calendar. However Dr Mitchell described delightfully the failing appetite over time for such an event:

> As the years passed, these June Dinners seemed to lose something of the spontaneity and informality which had made them so enjoyable … For many years the menu, too, was unchanging; vegetable soup, poached salmon with new potatoes and green peas, followed by strawberries and cream. With the abolition of the Friday fast, the menus, like the speeches, were longer and duller.[35]

Dr Mitchell's 'cri de coeur', if not from his digestive system, could be applied to countless dinners in countless institutions almost from time immemorial …

He took David Mitchell on an impromptu tour of the Belfast he had known in his youth.

> Like an inspecting officer, [Dickson] he studied the troops and the defence of the inhabitants over a wide area of the city. His colleague found it physically exhausting, but mentally quite fascinating. There was an almost continuous flow of information and wry comment on the political and social history of Belfast and of its citizens, famous or notorious, and of every political and doctrinal colour.
>
> The Registrar was on his own ground, literally and metaphorically. Of the other two, Freeman went to church and presumably prayed for the city, while the President Alan Thompson lay on his bed and read about it.[36]

The College met for a second time in Belfast in 1985, when the atmosphere was still difficult but less daunting than during the crises years around 1969.

Not Forgotten

While the College was busy addressing the considerable challenges of medicine in Ireland in the latter half of the twentieth century, the contribution of two of its outstanding pioneers in the nineteenth century was not forgotten.

In July 1978, the centenary of the death of William Stokes was commemorated with a two-day meeting at No 6 Kildare Street. Papers were read by Fellows of the College as well as a number of distinguished overseas visitors. One of the sessions was held at Stokes' old hospital, the Meath, and participants were given a tour of the hospital and a commentary on Stokes' life and career achievements.

During the next year it was decided that the College would also pay tribute to Sir Dominic Corrigan on the centenary of his death. A service was planned for St Andrew's Church in Dublin's Westland Row, where Corrigan was buried, and the intention was to lay wreaths, and that a cleric would conduct a short religious service.

There was only one snag. On the day, a priest was not available, and the President Dr Alan Grant, from Belfast, later described what happened next:

> There was shattering news – no priest would be attending. With the Secretary and the Librarian, a frantic search of the Library revealed a Book of Common Prayer, and a King James' Bible.
>
> There was no option: the President had to take the service. A short prayer followed by the Psalm, 'For the years of a man are threescore and ten', would give an introduction to [Corrigan's] achievements in the years most of us spend retired. The service could be finished off with the Lord's Prayer.
>
> The Vice-President, Dr Conor Ward, and Dr Eoin O'Brien, appeared, and we put on gowns and walked around to the church. It was a fine day. There were perhaps thirty people in the crypt, most of whom were not known to me. Nobody showed any sign that they realised the enormity of the situation. The occasion appeared to go smoothly, and with proper dignity.[37]

Corrigan was duly honoured with wreaths, and it was a suitable and touching tribute to one of the great men of Irish medicine, and one of the greatest – if not the greatest – in the history of the College.

Management of the College

There was a certain charm about the old regime where the Registrars Dr Kirkpatrick and Dr Dickson, as well as Miss Gardiner toiled away and did the best they could. However by May 1978 the work of the College had increased so much that a new management structure was necessary.

By this stage the Registrar was paid £500 plus expenses, the Treasurer £500, and the full-time Clerk £1,580. Extra posts were created including a new Assistant Clerk at £1,200 per annum, and two part-time secretaries at £11 a week. To meet this increased expenditiure, the Fellows' annual subscriptions were doubled – from £5 to £10 a year![38]

ROYAL COLLEGE OF SURGEONS IN IRELAND

Dr Harry O'Flanagan succeeded Dr Dickson as College Registrar, and was appointed on St Luke's Day, 1971. He held the post until 1975, and made an important contribution to the College of Physicians.

He was a Fellow of the College and also Registrar of the Royal College of Surgeons in Ireland, and was willing to undertake both appointments – an arrangement which was agreeable to both Colleges.

Harry O'Flanagan was a good administrator, and he was credited with many of the initiatives which led to the introduction of more modern management methods.[39]

Dr Alan Grant, was the first Northern President of the College, from 1977–80. He graphically described some of the difficulties of travelling regularly from the North across the Border during the Troubles, including 'suspect devices' on the roads and railway, and interrupted journeys.
RCPI

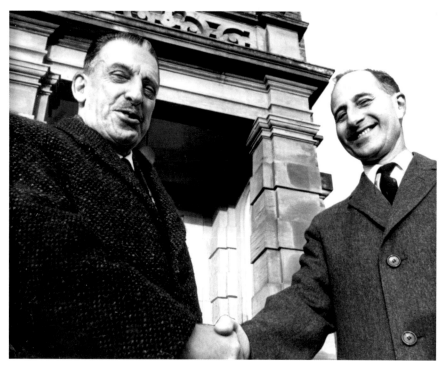

The truly historic – and previously unannounced – meeting of the Irish Taioseach Sean Lemass and the Northern Ireland Prime Minister Captain Terence O'Neill at Stormont in 1965 seemed to herald a new and progressive 'hands-across-the border' policy for both parts of the island which were experiencing better economic progress. Sadly, however, those hopes were dashed by the outbreak of the Troubles several years later.

Period of Change

This was also during a period of significant changes in society at large, as Ireland began to open itself out to greater challenges in the post-War world, and the economy improved enormously under the leadership of the Taoiseach Sean Lemass and an outstanding and visionary senior civil servant, TK Whitaker, the Secretary of the Department of Finance.

There was free secondary schooling from the mid-Sixties, while the medical profession was adjusting, not without pain, to the development of a National Health Service under central control. It was a period of enormous progress, and it helped to set the tone for those who were setting out to reform the College into a institution that could successfully meet the challenges of the second half of the twentieth century.

Opposition

The reforms advocated by Dr David Mitchell and others were not approved by everyone, however. In a delightfully phrased set of observations, he noted the reservations of the Old Guard. They included the long-term Registrar, Dr Dickson, whom he described in an affectionate though incisive pen-portrait. He paid tribute to Dickson's devotion to the College in his second career, after long service as the Chief Medical Officer of Ireland:

Bright Idea

Throughout most of its history, the College President had entertained the Fellows to dinner, usually at his own house. This could be an expensive exercise, and as the numbers of Fellows increased, this could become a financial burden – particularly as a special allowance for claret to fortify such entertaining by the President was abolished by the College in the early nineteenth century.

Such entertaining was expensive, and this deterred some of the less affluent Fellows from allowing their names to go forward for election as President. Accordingly, the custom of Presidential entertaining was abolished by the College in 1952.

A similar problem was presented by the traditional gifts which

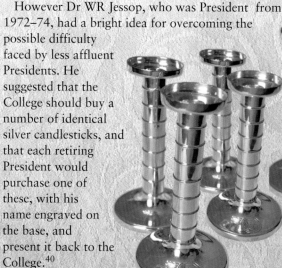

Dr WR Jessop

Presidents donated to the College at the end of their term of office. Some of these were elaborate, and expensive.

However Dr WR Jessop, who was President from 1972–74, had a bright idea for overcoming the possible difficulty faced by less affluent Presidents. He suggested that the College should buy a number of identical silver candlesticks, and that each retiring President would purchase one of these, with his name engraved on the base, and present it back to the College.[40]

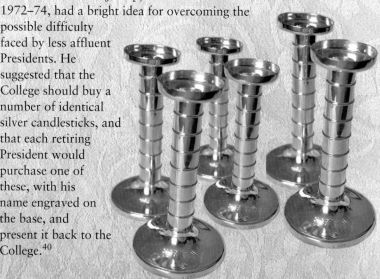

He controlled … the College … from the same chair in the library that Kirkpatrick had sat in for so long. He was there all day, every day, from nine o'clock. With a telephone and Miss Gardiner and her typewriter, he needed no other devices, electronic, mechanical or even human, to run the College.

Age and failing eyesight brought this second career to an end in 1971. He did nothing by halves, but as an ex-civil servant he was conservatively efficient, and rather disliked innovations. He was a custodian of all the 'ancient usages of the College', unenthusiastic about the expansion of its activities in the 1970s, and critical of some of the changes that resulted. He did not exert himself unduly to help would-be reformers.[41]

Modernisation

Nevertheless, it was clear to the younger generation of physicians that the College had to move with the times, because a policy of further stagnation would lead to continuing irrelevance, or even oblivion.

In 1968 the Institute of Obstetricians and Gynaecologists was established, and seven years later the Faculties of Pathology, Occupational Medicine and Community Health Medicine (later to collectively become Public Health Medicine) were founded. Then in 1982 the Faculty of Paediatrics was established.

During these decades there were also important developments in medical training and membership structures. In 1971 the Irish Committee on Higher Medical Training was established to monitor and develop the specialist training of doctors in Ireland, and in 1976, the General Purposes Committee was renamed the College Council, with the remit of becoming the College's advisory body.

A year later, Collegiate Membership was established to encourage greater involvement by the Members in helping to run the College. There were also significant developments concerning the replacement of the Membership Examination, which had scarcely changed since the 1880s.

From January 1971, candidates in Ireland would take the same Part I Multiple Choice Questions as their counterparts in the United Kingdom, and this was set in conjunction with the Royal Colleges of Physicians in Edinburgh, Glasgow and London. However, Part II (the clinical part) of the examination continued to be held in the traditional way by the Irish College for some years to come.

'Special Membership'

One important innovation was the establishment of 'Special Membership' examinations in the 1970s, to enable senior doctors who were not already involved with the College to be fast-tracked into Membership and Fellowships.

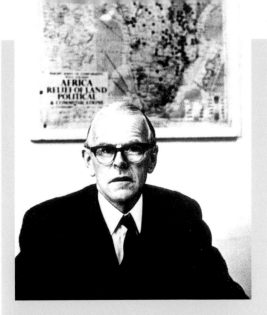

Dr Denis Burkitt
1911–93

Dr Denis Burkitt, who was born in Co Fermanagh and became a graduate of TCD was an outstanding figure in twentieth-century Irish medicine. He won many national and international awards for his work, and he was elected an Honorary Fellow of the Royal College of Physicians of Ireland, of the Royal College of Surgeons in Ireland, and of Trinity College Dublin.

A man of high Christian principles, he travelled widely in Africa – and particularly in Uganda – in an attempt to associate geographical locations with patterns of disease. He successfully found a pattern in the distribution of childhood tumours – Burkitt's Lymphoma – and among his many achievements was the development of chemotherapy.

Back in the United Kingdom, along with colleagues, he shared his knowledge of the role of a high-fibre diet and its role in helping to prevent various cancers. His 1979 book, *Don't Forget Fibre in Your Diet*, sold over 200,000 copies worldwide in its first few printings.

In his long and widely-travelled career, Dr Burkitt reminded students and young doctors that they should be prepared to work for long periods if they wanted to achieve something of significance in medicine.

When autographing his book, he frequently wrote the following words:

> Attitudes are more important than abilities,
> Motives are more important than methods,
> Character is more important than cleverness,
> And the heart takes precedence over the head.[42]

223

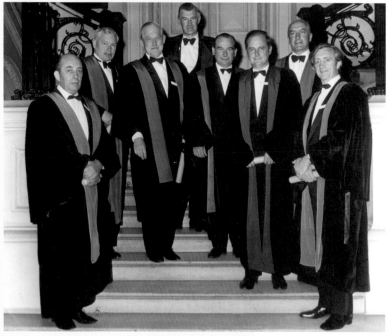

Risteárd Mulcahy, far right, with
colleagues at No 6 Kildare Street

The Cigarette
by WJ Leech

The cigarette was used as a
symbol of romance and
relaxation, until negative health
consequences were proved. The
addition of the cork tip was sold
as an aid to prevent irritation of
the throat – as the 1935
advertisement below says
'recommended by his doctor'.
In 1950 statisticians definitively
linked lung cancer and
smoking.[43] By 1965 the health
damage caused by smoking was
fully recognised by a television
advertising ban on tobacco.

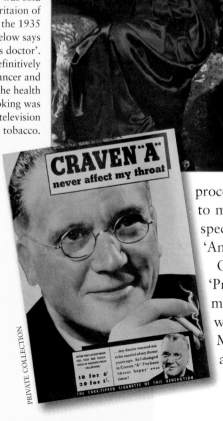

One such was Professor Risteárd Mulcahy, who
had already established a distinguished career as a
cardiologist, and had carried out important public
campaigns about smoking and heart disease.

Mulcahy was typical of many of the physicians
of his time, in that he became a member of the
Royal College of Physicians of London. He also
studied for an MD in his alma mater, University
College Dublin. When he returned from London to
medical practice in Dublin and joined the staff of
St Vincent's he did not see the need to join the
RCPI. He said:

By that time I had two senior qualifications and I
did not want to face further examinations. As the
two big Catholic hospitals – the Mater and St Vincent's – became more
prominent, it became obvious to many of us that we ought to join the
Irish College.

Senior colleagues in my team at St Vincent's were
already Members, and it would have been impossible for
me not to join with them. The College was aware that
we had not done their Membership examination, so
they devised a special one for us.

I remember going down to No 6 Kildare Street and
being examined by a three-man panel, including Dr
Bryan Alton. So I sat down and they obviously knew all
about my work on discouraging smoking, and I was also
well-known publicly about my views on smoking,
coronary disease and lung cancer.

The examiners asked me, 'Dr Mulcahy, do you think
smoking is a serious medical problem?' I replied, 'Yes',
and they said 'Thank you, you have passed the
examination.' It was almost like a miracle at Lourdes!

Though Professor Mulcahy recorded with typical
humour his examination for Special Membership of the
Irish College, there was a serious purpose behind the
procedure. A number of other outstanding physicians were admitted
to membership, in order to create a necessary balance across the
spectrum of an institution which had for too long retained its
'Anglican' trappings, because of its origin and long history.

Once this greater balance was achieved, and the image of
'Protestant' exclusivity had been erased by the touchstone of
medical excellence alone, the special membership examinations
were withdrawn. Between 1973 and 1978, a total of 53 'Special
Members' had been admitted, and elected Fellows 'as soon as
allowable'.[44]

CRAVEN "A"
never affect my throat

IN THE EASY-ACCESS INNER
FOIL PACK AND SEALED-
FRESH IN WEATHER-PROOF
"CELLOPHANE"

...my doctor warned me
to be careful of my throat
years ago. So I changed
to Craven "A". I've been
'throat happy' ever
since!

10 for 6⁴
20 for 1/-

THE CORK-TIPPED CIGARETTE OF THIS GENERATION

The need for such extraordinary measures was reflected in the background of those who were elected Presidents in that broad period of the College's history. As one medical historian, Tony Farmar, has pointed out:

> Edward Freeman, who was President of the College from 1952–55, was the first Catholic in the post since 1925, and the first UCD graduate, following eleven successive Trinity alumni.
>
> The next UCD man was Bryan Alton. As a result of this Trinity hegemony, for nearly two generations it was not customary for the senior men in St Vincent's to become Members or Fellows of the College, a situation which came to an end only in the 1970s.

Dr Bryan Alton
1919–91

Dr Bryan Alton is rightly regarded as another of the truly outstanding Presidents of the College. He was a greatly gifted individual and also a larger than life character, who travelled around in a Rolls-Royce, wore a diamond ring and diamond tie-pin, and incessantly smoked cigars inside and outside committee rooms and hospital corridors – much to the displeasure, no doubt, of some of his colleagues.

Behind the image, however, he was a shrewd operator, who did much for Irish medicine in general and for the College of Physicians in particular. He moved influentially among the corridors of power, and he was personal physician to a number of leading politicians, including Eamon de Valera, Erskine Childers, Charles Haughey and Brian Lenihan. He also served in the Irish Seanad from 1965–73.

He was extremely influential in medical circles, and he played a major role in the establishment of the Irish Committee on Higher Medical Training. He was also Chairman of the Medical Council, and the Postgraduate Medical and Dental Board, as well as being on the boards of several major hospitals and medical institutions.

Alton was particularly closely involved with the Mater Hospital where he was a physician. He became a co-founder of the highly successful Mater Hospital Pools, and he helped to raise large sums to establish a new Mater Hospital and the Mater Foundation.[45]

Alton had qualified as a dermatologist, but he also had a deep interest in cardiology and later developed his career in gastroenterology. He was elected a Fellow of the RCPI in 1947, and later served the College variously as Censor, Vice-President, Director of Education, and Treasurer. He was President from 1974–77.

One telling insight about Alton's style was illustrated during a meeting when a suggestion was made that the College might drop the 'Royal' title. Alton, who was an expert on gold and silver, was at that meeting and he reached out for a silver ornament on a nearby table. He turned it upside down and said, 'That

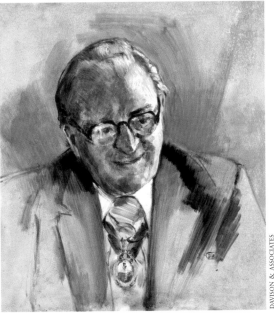

DAVISON & ASSOCIATES

Dr Bryan Alton,
portrait by Derek Hill
RCPI

Dr Bryan Alton was an outstanding College President from 1974–77. He was a flamboyant figure, who drove a Rolls-Royce and smoked Cuban cigars, but he was also a distinguished physician and College leader.
Dr Alan Grant, his successor as President, described him as 'a remarkable figure, transferring to our ancient institution the attitudes and methods of an industrial tycoon,... The Presidencies of David Mitchell and Bryan Alton were without doubt historic. It would be impossible, and impertinent, to make comparisons.'[46]

mark on the bottom is a Crown, and you can't buy a Royal title. It's worth its weight in gold, so you won't get rid of the 'Royal' title!'[47]

Professor John Crowe, who knew Dr Alton well, described him as an energetic and liberal man with a wide perspective:

> He could see far beyond the contemporary boundaries of Dublin medicine, and he was aware of the changes and developments in international medical practice ...
>
> He had sophisticated tastes with a wide spectrum of interests including fine art, antiques, porcelain and precious metals, and he was elected Master of the Company of Goldsmiths on three separate occasions.
>
> On a personal level, Bryan Alton was a kind man and a sympathetic doctor, warm and engaging with a relaxed sense of humour. He was never arrogant or aggressive, but was encouraging, generous and highly persuasive.
>
> Amusingly, he had a reputation for not requiring more than a few hours sleep, and he was usually at the hospital at 7.30 am or earlier, finishing a Cuban cigar presumably lit hours earlier. His intelligence, endless energy, these early starts and long days meant that he achieved far more than most during his very productive life.[48]

Professor Michael Ivo Francis Drury
1920–88

Another outstanding physician, and President of the College, from 1986–88 was Dr Ivo Drury who was a consultant physician, endocrinologist and a specialist in diabetes at the Mater Hospital and other hospitals. He was the recipient of many awards including the Fellowships of the American, Australian and Edinburgh Colleges of Physicians, and gained a high reputation as an international lecturer in his fields of medical expertise.

Drury was credited with helping to steer the College through the renovations of the interior of No 6 Kildare Street, after serious dry rot in the adjacent building owned by a Government department was also threatening their building. It took several years to gain a settlement of £250,000 for damages, and in the process the College made history. This was the first time that the owners of a building had been held liable for dry rot spreading into the adjoining premises. Despite the award for damages, the College also faced a considerable bill for refurbishment, however.

Under Ivo Drury's leadership, significant improvements were made to the College Building. As Dr Mitchell later noted:

> ... changes were made which altered and improved its ancient appearance. The re-decorated halls all lost their time-honoured names, and rooms were personalised in the modern fashion. The College Hall became the Corrigan Hall, the Statue Hall the Graves Hall, the Council Room the Stokes, the Middle Hall the Cheyne Room, and the Reading Room the Stearne Room.

The Library which had been badly affected by dry rot, was transformed and

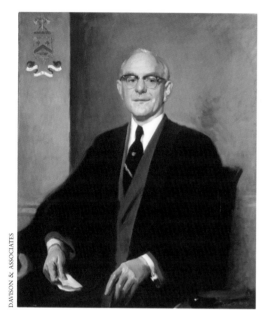

DAVISON & ASSOCIATES

Dr Ivo Drury, who was President from 1986–88. He was a highly regarded President of the College. He had a reputation as a reformer, who wished to continue the initiatives of his earlier colleagues and to continue with a wide programme of developments to ensure that the RCPI would remain at the forefront of the medical profession in Ireland and further afield. Sadly, he died suddenly in December 1988, during his term of office.

Dr Desmond Montgomery in an obituary in the *British Medical Journal* in February 1989, wrote:
It is not often given to a man to possess a high intellect and all the attributes of a scholarly and compassionate physician: when these are combined with a warm and friendly nature that man inspires admiration and love.

Portrait by John F Kelly

RCPI

impressively refurbished with considerable effort, and it remains one of the central attractions of the building.

Tragically, Dr Drury passed away suddenly in December 1988 during his term of office. His untimely death was mourned by a very wide range of his colleagues and friends, as well as his family.

Dr Drury had left the College in good shape. In the quarter-century leading up to 1988 he had witnessed and initiated many major developments, compared to the comparative stagnation of the previous half-century and more.

In 1963 there were only 155 Fellows, but by 1988 there were 1,650 Members and 550 Fellows. The College building had been renovated and refurbished, and was unrecognisable compared to the ramshackle structure of earlier years. A number of Faculties had been established; the membership examinations had been upgraded and modernised; postgraduate teaching continued to improve and advance, and a continuing programme of specialist lectures and social occasions had been developed.

Dr David Mitchell, one of the Presidents who had done so much to promote and sustain these vast improvement, noted modestly that 'the evidence is there to show that the College continues to extend its influence within the profession and beyond it'.[49]

This was good news after such a long period of stagnation, and there would be more good news in the years to come.

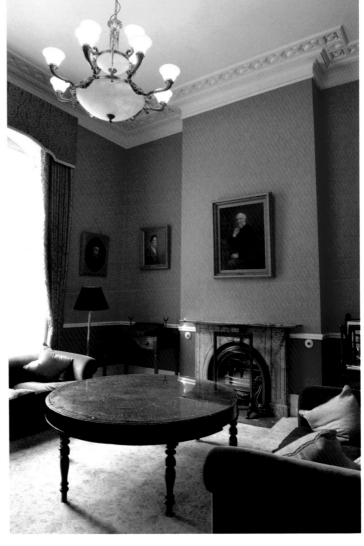

DERMOTT DUNBAR

The Stokes Room in the College

Lost Charter

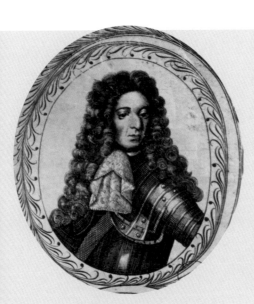

In 1977 the College decided to seek charity status and to achieve exemption from income tax. This required thirteen amendments to the College's Constitution, and to make these legal, the original Charter document was needed. Though several copies were readily available, the Irish Parliament would not accept one of these, unless the College could produce satisfactory evidence that the original had been lost or destroyed.

The College Secretary and Librarian then took matters into their own hands, and they made a search of all the banks' strong rooms – in one of which they found the Charter.

The College officers duly brought this priceless document before a joint Committee of both Houses of the Oireachtas, and in 1979, the Royal College of Physicians of Ireland Charter and Letters Patent Amendment Act became law.

Detail from the The Royal Charter granted by King William and Queen Mary in 1692
RCPI

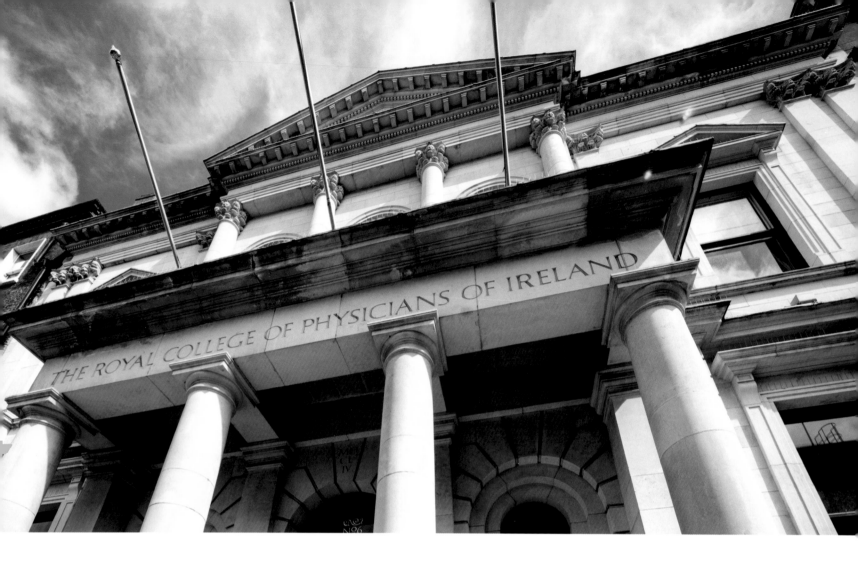

Full Circle

In the final decade of the twentieth century and well into the new Millennium, the Royal College of Physicians further consolidated its reputation and outreach. In many senses, the last 25 years have been one of the most productive periods in the College's long history.

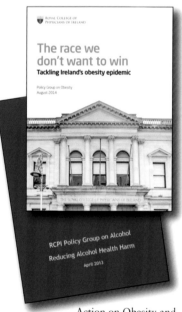

Action on Obesity and Alcohol – two current public health initiatives promoted by the College

RCPI

The headquarters at No 6 Kildare Street were extensively refurbished to a high standard, and two other offices and training centres were established nearby. Meanwhile the level of engagement on the part of the Fellows, Members and others associated with the College increased exponentially, and the RCPI developed an influential role helping to establish Government health policies and collaborating on national healthcare improvement initiatives. Raising public awareness of health issues and highlighting the need for individuals to take better care of their own health were key strategies.

Throughout these challenging times the College also maintained its historic mission of improving patient care and medical practice in Ireland – a policy which had inspired the founders more than 360 years previously.

In a real sense the College had come full circle. In the seventeenth century it had been established partly thanks to the expertise of medical outsiders who had come to Ireland through war and conquest. By the early twenty-first century, the College had achieved an international reputation for its excellence in medicine, healthcare, and post-graduate training. It was also exporting its expertise to many other parts of the world. All of this was a long way from the Fraternity of Physicians which John Stearne had established in 1654.

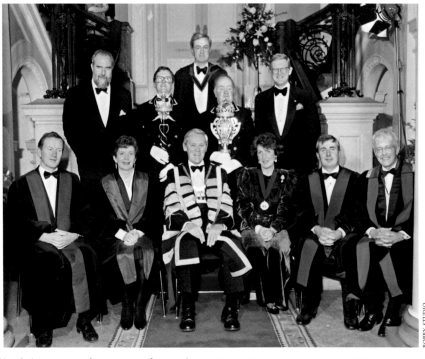

The 1992 Tercentenary of the College's Second Royal Charter: this photograph was taken in the College front hall after the Admission Ceremony at which HE Mary Robinson, President of Ireland was admitted as an Honorary Fellow and HRH Princess Margriet of the Netherlands was awarded the Stearne Medal.

SEATED FRONT ROW, LEFT TO RIGHT: Dr J Feely, Registrar, HE Mary Robinson, President of Ireland, Dr JS Doyle, President RCPI, HRH Princess Margriet of the Netherlands, Dr JAB Keogh, Treasurer and Dr ME Scott, Vice-President.

SECOND ROW LEFT TO RIGHT: Mr N Robinson, Mr M Gaughran, Caduceus, Mr J Farrell, Mace, Mr P van VollenhovenThird row: Mr JW Bailey, Secretary

Tercentenary 1992

In October 1992, the College celebrated the Tercentenary of the granting of the second Royal Charter by King William and Queen Mary. It seemed appropriate that one of the guests should be a member of the Dutch Royal Family, since King William had been the head of the House of Orange in Holland.

It was the intention of the College to bestow an Honorary Fellowship on Princess Margriet of the Netherlands. Others to be similarly honoured were to include the Irish President Mary Robinson, the Provost of Trinity College, Dr Tom Mitchell, and Dr Shaul Massry, Professor Emeritus of Medicine at the Keck School of Medicine at the University of Southern California.

However, the Fellows were informed in due course that it was the policy of the Dutch Royal Family not to accept Honorary Fellowships from overseas institutions, and so it was then decided to award the Dutch Royal guest with the prestigious Stearne Medal.[1]

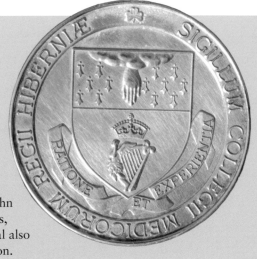

The Stearne Medal

In 1979, RCPI decided to create a medal which would be awarded 'from time to time to persons of distinction who have made a contribution to medicine in Ireland'.
Initially called the College Medal, it was first presented to Lady Valerie Goulding in 1979 for her contribution to establishing rehabilitation services in Ireland. In 1992 the medal was renamed The Stearne Medal, in recognition of John Stearne, who founded the Fraternity of Physicians, from which RCPI evolved. The remit of the medal also changed from national to international recognition.

Recipients of the Stearne Medal

1979	Lady Valerie Goulding
1992	Princess Margriet of the Netherlands (to mark the 300th anniversary of the founding of the King and Queen's of Physicians College in Ireland)
2005	Dr Catherine Molloy
2006	Mr Albert Reynolds
2007	Dr Stanley Roberts
2013	Professor T Joseph McKenna

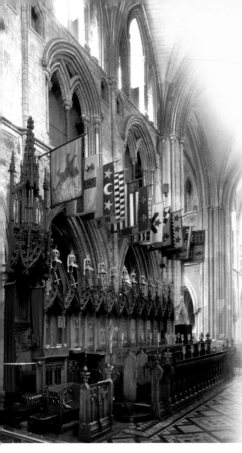

The tone of College Minutes for this period and for successive years became briskly businesslike, and therefore rather bland compared to those of earlier centuries. However, such a development is common to most institutions in the age of 'management language', where the avoidance of litigation and the implementation of that mysterious catch-all term, 'good governance', seems so important.

Nevertheless, reading between the lines, it is clear that the 1992 Tercentenary was an enjoyable affair. It proved so popular that the St Luke's Day Dinner was over-subscribed that year, and there even was a waiting list.

The celebrations also included various events held at St Patrick's Cathedral in Dublin which had a close connection with a College so steeped in Anglican tradition.

There was a series of scientific lectures, and the College donated £25,000 to the National Gallery of Ireland to help with the production of an impressive exhibition and handsome publication *The Anatomy Lesson: Art and Medicine*. However, just over a fortnight before the celebrations, the Minutes of 2 October, recorded that the Tercentenary Fund had brought in only £20,000 by that stage.

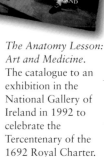

Interior of St Patrick's Cathedral where some of the events for the 1992 Tercentenary were held.
ST PATRICK'S CATHEDRAL, DUBLIN

As part of the celebrations, the Janssen Pharmaceutical company presented a new chain-of-office to the College President, Dr J Stephen Doyle, and there was an official State reception on 16 October. Three days later, at the routine monthly College meeting, Dr Doyle thanked everyone who had contributed to make the Tercentenary Celebrations 'such a success'. The Minutes noted formally that 'the reputation of the College had been greatly enhanced by these events, and the Fellows endorsed this sentiment'.[2]

The celebrations continued for a period after St Luke's Week, and in November 1992 the President was awarded an Honorary Fellowship from the Royal College of Surgeons in Ireland. A special joint dinner was held for the Councils of each College, and it was, by all accounts, 'a most enjoyable evening'. Surprisingly, this was the first time that the Councils of both Colleges had dined together, and this was an historic milestone in itself.

The Anatomy Lesson: Art and Medicine. The catalogue to an exhibition in the National Gallery of Ireland in 1992 to celebrate the Tercentenary of the 1692 Royal Charter.

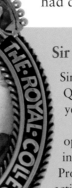

Sir Charles Edward Fitzgerald, 1843–1916

Sir Charles was 'Occulist-in-Ordinary in Ireland' to three British monarchs – Queen Victoria, King Edward VII and King George V – over a period of forty years.

He studied at Trinity and then in Paris. He returned to Dublin as an ophthalmic and aural surgeon, and worked with Sir Henry Swanzy as a surgeon in the National Eye and Ear Infirmary in Molesworth Street. He became joint Professor of Opthalmology at the Royal College of Surgeons, and took an active part in the amalgamation of the two Dublin ophthalmic hospitals, and in helping to establish the Royal Victoria Eye and Ear Hospital.

Fitzgerald was President of the College of Physicians from 1912–14, and donated the President's medal when he stepped down from office.[3]

The Travelling President's medal was presented to the College by Charles Fitzgerald in 1913.
RCPI

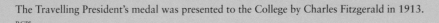

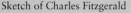

Sketch of Charles Fitzgerald
RCPI

Dr Stanley Roberts

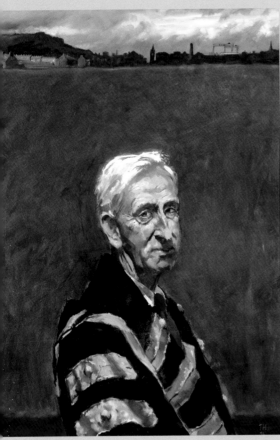

Dr Stanley Roberts was a consultant rheumatologist at the Royal Victoria and Musgrave Park Hospitals in Belfast. He was the second Ulsterman to become President of the College, from 1994–97. Earlier he had been Vice-President and Director of Examinations.

During his term in office, Dr Roberts led a sustained effort to affirm the high standard and international equivalence of the College examinations. He saw a need to foster harmony and a common purpose between the College, its Faculties and Institute. Of his election, he recalls:

> Before I could stand for the Presidency, I had to check with my employers. Rather too readily they agreed that I could easily be spared. There was a rumour that I brought down a busload of supporters to Dublin on the day. Actually, that was my 'election agent', a colleague who later himself became President. The interest stimulated a large attendance of Fellows, from whom a member of staff, strategically placed, was able to collect outstanding Annual subscriptions.

Though Dr Roberts enjoyed the role, the period was not without stress:

> I found that being President involved a lot of speaking, too many dinners and a good deal of travel. It meant driving up and down to Dublin two or three times a week and returning home around midnight to start work again next morning.
>
> In a Presidency lasting three years, my first was spent simply learning the job. In the middle years one tried not to do any irreversible damage, so that at the end the College could be returned intact to my successors.
>
> I was very busy during my term and when it ended, I soon suffered withdrawal. Fortunately (for me) I was offered chairmanship of the Committee at the centre of the hugely important extension of the College's responsibilities for postgraduate training. But after several years this position too had to be relinquished. At that time the then President, using a time-honoured phrase, 'we really don't know how we will manage without you', gave me a book and let me go. Of course it was I who would greatly miss an association which had been so crucial in my own medical career.[4]

In 1997 Dr Roberts was awarded an OBE 'for services to medicine', and in 2007, the Stearne Medal for his exceptional contribution to the College.

This portrait by Tom Halifax shows the Cave Hill overlooking Belfast's Albert Clock, and the distinctive yellow cranes of Harland & Wolff in the distance.
RCPI

The Tercentenary celebrations gradually faded into pleasant memory, as the everyday business of the College carried on. The Minutes of 19 October 1992 recorded a welcome report from the Treasurer, Dr Brian Keogh that the College had recorded a surplus of £60,000 for the year ending 31 July 1992, and that he had allocated £50,000 of this to the Building, Development and Maintenance Fund. The College would need all the money it could find to maintain its home at No 6 Kildare Street.

Raising Standards

However there were other major priorities in the development of the College, and not least in raising the examination standards to the highest level possible, and also reaching out to overseas medical institutions.

Dr Stanley Roberts, who took over from Dr Jim Fennelly, played an important role as Director of Examinations. He said:

> I prepared the papers, supervised the arrangements for the examiners and candidates with the assistance of a small staff.

He also talked about having been been an examiner himself:

> There were two members of staff in No 6 Kildare Street at that time. John and Alice Farrell lived in the basement, and they always welcomed us warmly with tea or coffee and biscuits. We examiners would work all day, and after the examinations were over, we had dinner. However there was always time for refreshments, and we used to go across to a nearby hotel for drinks.

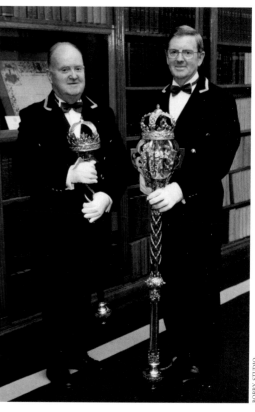

We used to sit in there relaxing, and then John would come across and say, 'Gentlemen, dinner is served'. So we would go back to the College where John was dressed in his grand uniform and holding the mace, and he would lead us in a procession into the room for dinner. It was such a warm and friendly place.

In these and subsequent years the College also took steps to successfully ensure that its Part Two examination measured up to the highest national and international standards. The required qualification to practise as a consultant was the MRCP, 'or its equivalent', which included the MRCPI.

Overseas Development

In 1992 there was another historic development when Dr Roberts and his senior colleague, Dr Brian Keogh travelled to Tabuk in Saudi Arabia to help administer the Part One examination, and to report to the College on the outcome. It was so successful that the Saudi authorities indicated their willingness to hold a similar examination in Tabuk a year later.

LEFT: John Farrell, College porter 1977–96 Michael Gaughran, College porter 1983–2001

During this period the College worked hard to maintain contacts with various overseas institutions, which led to the establishment of the RCPI examinations in several different countries. This in turn led to a significant rise in status for the College. There had been attempts to increase its overseas remit in earlier years, but despite good intentions expressed on all sides, these initiatives had achieved relatively little.[6]

By the early 1990s, however, the conditions for the development of permanent overseas contacts seemed more favourable. Dr Brian Keogh and Dr John Feely travelled to Oman to administer the Primary Membership examination of the College, and this initiative developed into a mutually beneficial relationship. A visit was also made to Egypt, but Keogh said later:

> We deferred that final decision. The general circumstances at the time did not seem right for us.[7]

In August 1992 the President of the College, Dr Stephen Doyle, travelled to South-East Asia to sign Memoranda of Understanding with the Academies of Medicine of Malaysia and Singapore. Later that year the Prime Minister of Malaysia and his wife visited the College in Dublin, and the Prime Minister was admitted as a 'ad eundem' Fellow of the Faculty of Public Health Medicine.

In March 1994 arrangements were being made for a joint meeting of the Royal Colleges in Dublin with the Academies of Medicine of Malaysia for June of that year.

In 1997 Dr Stanley Roberts, by that stage in his final year as President,

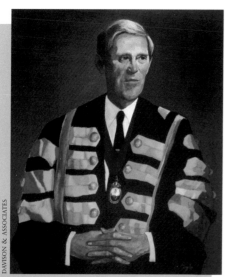

Portrait by John Timney Coyle
RCPI

Professor J Stephen Doyle

President of the College from 1991–94, Professor Doyle was a distinguished physician, and one of Ireland's leading gastroenterologists. He was one of the pioneers of modern endoscopy, and from 1975 until his retirement in 1993, he was Professor of Medicine at the Royal College of Surgeons in Ireland.

Following his retirement, he bought a small farm in Co Wexford, took up hunter breeding, and became a regular at the Dublin Horse Show. His obituarist in the *Irish Times* wrote:

> Professor Doyle is remembered as a kindly man, who discreetly helped those who were experiencing difficult times, and he was renowned for his integrity and honesty. A natural leader and excellent organiser, his aesthetic demeanour disguised a man who enjoyed life and a bit of craic.[5]

Professor Brian Keogh

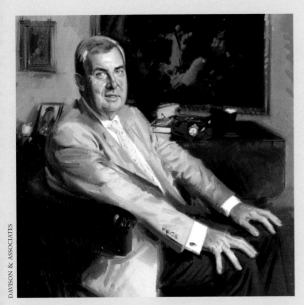

Portrait of Brian Keogh by AL Fisting
RCPI

Professor Brian Keogh, a consultant nephrologist, was President of the College from 1997–2000. He became a member of RCPI in 1972, and a Fellow in 1979. He is another College stalwart who gave exemplary service to RCPI, and was Treasurer from 1991–97.

Professor Keogh was involved with others, in the promotion of significant developments in training and examinations for the College, as well as its overseas outreach and also the extensive refurbishment of the headquarters building at No 6 Kildare Street. He said:

> As Treasurer of the College, it was imperative that expansion of the College activities both in Medical Education and Examination had to be a priority in the 1990s. For these reasons, examinations abroad were a major consideration, not withstanding our relationship with the UK Royal Colleges. Part of this process was the upgrading of standards in the Membership Examination and also continual professional development for our Fellows and Members.

Working closely with Stanley Roberts and John Feely, I believe these aims were achieved. I approached John Feely to stand for the Presidency of the College but he had many commitments to Trinity College and he would not have the time to serve in both positions. Sadly he died at an early age, and he was a great loss to the College.

As President, with the increased awareness of our reputation abroad and our growing expertise, I was very interested in developing the physical structure of the College, to accommodate the growing demand for College space. I worked closely with the Office of Public Works (OPW) to develop No 6 Kildare Street, at the rear of the College and the adjoining area, the property of the OPW. However, when I demitted the Office of Presidency, the incoming Officers at that time decided the plan would be too expensive. They decided to upgrade the building rather than to expand the College facilities, which was a great disappointment to me.[8]

travelled to Malaysia, and in Kuala Lumpur on 23 August, signed a Memorandum of Agreement between RCPI and the Malaysian Academy.

In his speech to the 31st Congress of the Academies of Medicine of Malaysia and Singapore, which was attended by the then Irish Ambassador to Malaysia Brendan Lyons, Dr Roberts said that the Memorandum:

> ... would have the effect of securing for doctors in Malaysia, as for postgraduate doctors in Ireland, identical and high standards of training which are internationally valid for physicians.
>
> This is not in any sense a short-term adventure for my College, but rather a natural extension of links already well-established at undergraduate level, and through the Irish universities' consortium, together with the activities of our sister College of Surgeons in Penang.[9]

As a memento of the occasion, Dr Roberts, on behalf of RCPI, presented to the Academy a solid silver George III 'Irish Loving Cup', made in Dublin in 1801 by Gustavus Byrne. He said that it was intended for use as a 'simple ceremony of friendship', and it was engraved with the crests of RCPI and the Malaysian Academy.

These overseas initiatives formed a strong base for an outreach which would broaden and deepen in the years to come.

Postgraduate Training

Another significant development during this period was the College's programme for Postgraduate Training. This was spearheaded by the President Stanley Roberts and a number of his senior colleagues, including John Feely, Brian Keogh and others, who worked closely with the Department of Health.

233

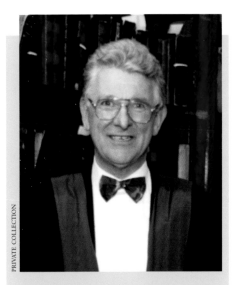

Dr George Murnaghan

Dr Murnaghan retired in December 2007 after more than nine years as Director of Higher Medical Training:

> I left a process that was up and running, and although it's for others to judge whether or not I had done a good job, I received great fulfillment from my role as Director.
>
> I had a long association with the College, going back to the time when it was run almost by the mythical 'man and a dog'. People did not want to upset the apple cart, and some believed that things were more or less fine as they were. However, when I left the College, it was in a much better position, because of the work and dedication of so many people. It had strategies, it had processes, and it was in a much better place.[10]

Roberts said later:

> We were required to give them certain guarantees about how we were going to work in a situation where they were delegating to the Royal Colleges the responsibility for post-graduate training for all the junior doctors in Medicine in the country. That was a huge undertaking.

Key Appointment

As a result, the College created the key position of Director of Higher Medical Training, and the first post-holder was Dr George Murnaghan. He had been a consultant obstetrician and gynaecologist in the Royal Maternity and Royal Victoria Hospitals in Belfast from 1974–87, but because of back problems he had to develop a new career in medical administration.

He became the Director of Risk and Litigation Management in the Royal Group of Hospitals Trust in Belfast, and gained a high level of expertise in administration, training and technology. This was precisely the kind of experience needed for the role he was about to undertake with the RCPI in Dublin.

Equally important, he was coming to Dublin as an 'outsider'. Although he was born in Dublin and had graduated in medicine from UCD, he had spent his professional life largely in the North, and therefore he carried no 'baggage' in a new role which required total independence from existing postgraduate training practices in the Republic. George Murnaghan was the right man, appointed to the right place, and at the right time. However, there were quite a few challenges for him along the way.

His wide brief included curriculum development, the introduction of a specialist registrar grade, the approval of training posts, and the recruitment and selection of specialist registrars. Another important role was the annual assessment of these appointees to ensure that progress was being made, and if not, to ensure remedial action was taken.

One of the greatest challenges was the human factor, because many consultants in the Irish Republic were opposed to the College taking over from them the management of the senior registrar posts. In the past, this had been done on a somewhat informal and personal basis.

Dr George Murnaghan recounts that during one of his first appointment procedures, a member of the panel was a close relative of one of the applicants for a specialist registrar's post.

> I told this senior consultant that he would have to withdraw from the panel during the interview for that particular post. His family member was appointed on merit, and rightly so, but the senior figure was not best pleased at what had happened, and he held it against me for quite some time.

Dr Murnaghan was greatly supported by Dr Stanley Roberts, and other senior figures, but he had to retain the independence of his post at all times, and also to develop a thick skin. He said:

I was not always welcomed with open arms when I went in to inspect a hospital. There were standards that had to be maintained, and if I was less than effusive about some of those places not coming up to scratch, I had to say so. People realised that if things did not change, they would be on their notice.[11]

During his time as Director, George Murnaghan visited every hospital in the Irish Republic and recalled:

The training developed from only six specialties to around 27 over time, and some were hugely impressive. Most impressive of all was the care taken by the people working in palliative medicine.[11]

More Building

For many decades in its earlier history, as we have seen, the College did not have a home of its own, and it was dependent on the willingness of successive Presidents to host functions in their homes. This was a costly business, particularly after the customary allowance of a supplement for claret was abolished in the early nineteenth century – during a period in which the institution which seemed invariably hard up.

The purchase and establishment of premises at No 6 during Sir Dominic Corrigan's time as President had been a breakthrough, but nearly a century later extensive refurbishments were needed.

By the early 1990s, it was time, yet again, to keep the building abreast of modern College developments and accommodation challenges.

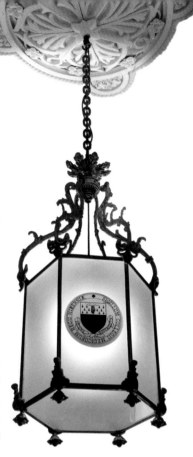

This ornate lamp with the College seal hangs in the entrance hall of No 6, and symbolises the retention of heritage at the heart of the building renovations.
DERMOTT DUNBAR

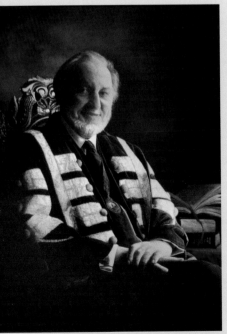

Dr Desmond Canavan

Dr Desmond Canavan, from Whitehouse in Co Antrim was the 136th President of the Royal College of Physicians, from 2000–03. His special expertise was in the treatment of infectious diseases.

He was educated at St Malachy's College Belfast, and graduated in medicine at Queen's University, Belfast in 1961.

His early training was at the Mater Hospital in Belfast, and he held senior posts at Purdysburn Fever Hospital and the Royal Victoria Hospital in Belfast.

Dr Canavan was closely involved with the College of Physicians and served on the examinations, education and training committees, and as a Censor. He was also a former Treasurer/Secretary and Chairman of the Corrigan Club.

He died in December 2004. In an *Irish Times* obituary, he was praised for his work with the College:

During his three-year term, there was a period of rapidly-accelerating development and expansion in the educational activity, with development of medical specialty programmes. With the popularity of the MRCPI or equivalent as a requirement of entry into training, the popularity of the examination grew at home and abroad.

As President, Dr Canavan significantly influenced these important developments for medicine. An inquiring mind, a profound interest in the subject, an ability to assemble and utilize the information available, so important for professional life, coloured everything he did.[12]

In 2006 RCPI named an award in memory of Desmond Canavan. This is presented annually by the Examinations department to candidates who have passed all parts of their Membership Exams, on the first attempt, within the year in question.

Professor T Joseph McKenna, who was Registrar from 1996–2003 and President from 2003–06 recalled:

> The refurbishing of the building had been coming into focus during the Presidency of Brian Keogh, and a lot of the decisions about how this would happen took place under the Presidency of Des Canavan. It continued during my Presidency, and the building was closed for a period while it was being renovated.
>
> Brian was an excellent Treasurer, and he became a very good President who pushed the developments. When his successors – Des Canavan, John Murphy and myself – took over, we continued. Brian and John invested a lot of time, counsel and energy, both executing the decisions and guiding the College, so I have nothing but very positive things to say about them.
>
> John Murphy and I were very much involved with the minutiae, agreeing the colour schemes, and the texture of the fabric and so on. It was a very interesting time.
>
> We wanted the College to be developed to a high specification, and to be versatile for all its functions. We realised that the office space was not going to be adequate to support the new College, and we wanted a building that would make a statement about our status. There is an old joke about a stranger asking a taxi-driver to take him to the College of Physicians, and ending up at the College of Surgeons. We wanted at least to bring the chances up to 50 per cent that the person might be actually brought to the College of Physicians![13]

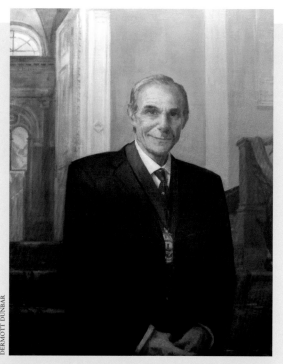

DERMOTT DUNBAR

Portrait of T Joseph McKenna by
Maeve McCarthy

RCPI

Professor T Joseph McKenna

Professor T. Joseph McKenna was Registrar of the College from 1996–2003, President from 2003–06, and a long-time member of the Council.

Widely regarded as one of the most successful Presidents in the history of the College, he was at the forefront of many of the important initiatives of recent times. These included the extensive refurbishment of the historic home at No 6 Kildare Street, the extension of the training programmes, and also the sweeping changes in the management structure and outreach to the wider world which better-equipped the College to meet the considerable challenges of the twenty-first century. He said:

> I was part of a group who had an opportunity to do something because of a momentum and a dynamic that was building up. European law required the setting up of a Specialist Register and the Medical Council asked us to set up a training programme roughly at the time when I became Registrar, and this coincided with a period when the College needed to be refurbished.
>
> So I had the opportunity to help front up for a short while during the refurbishment of the College and the development of the training programmes.
>
> I am happy where the College is today. I think the enemy would be to remain content with what we all have achieved, because in order to maintain a proper position of leadership and ensuring development, there is a dynamic that must be maintained.
>
> To preserve what is, would be a disservice. One must be pushing development. In doing that, there will always be mistakes, but there will always be the opportunity to correct them.[13]

In 2013 Professor McKenna was awarded the Stearne Medal for his outstanding contribution to the College of Physicians.

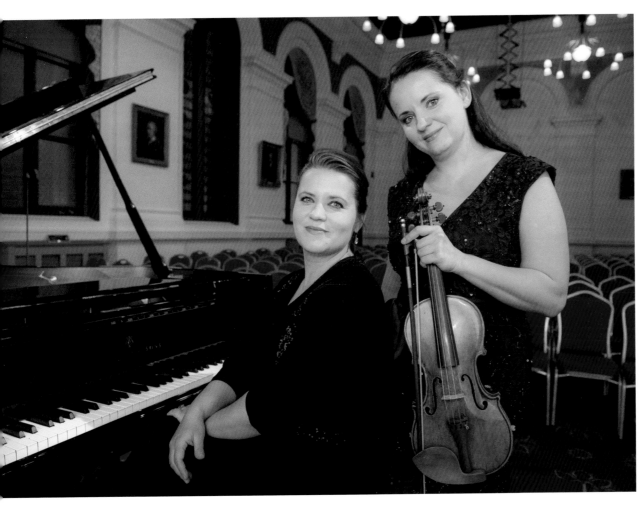

LEFT: The Skride Sisters, Balba (violin) and Lauma (piano), rehearsing for a recital in the Corrigan Hall in June 2015. This was staged in association with the Royal College of Physicians, the Latvian Embassy in Ireland, and the Royal Irish Academy of Music.

The recital was part of the KBC Great Music in Irish Houses Festival, featuring world-class musicians in beautiful buildings in Dublin, Wicklow and Kildare.

Alternative

Not everyone was happy with the new arrangements, and there had been elaborate plans to extend No 6 Kildare Street backwards towards Leinster House and to provide enough accommodation for proper office space as well. The complex negotiations continued with the Office of Public Works for several years, and the Minutes record an almost interminable series of meetings and reports to the College Council on the subject.

Finally it was decided to make No 6 Kildare Street the main function and corporate centre as well as the focus for important College ceremonies, and to rent space in a building nearby for administrative purposes. It was later necessary to rent space in another office building nearby.

Some people regarded this decision as 'a mistake', and in an ideal world it might have been better to have concentrated all the functions in one building, but that proved not to be possible.

The refurbishment of the College was costly and the building was reopened officially by the Tanaiste Mary Harney during St Luke's Week in 2005.

It was a project which had put a considerable strain on the College's finances at the time and for years afterwards, but the building has attracted a wide range of corporate and commercial events.

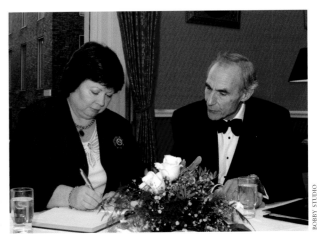

The Tanaiste Mary Harney with Professor T Joseph McKenna at the reopening of the refurbished College.
RCPI

237

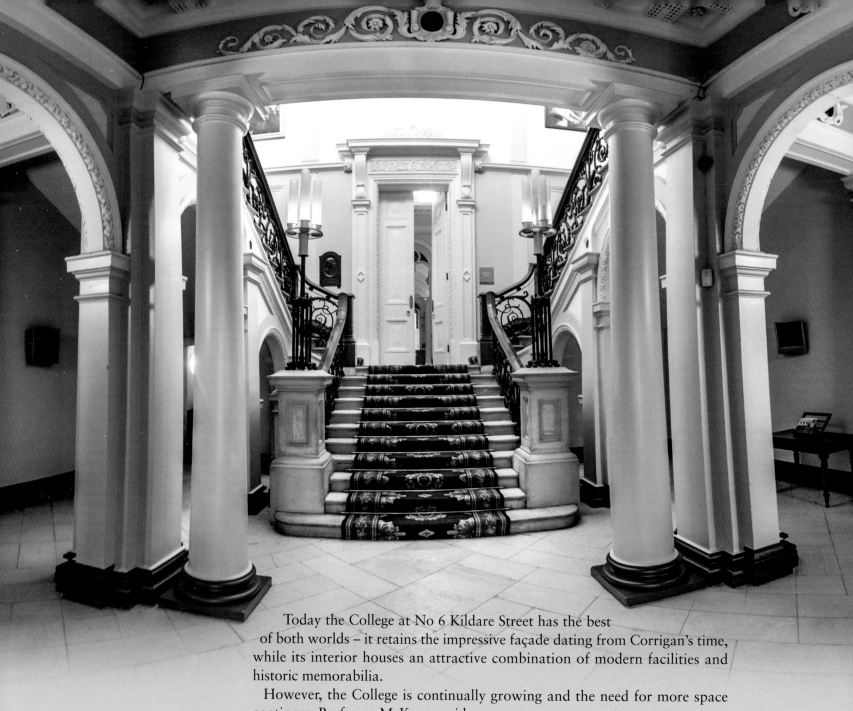

Today the College at No 6 Kildare Street has the best of both worlds – it retains the impressive façade dating from Corrigan's time, while its interior houses an attractive combination of modern facilities and historic memorabilia.

However, the College is continually growing and the need for more space continues. Professor McKenna said:

> When the major refurbishment of No 6 Kildare Street took place from 2003 onwards, it was not possible to envisage the requirement for space that developed even in the next five years. Therefore our estimated requirement for additional space was totally short of the reality.
>
> Now we would need a building, perhaps an office block, added on to this College, and I don't think that's the end of it. We are taking on more functions on behalf of the Department of Health and the HSE. I could see anything happening, and it may be that younger people may have less emotional attachment to No 6 Kildare Street than people of my generation. However I think that the history of the College is so strongly identified with this address that we should stay here, certainly as our main 'home'.[13]

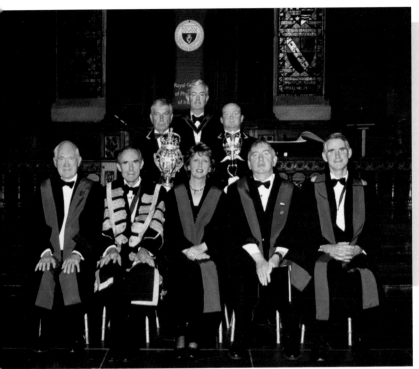

2004: Celebrating 350 Years

Mary McAleese was awarded an Honorary Fellowship as part of the 350th anniversary of the founding of the Fraternity of Physicians. Dr Gerry McElvaney, in his citation, said:

> That someone born in a working-class part of Belfast could some day become President of Ireland would have seemed a fantasy. Mary McAleese has achieved this. The President has made 'building bridges' one of her keystones in office. We are all familiar with the many ways she has sought to bring people of different traditions and beliefs together. Much of the work she does is unheralded and behind the scenes.

Dr McElvaney said that the College of Physicians 'was now at the centre of Irish Medical life and views itself in many ways, as similar to our President, as a servant of the people'.[14]

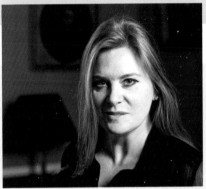

Joanna Holly

Joanna Holly, the Deputy CEO, joined RCPI in 2006, and brought with her a strong background in strategy development, organisational planning, change management and business focus. She developed this from her time spent working in the USA at Boston University Medical School and Harvard Medical School, and in Ireland at MMC Commercials Ltd and Trinity College Dublin Dental School and Hospital. Joanna holds a Master of Science in Organisational Behaviour from Trinity College Dublin.

> The College should be proud of its specialty training, education and healthcare improvement programmes and the esteem in which its graduates are held around the world. This training – developed and delivered by highly committed and enthusiastic Fellows of the College, Faculties and Institute – has served Ireland well.
>
> These people are the current and future leaders of Ireland's healthcare system, and their genuine commitment, compassion and energy to continually develop training, education and standards to meet the evolving needs of patients, is what drives progress within RCPI.

She also pays tribute to the role of the Government over many decades in promoting Ireland abroad.

> We have to give them credit because they really grounded *Ireland Inc.* so strongly that any organisation that had anything Irish to sell overseas was very well received. I am always amazed when I go to India, Malaysia, Australia and other countries to find that *Ireland Inc.* has such a brand of quality, particularly in education.

New Management Model

Within the first decade of the twenty-first century, the management structure was set on a new footing, to keep pace with the rapid development and outreach of the College.

Jonathan Bailey, who applied successfully for the new post of Secretary in 1990, was interviewed by a panel which included Dr Bryan Alton. Bailey recalls:

> The brief was amorphous and catch-all, and they did not seem to be clear about exactly what they wanted, though computerisation was high on the list. The College had been somewhat enclosed and they wanted to open it and broaden it out.
>
> I soon realised that it was important to balance different constituencies and mind-sets. It was not like a Chief Executive in a company, but rather like running a university.[15]

Bailey had a difficult start. Within a short period, two key figures had died – Brian Alton, the Treasurer, and Ciaran Barry, the President. Bailey says:

> ... by that stage we had an idea of the broad scaffolding, but the early deaths of these key figures caused great dislocation, and we had to fill in the gaps.[15]

The work of the College continued, but by 2006 Bailey knew that it was time for a change:

> This had been my fifth job and I knew in my bones that I did not want to continue in the College until my

Dr John Donohoe

Dr John Donohoe is a retired consultant nephrologist who was President of the College from 2007–11. He became a Member in 1981, and a Fellow in 1985. He has served on the Council since 1990 and was Registrar from 2006–07. He commented:

When I joined the College it seemed to lack direction and purpose, and at one point earlier on it had almost stalled. It's amazing that it survived, and that was due to people like Brian Alton who were able to find the money to keep it going.

In my early days, St Luke's Day had been reduced to a nice dinner on a Saturday night with a glittering guest list, but it was all a little bit shallow, and it seemed a pity that we would not develop it. Now it's beefed-up to a week-long exercise, with scientific, public and historical meetings. That's symbolic of the progress that we have made.

When I became President I was fortunate that this coincided with the appointment of Leo Kearns, our first professional CEO, and that was part of the catalyst needed to get the College on the right road.

We set about consolidating our financial basis, and our training and educational outreach, including Masterclasses which were streamed to around 25 hospitals throughout the country.

The RCPI had been regarded as a bit of an ivory tower, so we engaged in a programme of public seminars, including one on pregnancy, and the response was so great that people were queuing outside No 6 Kildare Street.

One important innovation was the updating of the database of Fellows and Members. It was chaotic, and required much hard work to modernise. However, out of that came the facility to pay subscriptions on-line, and to become part of the twenty-first century.

The College is a modern institution with a very long and distinguished history. It has weathered many storms, responding well to some of them, and not so well to others. Happily, it has survived and it has hit a new level of efficiency, achievement and purpose.

We cannot become complacent, and we probably need to broaden our income base to become less dependent on one source. As a former President, who has the privilege of still being on Council, I can see that the old vigour is still there, and it is heartening to realise that it's becoming even more vigorous as time goes by. It's this new involvement of Fellows and Members that is the lifeblood of the College, and this helps to guarantee its survival.[16]

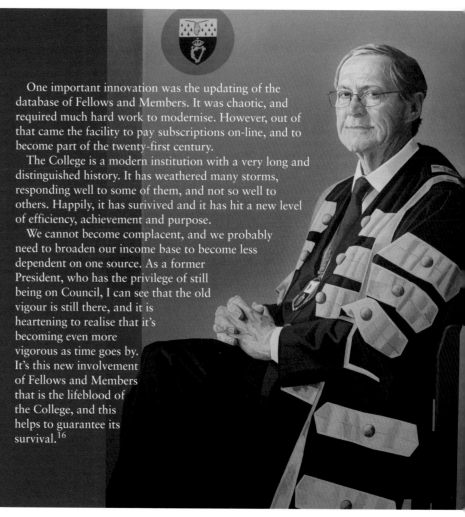

Portrait of John Donohoe by
James Hanley

retirement. I agreed with senior figures that it was time to bring in management consultants, and I made it clear to them that I did not want to be a long-term player as Secretary.[15]

Consultants

In 2004, the College appointed Deloitte to produce a Strategic Plan for the period from 2005–10, and the Report was delivered in May 2006. Professor McKenna was President during that period, and one of the drivers in producing the Report.

The Deloitte Report made a number of important recommendations, *inter alia*, to further develop the finances of the College, to raise and maintain training, education and examination standards in Ireland and overseas, to develop the crucial relationships with the Members and Fellows, encouraging their greater participation in the life of the College, and to improve overall the management and governance of RCPI.

The Report also recommended that the Council should be the Governing Body of the College, that a new Chief Executive Officer be appointed, and that a new Executive Committee should be established for setting and implementing strategy and ensuring the regular monitoring of the daily business of the College. The Executive Committee would consist of the President, the Treasurer, the Registrar and the new CEO.

The main recommendations of the Report were duly accepted, and the College moved into a new era of management, with a structure that was regarded as necessary for the challenges that lay ahead. Significantly, however, the delegation of authority from the Fellows to the Council is still a key item for discussion on the agenda each year at the Annual General Meeting on St Luke's Day. This is regarded as a necessary check and balance for the good governance of the College.

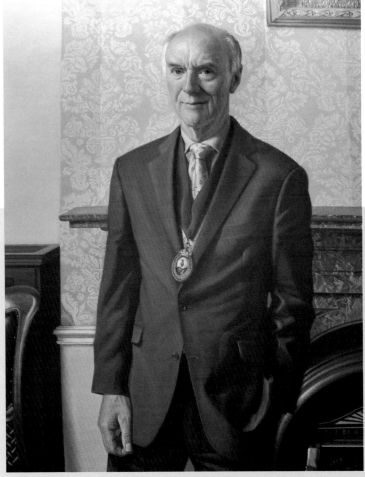

Portrait of John Crowe by
Alexander Carey Clarke
RCPI

DERMOTT DUNBAR

Professor John Crowe

Professor John Crowe, Consultant Gastroenterologist at the Mater University Hospital Dublin and Newman Professor at University College Dublin, was the College President from 2011–14. He became a Member of the College in 1974, a Fellow in 1980 and was Treasurer from 2005–10. He says of the College:

[RCPI] has a long heritage spanning five centuries of Irish life, from its foundation in 1654 by Dr John Stearne and his colleagues, to the present day. Right from its foundation, the College and its Fellows have played significant roles in Ireland, and today RCPI is a modern and innovative institution with an important role in modern Irish life.

RCPI always has been an important independent voice for high standards of medical practice, patient advocacy and public health in Ireland. Professional independence is one of its most important attributes of the Royal College of Physicians.

The core business of the College is the education and training of doctors for specialty practice, maintaining high standards of professional practice throughout a doctor's career, and conducting professional clinical examinations of a high international standard. I am pleased to say that all who work at RCPI are strongly committed to these objectives.

Modern medical practice is continuously evolving. The College considers external review and validation of its training and examinations to be fundamentally important and both have been subject to detailed international review within the last two years.

Public engagement is important. The College is not an island and engages with the public in an open and constructive way. It is certainly not reticent about making its views known on issues of public health, such as excess alcohol consumption, smoking and obesity and in doing so, has been effective at influencing government policy. No 6 Kildare Street opens its doors frequently during the year to the public for meetings on current topics of public interest which can be controversial and which are usually oversubscribed.

For the first time in its 361-year history there are lay members on Council, and the College is privileged to have the wisdom and advice of David Byrne a former Attorney General and EU Commissioner for Health, and Patricia Richard Clarke, a senior lawyer and Law Reform Commissioner.

Ireland is the College's home, but it has Members and Fellows all over the world and conducts its professional examinations in Australia, Dubai, India, Malaysia, Oman and Saudi Arabia.

RCPI has a significant international dimension and its overseas outreach is important and developing with international Chapters in Hong Kong, India, Malaysia, Oman and the United Arab Emirates. The College has recently established international training fellowships for senior trainees from Oman and Saudi Arabia. This excellent development is one that we would like to see extending to other countries, and particularly to Malaysia, where the RCPI Licentiate is awarded to the graduates of the RCSI Perdana and the RCSI/UCD Penang medical schools.[17]

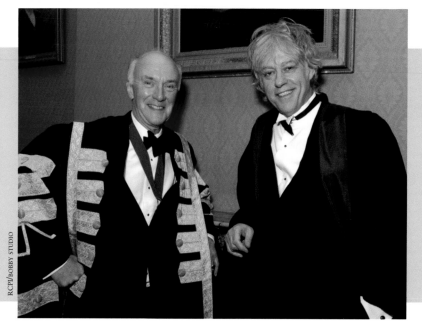

Sir Bob Geldof

Pictured here with Professor John Crowe, President of the College, during the award of an Honorary Fellowship in November 2011. In his citation Dr John Barragry paid tribute to Sir Bob Geldof's work for people in the developing world.

For most of his professional life, Bob Geldof has been an active, imaginative and dedicated crusader for Africa. In 1976 he said that he wanted to use his fame to do things, and he has. Unreservedly and with great pride, I as a Fellow of this College, recommend Sir Bob Geldof to be admitted to Honorary Fellowship of RCPI.[18]

First CEO appointed – Leo Kearns

Leo Kearns

'The College has transformed itself from where it was, in pretty much everything, and it will continue to do that. It's driven by the energy and commitment of its Officers, Fellows, Members, staff and trainees, and it has built very strong national and international connections. It's got a reputation as a voice that can be trusted in the health system, and it's now about continuing its mission of improving the quality of care to patients through training and education. While it will be constantly challenged to deal with a changing environment, I think it's now fit to take on that challenge.'[19]

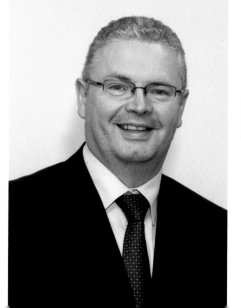

On 26 September 2006, the College announced the appointment of Leo Kearns as its first Chief Executive Officer. He had previously played a significant role in higher and medical education, particularly through the Working Group on Undergraduate Medical Education and Training, chaired by Professor Patrick Fottrell.

A number of major challenges faced the College at the time of Kearns' appointment. Fellows needed to become more engaged with the College, and the quality and scope of training and education needed to improve. The College also had to look outwards to engage more with the world, and also inwards, to improve its culture and capability. Kearns said:

Clinicians needed to have a voice in shaping national health policy, and the College embarked on a range of developments to help address these challenges. Led by senior clinicians with expert support from College staff, the Masterclass Educational Series was introduced and an Education Department formed; radical improvements occurred in postgraduate training; quality assurance programmes in histopathology and endoscopy were developed; and the College played a key part in the establishment of national clinical programmes, which have been critical in improving healthcare in Ireland.

We had to play an important role in bringing clinicians right back in to the centre of strategy and policy. I believe that the College became a conduit through which the health service was able to connect in a formal way with clinical leaders across the system.

Another important development was the establishment of the Forum of Irish Postgraduate Medical Training Bodies. The first Chairman was Professor McKenna, and Leo Kearns was the Secretary for six years.

The Forum allowed the medical professional bodies to work with the health system in a co-ordinated way. Joe McKenna provided the inspiration and leadership for its development, and demonstrated the need for the Colleges to act together rather than apart.

In mid-2013, Leo Kearns was seconded for a two-year period as the National Lead For Transformation and Change in the HSE.

Overseas Outreach

Later in 2013 the College appointed Dr Leonard JP O'Hagan, CBE as interim CEO. With his wide international business and marketing experience at the highest levels, he helped to greatly increase the overseas outreach of the College:

> Today we are all working together to create a world-class College, and we have developed a five-year plan that will ensure that the RCPI will be leading professional excellence for years to come. It will ensure the College continues to train doctors to the highest standards to cope with the health issues facing the Irish and international population, for at least the next 10 years. It is a powerful network and we are committed to fostering greater relationships in all corners of the globe.

Dr O'Hagan emphasised that the College has earned a reputation for training doctors to the highest international standards, and it is building on its success by developing international medical education and training programmes for doctors who wish to complete part of their training in the Irish healthcare system. At the same time, RCPI is using its expertise to develop global health policies and strategies to benefit developing countries.

> Embracing new technologies will enable us to deliver many of our strategic objectives, and the development of a digitally-enabled Global Medical Knowledge Platform will form a key part of our future activities. I am confident that the five-year strategic plan will position RCPI as a significant global presence in the medical knowledge and collaboration space in the years ahead.
>
> It has been my pleasure to work with so many dedicated doctors who care deeply for their patients and for the health and well-being of people in Ireland and beyond. I am also indebted to the dedicated staff who so ably support the work of the Royal College of Physicians of Ireland.

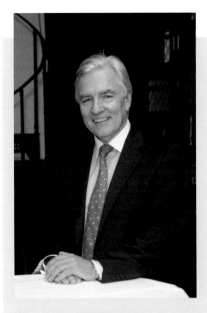

Dr Len O'Hagan

Dr Len O'Hagan was interim CEO of the College from 2013–15. In 2015 he became Vice President of Global Affairs.

He is Chairman of Northern Ireland Water, Chairman of the all-island Congenital Heart Disease Network board, and a non-executive director of Independent News and Media plc.

He is a former Chairman of Belfast Harbour Commissioners and of the Metropolitan Arts Centre. He was awarded honorary degrees from the University of Ulster in 2011 and Queen's University in 2012. Her Majesty the Queen awarded Len a CBE in 2013, and appointed him a Deputy Lieutenant for Co Down.

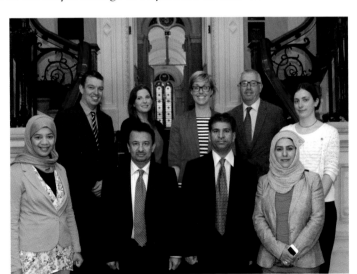

Overseas visitors at the College

BACK ROW, LEFT TO RIGHT: Staff from RCPI – Mr Martin McCormack, Head of Operations; Ms Ciara O'Donohoe, Programme Coordinator, International Affairs; Ms Ciara Buckley, Manager, International Affairs; Mr John Magner, Head of International Affairs; Ms Harriet Wheelock, Keeper of Collections

FRONT ROW, LEFT TO RIGHT: Staff from Sultan Qaboos University Hospital, Oman – Ms Samira Al Rabsi, Nurse Educator/Administrator; Dr Saif Al-Yaarubi, Paediatric Endocrinologist/Chairman Hospital Training Committee; Dr Abdullah Al Mujaini Ophthalmologist/Director Training & Continuing Professional Development; Dr Huda Al Uwaisi, Nurse Educator/Administrator
RCPI

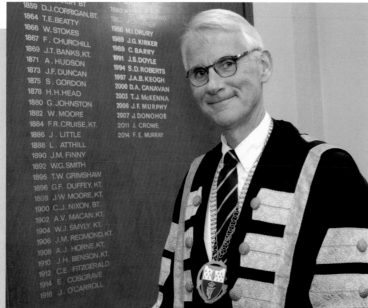

Professor Frank Murray

A distinguished consultant gastroenterologist in Dublin with family roots in Northern Ireland, Professor Murray was installed as President of the College on St Luke's Day, 2014. He became a Member in 1982 and a Fellow in 1994. From 2007–14 he was Registrar of the College. Professor Murray comments:

It is a great honour to be President of the Royal College of Physicians of Ireland and to continue the great work of my many distinguished predecessors.

Medicine constantly changes but the mission of the College remains essentially the same – to care for the health of the nation.

Since I became involved with RCPI in 1982, I have taken an active part in the work of the College to enhance medical training and in other areas, particularly advocacy around alcohol.

I feel that I am part of the College and the College is part of me. The College can help all of its trainees, Members and Fellows to make a difference.

It is a great challenge and privilege to serve this great College as best I can.

Training and Help for Doctors

Professor Frank Murray, who was installed as President in 2014 sees his main priorities as being to further develop medical training:

This is at the heart of RCPI's activities, and I am also focused on supporting the health and well-being of the doctors on our medical training programmes, and that of our Members and Fellows.

Promoting and advocating for the health of the Irish population has long been part of our mission and is something that I am proud to continue. I also am committed to developing a philanthropic role for RCPI, to do good where we can.

It would be foolish to claim that we in the College could end world poverty, for example, but we can do much to provide help in the developing world in a focused manner, particularly by helping to develop medical training.

The Developing World

The EQUALS initiative, which is chaired by David Weakliam, is currently sending out medical equipment to Zambia for use in hospitals there.

I am very much part of this bigger team and I look forward to providing direction and support where I can. EQUALS is also helping to train staff in Zambia to maintain this equipment, which can make a difference to the provision of healthcare in that country. We are also taking steps along with the Government of Zambia to help them to develop a modern training programme for their doctors, using much of the experience and expertise developed in Ireland

Today RCPI is delivering postgraduate medical examinations beyond Ireland in centres in the Middle East and Asia. The College has also developed international medical graduate programmes, that attract doctors from Oman, United Arab Emirates, Saudi Arabia, Kuwait and Pakistan and India.

Much of our international reputation is a testament to the enormous contribution that so many of our more than 10,000 trainees, Members and Fellows are making in 85 countries in all corners of the world.

We are proud of them and keep in touch with them through our international Chapters and other events, particularly around our annual St Luke's Symposium each October.

Public Health

In tandem with these initiatives, the College is also a strong advocate for public health measures that will ease the burden of chronic illness in the future, and improve the quality of life for the population in general. RCPI has brought together groups of healthcare professionals to craft evidence-based policies around tobacco, alcohol and obesity. From 2015, two new policy groups will focus on physical activity and ageing:

> These groups are formulating policy measures and are actively engaging with the Government and others to have them implemented. We have enjoyed some success and I am confident we will continue to inform the public health debate, new legislation, and other measures that can be beneficial for the Irish population.

Strong Voice

Professor Murray stresses that:

End the sale of cheap alcohol, expert urges
Country's relationship with drink 'now at crisis point'

Irish Daily Mail, 11 March 2015: headline to an article by Jennifer Bray on Professor Frank Murray's report to the Oireachtas health committee.

> As a College we have a strong voice and we are making it heard where it matters.
>
> Our call for an end to Diageo's drinking festival, 'Arthur's Day', in 2014, led to its demise. RCPI is also lending its support to the Public Health (Alcohol) Bill 2015 that is an important first step in addressing Ireland's unhealthy relationship with alcohol. [The Bill] contains important measures, such the introduction of a minimum unit price for alcohol (MUP), which has the potential to reduce the harm that alcohol is increasingly causing in our society. We are strong advocates in this arena, and we can make a difference.
>
> Our clinicians are also leading many changes and initiatives within the Irish healthcare system through the 24 National Clinical Care Programmes (being) developed with the Health Service Executive. These programmes are saving lives, facilitating greater access to the health services for patients and creating consistent models of care.

Turning Point

The President believes that placing medical training at the heart of the College's activities, and creating a professional management structure to support it, was the biggest development in the history of the College:

> The Deloitte Report was a turning point for RCPI. The new CEO, Leo Kearns then helped greatly to modernise the College, and to help us to work more closely with the national authorities in tackling Ireland's complex health challenges.
>
> More recently Dr Len O'Hagan, who has been CEO during Leo's secondment, has helped to give us a sharp focus on strategy, and to develop a world-class service in everything we do.
>
> I also believe that Professor Joe McKenna, previous Registrar and President of RCPI was the major driving force in our modernisation. The emphasis on medical training is what has really made the College what it is today, and has made it fit for purpose for the twenty-first century.

245

Changing Times at RCPI

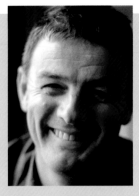

Dr Ronan Kavanagh is a consultant rheumatologist at the Galway Clinic, and a Member of the College. He comments:

For the last couple of decades, like most of the physician colleagues of my generation, I have not had a whole lot to do with the Royal College of Physicians of Ireland. Having passed the MRCP examination in 1993, my only regular dealings with them have been an annual, last-minute scramble to enter CPD activities on their website. My only reminder of their activities was photographs of conferring ceremonies in the Events sections of medical press publications.

These were pictures of established-looking and slightly older physicians in College gowns and ties, looking rather pleased with themselves as they handed out scrolls to new Members or Fellows. Thoreau once said, 'Beware of any venture that requires new clothes'.

Overall, my impression of the RCPI was one of a rather austere, conservative and Dublin-centric sort of establishment without a whole lot to offer a physician like me. The 'culchie' in me also admits to being a little intimidated by portraits of the elder lemons of Irish medicine that adorn the walls of its imposing building at No 6 Kildare Street.

The physicians captured in those oil paintings looked how I might have imagined my MRCP examiners to have looked (before I had actually met them): imposing, aristocratic, intolerant of imperfection (I had more than one attempt at the MRCP!), and a little stuffy.

However, things have been changing, as Dr Kavanagh confirms:

It has become increasingly obvious to me (largely through their active and engaging Twitter account and newly-revamped website) that the College appears to have been busy reinventing itself, in terms of what it had to offer to Irish physicians twenty years ago (for example, the Membership examination). RCPI is now almost unrecognisable.

Under the direction of their VP of Education, Dr Diarmuid O'Shea, they now offer an almost bewildering variety of educational programmes – highly relevant to those practising modern medicine.

They have also started to engage with the general public through their annual St Luke's Day meeting. Their recent well-publicised campaigns on alcohol harm to health and their 'Let's Talk About Sex Awareness' campaign are other good examples of the College using its profile to engage with the general public on important health-related issues. It is also nice, for a change, to see doctors being reflected in such a positive light in the media.

Recently, the prospect of becoming a Fellow of the College came up with a few of my younger medical colleagues, over coffee.

'You've been knocking around for a while, Ronan,' one of them asked. 'Have you ever thought of becoming a Fellow?'

'I'm beginning to think that I might be too old…'[20]

Past Present and Future

The College survived many tumultuous periods of history. This entry in the Minute Book notes the postponement of the annual St Luke's Day Dinner of 1914, just weeks after the outbreak of the First World War.
RCPI

The College of Physicians of Ireland has come a long way since it was established in 1654 by John Stearne as a Fraternity of Physicians. Its story is one of great survival through all the vicissitudes of history, including conflict and war, financial crises, clinical challenges, and political upheavals. Not least of these was the Partition of the island, in the early twentieth century. In the aftermath of this, both parts of Ireland succumbed to virtual nervous breakdowns, and the College very nearly ceased to exist.

As a former President noted:

Non-teaching and almost homeless, the College of Physicians remained for too many of its early years a small, high-grade, exclusive Protestant club.[21]

All that has changed, however, and the College is now an interdenominational and multi-cultural institution. A great deal has been achieved, particularly in recent years. Dr Alan Grant, President from 1977–80 made a heartfelt plea, when he said he had only three wishes:

… that the College will continue to thrive, that it will expand its influence in Ireland, and that it will increase its repute beyond these shores.[22]

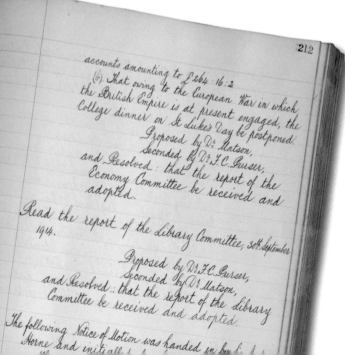

212

accounts amounting to £264 : 16 : 2

(b). That owing to the European War in which the British Empire is at present engaged, the College dinner on St Luke's Day be postponed.
Proposed by Dr Matson,
Seconded by Dr F.C. Purser,
and Resolved: that the report of the Economy Committee be received and adopted.

Read the report of the Library Committee, 30th September 1914.

Proposed by Dr F.C. Purser,
Seconded by Dr Matson,
and Resolved: that the report of the Library Committee be received and adopted.

The following Notice of Motion was handed in by

In all three counts, the College has been successful, and doubtless this success will continue. The achievements of the past 360 years and more have been due to the hard work and vision of so many people, and not just those mentioned in this publication. The bland language of modern management, the speed of current technology and the complex implementation of healthcare systems, are just three factors that have radically changed the face of medicine since the days of the early pioneers.

The approach within the College itself has also changed for the better, from the somewhat ramshackle management of earlier times, when money to keep it going was extremely scarce, and when – on at least one infamous occasion – personal animosities were settled by a sword duel on a Dublin street! Nevertheless, one of the duellists, Sir Patrick Dun, is still fondly remembered as a major figure in the history of the College.

Doubtless there are still differences of opinion today, as there are in every institution run by human beings, but these are handled in a much more professional manner – though perhaps not as colourfully as on occasion in the old days, when many larger-than-life characters dominated the scene.

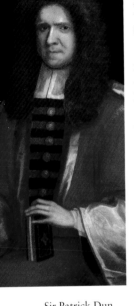

Sir Patrick Dun,
1642–1713 – one of
the truly great figures
in the history of the
College
RCPI

DAVISON & ASSOCIATES

Huge Changes

The College has changed out of all recognition during its long journey. Dr John Fleetwood, one of the pioneering medical historians, wrote in 1951:

> We have come a long way since Dian Cécht founded the Irish medical profession. Witchcraft and religion, reason and superstition, prejudice and magnaminity, have all played their part in making us what we are today. But they were only influences. The big thing in any community is the men (and women) who make it up. The lesser are just as important as the greater. And so it is today.[23]

This is the voice of wisdom, but perhaps the last words should lie with Robert James Graves, 1796–1853, an outstanding pioneer of modern medical practice. He wrote:

> A short and transitory existence has been allotted to our bodies; individuals die, generations pass away, but the common intellect of mankind fears not the same fate, nor shares the same brief mortality.[24]

The story of the College of Physicians will continue, progress in medicine will continue, and the healing touch of physicians and their colleagues will continue, to bring comfort and hope where it is needed.

This lies at the heart of the important and eventful story of the Royal College of Physicians of Ireland, and will continue to do so, as long as the welfare of the patient remains at the centre of all it sets out to achieve.

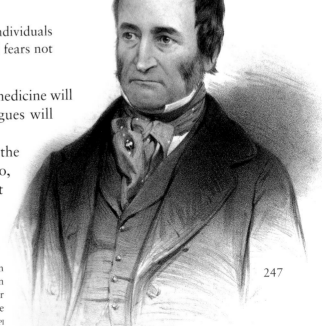

Robert Graves, 1796–1853 – an
outstanding pioneer of modern
medical practice, and a former
President of the College
RCPI

247

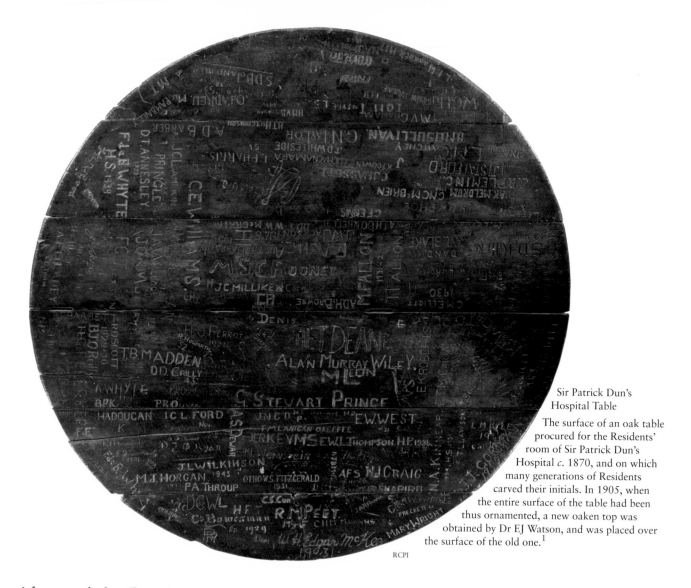

Sir Patrick Dun's Hospital Table

The surface of an oak table procured for the Residents' room of Sir Patrick Dun's Hospital *c.* 1870, and on which many generations of Residents carved their initials. In 1905, when the entire surface of the table had been thus ornamented, a new oaken top was obtained by Dr EJ Watson, and was placed over the surface of the old one.[1]

RCPI

Presidents of the Royal College of Physicians of Ireland

The Presidents were elected on St Luke's Day, 18 October, unless otherwise stated

FRATERNITY OF PHYSICIANS OF TRINITY HALL

1654–67	John Stearne

COLLEGE OF PHYSICIANS IN DUBLIN

1667–69	John Stearne. (Died in office)
1672–74	Sir Abraham Yarner
1674–75	Ralph Howard
1675–77	Charles Willoughby
1677–81	Robert Waller
1681–87	Patrick Dun
1687–89	John Crosby (Election not approved by TCD, no further election made until 1690)
1690–92	Patrick Dun

KING AND QUEEN'S COLLEGE OF PHYSICIANS IN IRELAND

1692–94	Patrick Dun
1694–95	John Madden
1695–96	Ralph Howard
1696–97	Sir Patrick Dun, Kt.
1697–98	John Madden
1698–99	Patrick Dun
1699–1700	D Comyng
1700–01	John Madden
1701–02	Ralph Howard
1702–03	Thomas Molyneux
1703–04	Richard Steevens
1704–05	William Smyth
1705–06	Robert Griffith
1706–07	Sir Patrick Dun
1707–08	Ralph Howard
1708–09	William Smyth
1709–10	Sir Thomas Molyneux, Bart.
1710	Richard Steevens (Died in office)
1710–11	William Smyth (Dec. 19)
1711–12	Robert Griffith
1712–13	Patrick Mitchell
1713–14	Sir Thomas Molyneux
1714–15	James Grattan
1715–16	Richard Hoyle
1716–17	Richard Helsham
1717–18	Samuel Jemmatt
1718–19	Bryan Robinson
1719–20	William Smyth
1720–21	Sir Thomas Molyneux
1721–22	William Smyth
1722–23	James Grattan
1723–24	Patrick Mitchell
1724–25	Patrick Hoyle
1725–26	Richard Helsham
1726–27	Samuel Jemmat
1727–28	Bryan Robinson
1728–29	Henry Cope
1729–30	Francis Le Hunt

1730–31	Samuel Arnoldi	1790–91	Arthur Saunders	1873–75	James Foulis Duncan
1731–32	Thomas Madden	1791–92	William Harvey	1875–78	Samuel Gordon
1732–33	Alexander McNaughton	1792–93	Francis Hopkins	1878–80	Henry Haswell Head
1733–34	William Stephens	1793–94	Patrick Plunket	1880–82	George Johnston
1734–35	John van Lewen	1794–95	Edmund Cullen	1882–84	William Moore
1735–36	John Hemsworth	1795–96	Edward Hill	1884–86	Francis Richard Cruise
1736–37	Thomas Kingsbury	1796–97	Arthur Saunders	1886–88	James Little
1737–38	Francis Foreside	1797–98	William Harvey	1888–90	Lombe Atthill
1738–39	James Grattan	1798–99	Francis Hopkins	1890–92	John Magee Finny
1739–40	Bryan Robinson	1799–1800	Robert Perceval (Nov 4)	1892–95	Walter George Smith
1740–41	Henry Cope	1800	William Harvey (Aug 4)	1895–96	Thomas Wrigley Grimshaw
1741–42	Francis Le Hunt	1800–01	Patrick Plunkett	1896–98	Sir George Duffey
1742–43	William Stephens	1801–02	Edward Hill	1898–99	Sir John William Moore
1743–44	John Hemsworth	1802–03	William Harvey	1900–02	Sir Christopher J Nixon
1744–45	Thomas Kingsbury	1803–04	Francis Hopkins	1902–04	Sir Arthur Vernon Macan
1745–46	Patrick Hewetson	1804–05	Alexander Pellisier	1904–06	Sir William Josiah Smiley
1746–47	Edward Aston	1805–07	James Cleghorn	1906–08	Sir Joseph Michael Redmond
1747–48	Edward Smyth	1807–08	Daniel Mills	1908–10	Sir Andrew John Horne
1748–49	Robert Robinson	1808–09	Edward Hill	1910–12	Sir J Hawtrey Benson
1749–50	Sir Edward Barry, Bart.	1809–10	William Harvey	1912–14	Charles Edward Fitzgerald
1750–51	Thomas Lloyd	1810–11	Francis Hopkins	1914–16	Ephraim MacDowel Cosgrave
1751–52	John Anderson	1811–12	James Cleghorn	1916–19	Joseph Francis O'Carroll
1752–53	John Ferrall	1812–13	Thomas Herbert Orpen	1919–22	Sir James Craig
1753–54	Ezekiel Nesbit	1813–14	Edward Hill	1922–23	Michael Francis Cox
1754–55	Constantine Barbor	1814–15	William Harvey	1924–25	Sir William John Thompson
1755–56	Anthony Relhan	1815–16	Francis Hopkins	1925–27	Henry Thomas Wilson
1756–57	Richard Wood	1816–17	James Cleghorn	1927–30	William Arthur Winter
1757–58	Adam Humble	1817–18	Anthony Gilholy	1930–33	Thomas Gillman Moorhead
1758–59	Henry Quin	1818–19	Thomas Herbert Orpen	1933–34	Francis Carmichael Purser
1759–60	William Stephens	1819–20	Hugh Ferguson	(Died	in office.
1760–61	Robert Robinson	1820–21	James Callenan	1934–36	John Agar Matson
1761–62	Patrick Hewetson	1821–22	George Francis Todderick	1937–40	William Boxwell
1762–63	John Ferrall	1822–23	Robert Bredin	1940–43	Robert James Rowlette
1763–64	Ezekiel Nesbit	1823–24	Samuel Litton	1943–46	William Geoffrey Harvey
1764–65	Constantine Barbor	1824–25	John O'Brien	1946–49	Bethel Solomons
1765–66	Richard Wood	1825–26	James John Leahy	1949–52	Leonard Abrahamson
1766–67	Henry Quin	1826–27	William Brooke (Feb 20)	1952–55	Edward Thomas Freeman
1767–68	Sir Nathaniel Barry, Bart.	1827–28	Hugh Ferguson	1955–58	Francis Joseph O'Donnell
1768–69	Clement Archer	1828–29	Charles Richard A Lendrick	1958–60	Patrick Theo Joseph O'Farrell
1769–70	Constantine Barbor	1829–31	Samuel Litton	1960–63	Robert Elsworth Steen
1770–71	John Ferrall	1831–33	Hugh Ferguson	1963–66	Brian Pringle
1771–72	Henry Quin	1834–35	Jonathan Osborne	1966–69	Alan Thompson
1772–73	Sir Nathaniel Barry	1836–37	Charles Philips Croker	1969–72	David Mitchell
1773–74	John Ferrall	1838–41	George Alexander Kennedy	1972–74	William Jessop
1774–75	Henry Quin	1841–43	Sir Henry Marsh, Bart.	1974–77	Bryan Alton
1775–76	Sir Nathaniel Barry	1843–45	Robert James Graves	1977–80	Alan Grant
1776–77	Clement Archer	1845–47	Sir Henry Marsh	1980–83	Dermot Holland
1777—78	Francis Hutcheson	1847–49	Robert Collins	1983–86	John Kirker
1778–79	John Ferrall (died in office)	1849–51	William Stokes	1986–88	Ivo Drury
1779–80	Henry Quin (Sept 20)	1851–53	William Fetherston-Haugh	1988–91	Ciaran Barry
1780–81	Francis Hutcheson		Montgomery	1991–94	Stephen Doyle
1781–82	Henry Quin	1853–55	Evory Kennedy	1994–97	Stanley Roberts
1782–83	Edward Hill	1855–56	John Mollan	1997–2000	Brian Keogh
1783–84	Arthur Saunders	1857–59	Sir Henry Marsh	2000–03	Desmond Canavan
1784–85	William Harvey	1859–64	Dominic John Corrigan	2003–06	T Joseph McKenna
1785–86	Francis Hopkins	1864–66	Thomas Edward Beatty	2006–07	JF Murphy
1786–87	Patrick Plunket	1866–67	William Stokes	2007–11	John Donohoe
1787–88	Edmund Cullen	1867–69	Fleetwood Churchill	2011–14	John Crowe
1788–89	Charles William Quin	1869–71	John Thomas Banks	2014–	Frank Murray
1789–90	Edward Hill	1871–73	Alfreds Hudson		

Vice-Presidents of the Royal College of Physicians of Ireland

Elected 18 October each year unless otherwise stated

The role of Vice-President is mentioned in the 1692 Charter, and was to be held by one of the Censors of the College. Following the election of John Madden as Vice-President in 1693, no other Vice-President is identified in the Officer's Role or Minute Books until 1812.

1693–94	John Madden (January)	1885–87	J Magee Finny	1962–64	BE O'Brien
1694–1811	*Not identified*	1887–89	Arthur Wynne Foot	1964–65	WJE Jessop
1812–13	James Callanan	1889–91	George F Duffey	1965–66	PA McNally
1813–14	James John Leahy	*1891–92*	*Not identified*	1966–67	JA Wallace
1814–17	George Todderick	1892–94	John William Moore	1967–68	BG Alton
1817–22	Samuel Litton	1894–96	Andrew J Horne	1968–70	M Abrahamson
1822–23	John O'Brien	*1896–97*	*Not identified*	1970–71	Harry O'Flanagan
1823–25	W Stack	1897–98	William Beatty	1971–72	JG Kirker
1825–26	Robert J Graves	1898–1900	William J Smyly	1972–73	Patrick Sweeney
1826–27	Samuel Litton	1900–02	Joseph Redmond	1973–75	P Holland
1827–28	John O'Brien	1902–04	Henry T Bewley	1975–77	Alan Proctor Grant
1828–29	George Alexander Kennedy	1904–06	Edward Lennon	1977–78	Douglas Mellor
1829–31	John O'Brien	1906–08	Conolly Norman	1978–79	T Dundan
1831–33	James Henry	1908–10	Ephraim MacDowel Cosgrave	1979–80	OC Ward
1833–34	W J Morgan	1910–12	George Peacock	1980–82	J Stephen Doyle
1834–35	John O'Brien	1912–14	James Craig	1982–83	LG McElearney
1835–36	Charles P Croker	1914–16	Joseph O'Carroll	1983–84	Ivor Drury
1836–38	William F Montgomery	1916–18	Henry T Bewley	1984–85	SD Roberts
1838–39	Jonathan Osborne	1918–19	Alfred R Parsons	1985–86	Oliver FitzGerald
1839–40	John O'Brien	1919–20	ST Gordon	1986–87	Conor McCarthy
1840–41	William F Montgomery	1920–22	Ninian M Falkner	1987–88	K O'Malley
1841–46	George Alexander Kennedy	1922–24	Sir WJ Thompson	1988–90	John F Murphy
1846–47	Aquilla Smith	1924–26	William A Winter	1990–91	Michael Buckley
1847–48	Percival [Head]	1926–28	Bethel Solomons	1991–92	Michael Scott
1848–49	William Stokes (March)	1928–30	John A Matson	1992–93	G Bourke
1849–50	Cathcart Lees	1930–32	WJ Dargan	1993–94	Dermot MacDonald
1850–51	Henry Law Dwyer	1932–33	FC Purser	1994–95	D Keelan (December)
1851–53	Aquilla Smith	1933–35	W Boxwell	1995–96	J Fennelly
1853–54	[ ] Brady	1935–36	FJ O'Donnell	1996–97	P McKiernan
1854–55	William Barker	1936–38	WG Harvey	1997–98	F Gleeson
1855–56	James F Duncan	1938–40	RJ Rowlette	1998–99	B McDonagh
1856–57	Fleetwood Churchill	1940–42	VM Synge	1999–2000	C Burke
1857–59	Aquilla Smith	1942–43	TM Healy	2000–01	E Egan
1859–61	John Moore Neligan	1943–44	R E Steen	2001–02	John Donohoe
1861–64	*Not identified*	1944–45	CJ Murphy	2002–03	George Mellotte
1865–66	George Johnson	*1945–46*	*Not identified*	2003–04	Frank Murray
1866–67	William Moore	1946–47	Alan Thompson	2004–05	John Crowe
1867–68	Samuel Gordon	1947–49	Edward A Keelan	2005–06	Kathleen McGarry
1868–70	Henry Freke	1949–50	PT O'Farrell	2006–07	Bernadette Herity
1871–72	Samuel Gordon	1950–52	GT O'Brien	2007–08	Mick Molloy
1872–73	Robert D Lyons	1952–54	JA Wallace	2008–09	John Barragry
1873–77	*Not identified*	1954–56	DM Mitchell	2009–10	Randal Hayes
1877–78	James Little	1956–58	RB Pringle	2010–11	Mary Holohan
1878–84	*Not identified*	1958–59	Morgan Crowe	2011–12	Donal Reddan
1884–85	George F Duffey	1959–61	Anna M E McCabe	2012–13	Hilary Humphreys
		1961–62	RS W Baker	2013–14	Hilary Hoey
				2014–15	Michael O'Connell

Registrars of the Royal College of Physicians of Ireland

Elected 18 October each year unless otherwise stated

1693–94	Duncan Cuming	1774–76	James Thornton
1694–95	Thomas Molyneux	1776–77	Edward Hill
1695–97	William Smyth	1777–80	William Harvey
1697–1700	Joseph Pratt	1780–82	Francis Hopkins
1700–01	Richard Steevens	1782–83	Edmond Cullen
1701–02	Edward Wetenhall	1783–84	Charles William Quin
1702–03	William Smyth	1784–87	Stephen Dickson
1703–04	Robert Griffith	1787–90	John William Boyton
1704–05	Patrick Mitchell	1790–93	Alexander Pellisier
1705–10	James Gratton	1793–96	James Cleghorn
1710–12	Richard Hoyle	1796–98	Matthew Stritch
1712–13	Samuel Jemmat	1798–99	Anthony Gilholy
1713–16	Bryan Robinson	1799-1800	Thomas J Bryanton
1716–17	Samuel Jemmat	1800–03	Daniel Mills
1717–19	William Smyth	1803–04	Thomas Herbert Orpen
1719–22	Samuel Singleton	1804–07	Hugh Ferguson
1722–24	Richard Hoyle	1807–08	Francis Barker
1724–25	Henry Cope	1808–09	James John Leahy
1725–26	Constantine Ormsby	1809–10	Martin Tuomy
1726–27	Francis Le Hunt	1810–12	Peter Edward McLoghlin
1727–28	Samuel Arnoldi	1812–14	George Todderick
1728–29	James Grattan	1814–17	Samuel Litton
1729–30	Alexander McNaughton	1817–20	James Clarke
1730–31	William Stephens	1820–22	William Stack
1731–32	John Van Lewen	1822–23	Charles Richard A Lendrick
1732–33	Charles Kemys	1823–29	Jonathan Osborne
1733–34	John Hemsworth	1829–32	David Brereton
1734–35	Thomas Kingsbury	1832–38	George Alexander Kennedy
1735–37	Francis Foreside	1838–41	William O'Brien Adams
1737–38	Edward Aston	1841–51	Jonathan Labatt
1738–40	Edward Smyth	1851–60	William Edward Steele
1740–41	Thomas Lloyd	1860–61	William Moore
1741–42	Edward Barry	1861–68	Lombe Atthill
1742–43	Thomas Lloyd	1868–71	James Little
1743–45	John Anderson	1871–82	John Magee Finney
1745–46	John Ferrall	1882–92	John William Moore
1746–47	Ezekiel Nesbit	1892–97	Guy P L Nugent (May)
1747–48	Constantine Barbor	1897–10	James Craig (June)
1748–49	Anthony Relhan	1910–54	T Percy C Kirkpatrick (July)
1749–54	Richard Wood	1954–71	Charles Dickson
1754–55	Adam Humble	1971–75	Harry O'Flanagan
1755–58	Henry Quin	1975–89	Ciaran Barry
1758–61	Nathaniel Barry	1989–96	John Feely
1761–62	Clement Archer	1996-2003	T Joseph McKenna
1762–66	Archibald Hamilton	2003–06	N Gerard McElvaney
1766–68	John Vicars	2006–07	John Donohoe
1768–69	Francis Hutcheson	2007–14	Frank Murray
1769–73	William Lloyd	2014–	Diarmuid O'Shea
1773–74	Francis Hutcheson		

Treasurers of the Royal College of Physicians of Ireland

Elected 18 October each year unless otherwise stated

1695-1728	Thomas Molyneux	1811–12	Thomas Herbert Orpen
1728-1737	Samuel Jemmat	1812–13	Francis Hopkins
1737-1740	James Grattan	1813–15	Peter Edward McLoghlin
1740-1749	Bryan Robinson (Feb)	1815–19	George Todderick
1749	William Stephens (Feb – Oct)	1819–42	Thomas Herbert Orpen
1749–50	Robert Robinson	1842–47	Robert Collins
1750–51	Edward Barry	1847–55	John Mollan
1751–52	Bryan Robinson	1855–72	Henry L Dwyer
1752–54	Edward Barry	1872–90	Aquilla Smith
1754–55	Ezekiel Nesbit	1890–02	Lombe Atthil (Nov)
1755–56	Constantine Barbor	1902–44	Henry Theodore Bewley (Feb)
1756–57	Anthony Relhan	1944–74	Geoffrey Bewley
1757–67	Ezekiel Nesbit	1974–84	David Michael Mitchell
1767–68	Henry Quin	1984–91	Bryan Gerard Alton
1768–69	Nathaniel Barry	1991–97	J A Brian Keogh
1769–70	Clement Archer	1997–2006	John F Murphy
1770–71	Constantine Barbour	2006–10	John Crowe
1771–72	John Ferrall	2011–	J Conor O'Keane
1772–73	Henry Quin		
1773–74	Nathaniel Barry		
1774–75	John Ferrall		
1775–76	Henry Quin		
1776–77	Nathaniel Barry		
1777–78	Clement Archer		
1778–80	Francis Hutcheson		
1780–81	Henry Quin		
1781–83	Francis Hutcheson		
1783–84	Edward Hill		
1784–85	Arthur Saunders		
1785–86	William Harvey		
1786–87	Francis Hopkins		
1787–88	Patrick Plunket		
1788–89	Edmond Cullen		
1789–90	Charles William Quin		
1790–91	Edward Hill		
1791–92	Arthur Saunders		
1792–93	William Harvey		
1793–94	Francis Hopkins		
1794–95	Patrick Plkunket		
1795–96	Edmond Cullen		
1796–97	Edward Hill		
1797–98	Arthur Saunders		
1798	Francis Hopkins (Oct–Nov)		
1798–99	William Harvey (Nov)		
1799–1802	Francis Hopkins		
1802–03	Edward Hill		
1803–04	James Cleghorn		
1804–08	Francis Hopkins		
1808–11	Daniel Mills		

Endnotes

Arts and Science
1 Seamus Heaney, 'Out of the Bag': *Electric Light* (Faber and Faber, 2001)

The Early Days
1 Aidan Clarke, in Martin and Moody, *The Course of Irish History*, ed. Keogh (The Mercier Press, 2011), p. 152.
2 Tony Farmar, *Patients, Potions and Physicians – A Social History of Medicine in Ireland, 1654–2004* (A & A Farmar, in association with the Royal College of Physicians in Ireland, 2004), p. 4.
3 JDH Widdess, *A History of the Royal College of Physicians of Ireland, 1654–1963* (E & S Livingstone, Edinburgh and London, 1963), p. 3.
4 Mary Ann Lyons, 'The Role of Graduate Physicians in Professionalising Medical Practice in Ireland, c. 1619–54' in *Ireland and Medicine in the Seventeenth and Eighteenth Centuries*, James Kelly and Fiona Clark (Ashgate, 2010), pp 22–23.
5 Lyons, in op. cit., pp 26–27.
6 John Bergin in *Dictionary of Irish Biography: From the Earliest Times to the Year 2002*, ed. James McGuire and James Quinn (Royal Irish Academy, published in nine volumes, 2009).
7 Widdess, op. cit., pp14–16.
8 TC Barnard in *Dictionary of Irish Biography*.
9 Barnard in op. cit.
10 Widdess, op. cit., p. 19.
11 Widdess, op. cit., p. 22.
12 Jonathan Bardon, *A History of Ireland in 250 Episodes* (Gill & Macmillan, 2009), p. 209.
13 O'Brien and Widdess, *A Portrait of Irish Medicine*, RCPI and Ward River Press, p. 64.
14 Lyons, op. cit., pp 36–37.
15 Farmer, op. cit., p. 7.

The Life and Times of Sir Patrick Dun
1 Farmar, op. cit., p. 33; TW Belcher, *Memoir of Sir Patrick Dun . . .* (Hodges, Smith, 1866).
2 Helen Andrews in *Dictionary of Irish Biography*.
3 Widdess, op. cit., p24.
4 Sir John Dalrymple *Memoirs of Great Britain and Ireland, . . .* (1773), pp 114–129.
5 Widdess, op. cit., p. 31.
6 Widdess, op. cit., pp31–2.
7 Widdess, op. cit., p. 33.
8 Widdess, op. cit., p. 35.
9 Harmen Beukers, *The Anatomy Lesson* (National Gallery of Ireland, 1992) p. 121.
10 Widdess, op. cit., p. 21.
11 Helen Andrews in *Dictionary of Irish Biography*.
12 Enda Leaney in *Dictionary of Irish Biography*, pp 760–61.
13 Davis Coakley, *Irish Masters of Medicine* (Town House, 1992), pp 7–13.
14 Widdess, op. cit., pp 40–41.
15 Eoin O'Brien and Anne Crookshank, *A Portrait of Irish Medicine* (Ward River Press, 1983), p. 69, op. cit.
16 Coakley, *The Anatomy Lesson* (National Gallery of Ireland, 1992) p. 59.
17 Eileen Kane, *An Irish Giant* in Irish Arts Review, 1990–1, p. 96.
18 Coakley, *The Anatomy Lesson* (National Gallery of Ireland, 1992) p. 61.

The Age of Reason and Unreason
1 O'Brien and Crookshank, op. cit., p. 77.
2 James Malton, Notes to the Engravings, 1797 in *The Irish Prints of James Malton* (Andrew and Charlotte Bonar Law, 1999), p. 72.
3 The Dun Estate, Harriet Wheelock, RCPIblog.ie.
4 Widdess, op. cit., p. 50.
5 Widdess, op. cit., p. 50.
6 RF Foster (ed.), *The Oxford Illustrated History of Ireland* (Oxford University Press, 1989), p. 163.
7 Farmer, op. cit., p. 33.
8 Farmer, op. cit., p. 45.
9 Farmer, op. cit., p. 46–7.
10 Widdess, op. cit., pp96–7.
11 Trinity College Dublin website: www.tcd.ie
12 Chelsea Medicine Garden website: www.chelseaphysicgarden.co.uk
13 Widdess, op. cit., pp89–91.
14 Widdess, op. cit., p.98.
15 Widdess, op. cit., pp94–5.
16 James Malton, Notes to the Engravings, 1797, in *The Irish Prints of James Malton*, p. 33.

Hospitals, Healing and Hope
1 Richard Killeen, *A Brief History of Ireland: Land, People, History* (Constable & Robinson, 2012), p. 105.
2 Bardon, *A History of Ireland in 250 Episodes*, p. 259.
3 John F Fleetwood, *History of Medicine in Ireland* (Skellig Press, 1983), pp 95–96.
4 Ibid, p.103.
5 Brooking's *City of Dublin, 1728*, ed. Maurice James Craig (The Irish Architectural Archive & the Friends of the Library, Trinity College, Dublin, 1983).
6 James Malton, Notes to the Engravings, 1797, in *The Irish Prints of James Malton*, p. 57.
7 Ibid.
8 Widdess, op. cit., pp103–4.
9 Southwell, op. cit., pp97–98.
10 Southwell, op. cit., p. 99.
11 Op. cit., p. 106.
12 The Edward Worth Library
13 Widdess, op. cit., p.105.
14 Widdess, op. cit., p.106.
15 Fleetwood op. cit., p. 103.
16 Ibid., p.103.
17 James Kelly in Dictionary of Irish Biography.
18 Charles Lucas, RCPI blog.ie
19 Ibid
20 Alan Browne, *Masters, Midwives and Ladies-in-Waiting: Rotunda Hospital, 1745–1995* (A & A Farmar, 1995), p. 8.
21 James Malton, Notes to the Engravings, 1797 in *The Irish Prints of James Malton*, p. 61.
22 *British Medical Journal*, 5 July 1947.
23 Thomas Campbell, *A Philosophical Survey of the South of Ireland, in a Series of Letters to John Watkinson MD* (1778), ex Libris of the Belfast Harbour Commissioners, pp26–27.
24 Coakley, op. cit., p. 31.
25 Widdess, op. cit., pp 108–9.
26 Widdess, op. cit., pp 72–3.
27 Ibid., pp72–3.
28 Carmel Doyle in *Dictionary of Irish Biography*, pp 349–50.
29 Widdess, op. cit., p. 102.
30 Ibid., DIB., pp 349–50.
31 Widdess, op. cit., pp 73–5.
32 Widdess, pp 107–8.
33 Ibid., pp 107–8.
34 Marsh's Library, Dublin.

Dun's Library
1 Widdess, op.cit., p. 53.
2 The author is indebted to Harriet Wheelock for the information contained in her lecture on Dun's Library, presented at a Symposium at the Royal College of Physicians of Ireland on 16 October 2013. In this talk, she paid tribute to Robert Mills, who was the College Librarian for 35 years, until his retirement in May 2013.
3 1785 Act of Parliament (25 Geo III. C.42).
4 Harriet Wheelock lecture to the RCPI Symposium, 2013, op. cit.
5 Harriet Wheelock lecture to the RCPI Symposium, 2013, op. cit.
6 Coakley, op. cit., p. 178

New Century, New Challenges
1 Cecil Woodham-Smith, *The Great Hunger: Ireland 1845–1849* (Hamish Hamilton, 1962), pp 15–16.
2 Beckett, op. cit., pp 284–5.
3 TW Moorhead, *A Short History of Sir Patrick Dun's Hospital* (Hodges, Figgis and Co., 1942), p. 12.
4 Ibid., pp 19–23.
5 Widdess, op. cit., p. 140.
6 Widdess, op. cit., p. 206.
7 JF Maher and JAB Keogh, 'Osborne of Dublin and the Origin of Nephrology in Ireland', *Irish Journal of Medical Science*, 161, No. 6, June 1992, pp 420–22.
8 Widdess, pp 206–7.
9 Widdess, Ibid., p. 144.
10 Widdess, Ibid., p. 144.
11 Widdess, Ibid., pp 144–5.
12 Widdess, Ibid., p. 120.
13 Widdess, Ibid., p.122.
14 Widdess, Ibid., p. 124.
15 Widdess, Ibid., p.126.
16 Cork Street Fever Hospital Committee Proceedings, 23 October 1801.
17 Cork Street Fever Hospital, RCPIblog.ie
18 Widdess, Ibid., pp 138–142.
19 Moorhead, op. cit., pp 28–33.
20 Ibid., pp 45–49.
21 Op. cit., p. 24.
22 Op. cit., Preface.
23 Coakley, Anatomy and Art: Irish dimensions; *The Anatomy Lesson: Art and Medicine*, (National Gallery of Ireland, 1992) p. 57.
24 Murray, Peter, *Daniel Maclise*, Crawford Art Gallery, Gandon Editions.
25 Coakley, *Anatomy and Art . . .* (National Gallery of Ireland, 1992).
26 Ibid.

Laying the Foundations
1 Beckett, op. cit., p. 284.
2 Foster, RF, op. cit. p. 183.
3 Widdess, op. cit., p. 150.
4 Kevin Flude, *Divorced, Beheaded, Died . . .* (Michael O'Mara Books, 2009), pp 130–130.
5 Widdess, op. cit., p. 155.
6 Farmer, op. cit., p. 64.
7 Widdess, op. cit., pp. 155–6.
8 *The Anatomy Lesson*, op. cit., p. 29.
9 Widdess op. cit., p. 152.

10 www.workhouses.org/DublinNorth/.

11 Moylan, Thomas King (1938). *Vagabonds and sturdy beggars.* Dublin Historical Record 1 (2): 66–9.

12 Eoin O'Brien, *The House of Industry Hospitals, 1772–1987* (Anniversary Press, Dublin, 1987).

13 *Journal of the Irish Colleges of Physicians and Surgeons,* Vol. 3, No. 3, Jan 1974.

14 Widdess, op. cit., pp 150–155.

15 John Cheyne, *Essays on the Partial Derangement of the Mind in Supposed Connection with Religion* (1843), p. 28.

16 Coakley, *Irish masters of Medicine,* op. cit., p. 68.

Robert Graves and William Stokes

1 *The Anatomy Lesson,* (National Gallery of Ireland, 1992), p. 97.

2 Coakley, op. cit., p. 89.

3 Widdess, op. cit., pp 161–2.

4 Widdess, op. cit., p. 159–161.

5 Widdess, op. cit., p. 165.

6 Graves Lecture 1, p. 1, from *Robert Graves, Evangelist of Clinical Medicine,* Coakley, p49.

7 Sir Frederick Conway Dwyer, RCPI blog.ie

8 Widdess, op. cit., pp 161–5.

9 William Wilde, 'Portrait of Graves', *Dublin University Magazine,* Vol. XXVII, pp 260–73.

10 Coakley, *Irish Masters of Medicine,* p. 96.

11 Coakley, op. cit., p. 98.

12 Farmar, *Patients, Potions & Physicians,* p. 81.

13 *The Lancet,* Vol. 357, June 2001.

14 RCPIblog.ie

15 Fleetwood, *History of Medicine in Ireland,* p. 1920.

16 Coakley, op. cit., pp 83–4.

17 Coakley, op. cit., p. 134.

Sir Dominic Corrigan

1 Widdess, op. cit., pp 184–5.

2 Widdess, op. cit., p. 186.

3 RCPI blog.ie

4 O'Brien, *Conscience and Conflict: A Biography of Sir Desmond Corrigan, 1802–1880* (Glendale Press, Dublin, 1983), p. 64.

5 Op. cit., p. 75.

6 Coakley, op. cit., p. 108.

7 Coakley, op. cit., p. 109.

8 Coakley, op. cit., pp 110–111 and Lyons, *Dictionary of Irish Biography.*

9 Lyons, op. cit., p. 863.

10 Some modern historians refer to period of the Great Famine as 1845–52, arguing that its effects were still manifest some two years after the previously accepted end date of 1850.

11 Beckett, op. cit., p. 343.

12 Beckett, op. cit., p. 343.

13 *Dublin Quarterly Journal of Medicine,* Vol. IV, No. 7, August and November, pp 134–145.

14 Op. cit., p. 139.

15 'On the Mortality of Medical Practitioners in Ireland' (second article, *Dublin Quarterly Journal of Medical Science*), Vol. V, February 1848, p. 119.

16 Tony Farmar, *Patients, Potions & Physicians,* (A & A Farmar, 2004), p. 94.

17 *Dublin Quarterly Journal of Medical Science,* op. cit., p. 119.

18 O'Brien and Crookshank, *A Portrait of Irish Medicine,* pp. 130–1.

19 Op. cit., p. 129.

20 *Dublin Quarterly Journal of Medical Science,* op. cit., p. 525.

21 Peter Gray, *The Irish Famine,* (Thames and Hudson, 1995).

22 TJ McKenna, in an interview with the author at the RCPI, 24 June, 2014.

23 Mike Corbishley and John Gillingham, *The Young Oxford History of Britain and Ireland* (Oxford University Press, 1997), p. 316.

24 Coakley, *Irish Masters of Medicine,* p. xiii.

25 Beckett, p. cit., p. 350.

At Home, No 6 Kildare Street

1 Farmer, op. cit., p. 100.

2 Widdess, pp 139–140.

3 Coakley, op. cit., p. 121 and O'Brien, *op. cit.,* p. 225.

4 Helen Andrews in *Dictionary of Irish National Biography,* pp 368–9.

5 Design brief for No 6 Kildare Street, RCPIblog.ie.

6 James McDowell, *No. 6 Kildare Street. An Architectural History, 1859–1875,* The royal College of Physicians of Ireland.

7 Widdess, op. cit., pp 196–7 (working on material from Belcher and earlier sources).

8 Widdess, op. cit., p. 198.

9 Eoin O'Brien, from a booklet, 'The Royal College of Physicians of Ireland' (The Anniversary Press, Dublin, 1989).

10 Widdess, p. 200.

11 Widdess, pp 200–1.

12 Widdess, op. cit., pp 200–201.

13 Widdess, op. cit., p. 203.

14 www.Dublin's Great Estates – www.dublinestates.blogspot.co.uk

15 Obituary from *British Medical Journal,* 1880, Vol. I, p. 219, and also O'Brien, *Conscience and Conflict,* pp 328–9.

16 Widdess, p. 191.

17 *The Lancet,* 1880, pp 268–9, also quoted by O'Brien, op. cit., p. 329.

18 Coakley, op. cit., p 11.

Reform, Recognition, Revolution

1 National Gallery of Ireland

2 Marian Broderick, *Wild Irish Women* (O'Brien Press, 2002), pp124–8.

3 Widdess, op. cit., pp 226–7.

4 Widdess, op. cit., p. 228.

5 Widdess, op. cit., p. 199.

6 O'Brien, op. cit., p. 240.

7 Mary Mulvihill, *Ingenious Dublin: A Guide to the City's Marvels, Discoveries and Inventions* (Ingenious Guides, 2012).

8 Women in Stone, Edinburgh blog. Womeninstoneedinburgh.blogspot.co.uk

9 Laura Kelly, *Irish Women in Medicine, c. 1880–1920s: Origins, education and careers* (Manchester University Press, 2013).

10 RCPI Adopt a portrait.

11 Sir Charles Cameron, RCPI blog.ie

12 Kelly, op. cit., p. 39.

13 Op. cit., p. 39.

14 Op. cit., p. 37.

15 *British Medical Journal,* 7 May 1898, pp 1236–7.

16 *BMJ,* as above.

17 David Murphy in *Dictionary of Irish Biography,* p. 1012.

18 Kelly, op. cit., pp 38–9.

19 Carol M Martel, *Historical Dictionary of the British Empire,* Vol. II (Greenwood Press, 1996), pp 874–5.

20 Kelly, op. cit., pp 41–3.

21 Kelly, op. cit., p. 43 and *Dublin Medical Press,* 23 May 1877, p. 417.

22 Kelly, op. cit., p. 46.

23 Widdess, pp 212–13.

24 *Minutes,* Vol. 25, 1 March 1912, pp 7–8.

25 Kelly, op. cit., p. 11.

26 Kelly, op. cit., p. 9.

27 *Minutes,* 29 August 1914, pp 201–2.

28 *Minutes,* 1915, pp 246–7.

29 Kelly, op. cit., p. 4.

30 Kelly, op. cit., p. 35.

31 Surgeon-General Charles Sibthorpe RCPIblog.ie.

32 *National Gallery of Ireland: The Essential Guide,* 2008.

33 Bardon, op. cit., p. 395.

34 Widdess, op. cit., p. 234.

35 *Minutes,* Vol. 20, 1889–93, pp 179–80.

Violence … and more Violence

1 JB Lyons in *A Portrait of Irish Medicine,* O'Brien and Crookshank: Chapter 5, pp 147–149.

2 *Disease and Dirt: Public health in Dublin,* Dublin City Library.

3 CSFH/1/5/1

4 *RCPI Journal,* Vol. XXV, p. 35 (RCPI/2/1/1/27).

5 *RCPI Journal,* Vol. XXV, pp 74–93 (RCPI/2/1/1/27).

6 John Keegan, *The First World War* (Hutchinson, 1998), p. 3. Keegan's father served in the conflict.

7 *RCPI Journal,* Vol. XXV, pp 14–5 (RCPI/2/1/1/27).

8 *RCPI Journal,* Vol. XXV, pp 100–2 (RCPI/2/1/1/27).

9 RCPI 1/2/3/2/14.

10 Peter Costello: Appendix 3 in *Holles Street, 1894–1994: The National Maternity Hospital – a Centenary History,* Tony Farmar, (A & A Farmar, 1994), pp 208–9.

11 Helen Andrews in *Dictionary of Irish Biography.*

12 *RCPI Journal,* Vol. XXV, p. 212 (RCPI/2/1/1/27).

13 Fergus Brady, 'The Belgium Doctors' and Pharmacists' Relief Fund', RCPI Heritage Centre Blog (http://rcpilibrary.blogspot.ie/2014/08/the-belgium-doctors-and-pharmacists.html).

14 *RCPI Journal,* Vol. XXV, p. 240 (RCPI/2/1/1/27).

15 *RCPI Journal,* Vol. XXV, p. 251 (RCPI/2/1/1/27).

16 *RCPI Journal,* Vol. XXV, pp 295–6 (RCPI/2/1/1/27).

17 *RCPI Journal,* Vol. XXV, p. 313 (RCPI/2/1/1/27).

18 *Reveille: Telling Ireland's Military Story,* ed. Wesley Bourke and Billy Galligan, Winter 2014, p. 20.

19 EE O'Donnell SJ, *Father Browne's First World War,* 1914, Messenger Publications.

20 *RCPI Journal,* Vol. XXV, p. 321 (RCPI/2/1/1/27).

21 Erich Maria Remarque, *All Quiet on the Western Front* (first published in German in 1929, and in English translation later in 1929 by Putnam and Co.).

22 Thomas McCreary, the author's grandfather, served as a stretcher-bearer at the Battle of the Somme in 1916. Like many men who had been to the Front, he rarely talked about this throughout the rest of his life. However, on one occasion he told his family about having been present at an operation to amputate the leg of a wounded soldier, when the only 'anaesthetic' available was a draught of strong Irish whiskey.

23 *Reveille: Telling Ireland's Military Story,* Winter 2014, p. 29, and Archives HW/FB.

24 Helen Andrews in *Dictionary of Irish Biography.*

25 Dominic Hayhoe (Chief Executive, Forces War Records), *Trench Traumas and Medical Miracles* (Forces War Records publication), p. 3. (www.forces-war-records.co.uk.)

26 Moorhead, *A Short History of Sir Patrick Dun's Hospital,* pp 185–7.

27 David Durnin, 'Irish Doctors in the First World War', History of Medicine in Ireland Blog (http://historyofmedicineinireland.blogspot.co.uk/2013/04/irish-doctors-in-first-world-war-by_10.html).

28 Harriet Wheelock, 'World War I and Robertson Stewart Smyth', RCPI Heritage Centre Blog (http://rcpilibrary.blogspot.ie/2010/11/world-war-i-and-robertson-stewart-smyth.htm).

29 Sir Max Hastings, The *Sunday Times,* 25 January, 2015.

30 Lyons in *Dictionary of Irish Biography,* and Lyons, *Brief Lives of Irish Doctors* (Blackwater Press), 1978.

31 'Some Experiences in a Base Hospital in Egypt', *Dublin Journal of Medical Science* civil (1916), Part Three, pp 411–416.

32 *The Times Great Irish Lives* (Times Books, 2009) with a Foreword by Dr Garret Fitzgerald, ed. Charles Lysaght, p. 164.

33 Lyons, *Brief Lives of Irish Doctors*, p. 141, and RCPI Archive.

34 Foster (ed.), *The Oxford Illustrated History of Ireland*, p. 239.

35 *History Ireland*, Vol. 22, No. 4 (July/August 2014), pp 14–17.

36 Moorhead, op. cit., pp 187–189.

37 Margaret Ó hÓgartaigh, *Kathleen Lynn: Irishwoman, Patriot, Doctor* (Irish Academic Press, 2006).

38 Ó hÓgartaigh, *Dictionary of Irish Biography*, pp 659–60.

39 Willian Lawsoist, President's Address, 'Infant Mortality and The Notification Of Births Acts, 1907, 1915', *Journal of the Statistical and Social Inquiry Society of Ireland*, Part XCVII.

40 Article about Airfield House, *The Forum Newsletter for Dun Laoghaire – Rathdown Community Forum*, Vol. 7, Issue 1 (March 2006) http://www.dlrcommunityforum.ie/Forum-March-06.pdf. http://www.dlrcommunityforum.ie/Forum-March-06.pdf.

41 Letter to the President of the Council of the Irish Free State from Sir John Lumsden, British Red Cross Society and the Order of St John of Jerusalem, Vice Chairman, Joint Committee, Leinster, Munster and Connaught, 10 December 1923. (http://www.nationalarchives.ie.)

41 www.earlscliffe.com, memories of Sir Lumsden's granddaughter, Margery Stratton.

42 David Mitchell, *A 'Peculiar' Place: The Adelaide Hospital, Dublin; Its Times, Places and Personalities, 1839–1989* (Blackwater Press, 1990).

43 Lyons, op. cit., p. 158.

44 Obituary in *The Times*, 16 July 1927, from *The Times Great Irish Lives*, p. 108.

45 Widdess, *The Royal College of Surgeons in Ireland and Its Medical School, 1784–1984* (RCSI, 1984), Appendix III, pp 153–156.

46 *RCPI Journal*, Vol. XXV, p. 339 (RCPI/2/1/1/27).

47 *RCPI Journal*, Vol. XXV, p. 339 (RCPI/2/1/1/27).

48 *RCPI Journal*, Vol. XXVI, pp 4-6 (RCPI/2/1/1/28).

49 *BMJ* (1918), Vol. II, pp 491–492), and the College Annals, Vol. L, 19189–21, p. 49.

50 AM Cooke, The College of Physicians of London, (Clarendon Press and the Royal College of Physicians of London, 1972) pp 1030–31.

51 *BMJ*, op. cit., p. 492.

52 Annals of the Royal College of Physicians of London, MS 1042/22.

Into the Unknown

1 *RCPI Journal*, Vol. XXVI, p. 90 (RCPI/2/1/1/28).

2 Winston Churchill, *The Aftermath: The World Crisis, 1918–1928* (Macmillan, 1929), p. 319.

3 St Ultan's Hospital, RCPIblog.ie

4 *History Ireland*, No. 4, Jul/Aug 2005.

5 *RCPI Journal*, Vol. XXVI, p.42 (RCPI/2/1/1/28).

6 TCD.ie.

7 Anne Mac Lellan, *Dorothy Stopford-Price: Rebel Doctor* (Irish Academic Press).

8 *RCPI Journal*, Vol. XXVI, pp.75–6 (RCPI/2/1/1/28).

9 *RCPI Journal*, Vol XXVI, p.164 (RCPI/2/1/1/28).

10 *RCPI Journal*, Vol XXVI, p.108 (RCPI/2/1/1/28).

11 *RCPI Journal*, Vol XXVI, p.170 (RCPI/2/1/1/28).

12 *RCPI Journal*, Vol XXVI, p.181 (RCPI/2/1/1/28).

13 *RCPI Journal*, Vol XXVI, pp.205–6 (RCPI/2/1/1/28).

14 Richard Hawkins, *Dictionary of Irish Biography*, Vol 1, pp. 139–40.

15 *RCPI Journal*, Vol XXVI, p.254 (RCPI/2/1/1/28).

16 *RCPI Journal*, Vol XXVI, p. 292–3 (RCPI/2/1/1/28).

17 Coakley, *Masters of Irish Medicine*, pp 241–252.

18 *RCPI Journal*, Vol XXVI, p. 293 (RCPI/2/1/1/28).

19 *RCPI Journal*, Vol XXVI, p. 294–5 (RCPI/2/1/1/28).

20 *RCPI Journal*, Vol XXVIII, p. 38 (RCPI/2/1/1/30).

21 Dr Charles Dickson, *Dictionary of Irish Biography*, by CJ Woods.

22 Fergus Brady, Cork Street Medical Reports, 1938–48, RCPI Blog.

23 Feely, *The Anatomy Lesson*, p. 101.

24 Obituary in *The Times*, London, 30 August 1975, reprinted in *Great Irish Lives*, pp 192–201.

25 Tom Garvin, *Preventing the Future: Why was Ireland so poor for so long?* (Gill and Macmillan, 2004).

26 From an interview with the author, February 2015.

27 From an interview with the author in Dublin, 19 November 2014. Professor Mulcahy has also written a book, *My Father, the General: Richard Mulcahy and the Military History of the Revolution* (Liberties Press, 2009).

28 *RCPI Journal*, Vol XXVII, p. 372 (RCPI/2/1/1/29).

29 *RCPI Journal*, Vol XXVII, p. 282 (RCPI/2/1/1/29).

30 Bardon, op. cit., pp 495–496.

31 Bardon, op. cit., p. 496.

32 *RCPI Journal*, Vol XXVIII, p. 186 (RCPI/2/1/1/30)

33 *RCPI Journal*, Vol XXVIII, p. 200 (RCPI/2/1/1/30).

34 RCPI Archive, p. 25 (FJO/3/3).

35 Op cit., p. 28.

36 Op cit., p. 29.

37 FJO/3/2, p. 3.

38 FJO/3/3, pp 21–22.

39 Wheelock, Collection List for the Major General O'Meara Papers, RCPI, 2013.

40 William Murphy in *Irish Dictionary of Biography*.

41 Widdess, op. cit., p. 218.

42 Bardon, op. cit., p. 497.

43 Alf McCreary, *Titanic Port. The Illustrated History of Belfast Harbour* (Booklink, 2010), pp 221–225.

44 *RCPI Journal*, Vol XXVIII, p. 406 (RCPI/2/1/1/30)..

45 Killeen, op. cit., *A Brief History of Ireland*, p. 274.

46 Brian Barton, *The Belfast Blitz: The City in the War Years*, (Ulster Historical Foundation, 2015).

47 Widdess, op. cit., p. 218.

48 Lyons in *Dictionary of Irish Biography*.

49 *RCPI Journal*, Vol. XXVII, p. 229 (RCPI/2/1/1/29).

Brave New World

1 *RCPI Journal*, Vol XXIX, p. 231 (RCPI/2/1/1/31).

2 RCPI/9/5/3.

3 Malan Marais, *Heart Transplant: The Story of Barnard and the Ultimate in Cardiac Surgery* (Voortrekkerpers, 1968).

4 John Horgan, *Noel Browne: Passionate Outsider* (Gill & Macmillan, 2009), p. 294.

5 Widdess, op. cit., pp 237–238.

6 David Mitchell, *25 Years: An Interim History of the Royal College of Physicians of Ireland, 1963–88* (RCPI, 1992), p. 83.

7 Op. cit., p. 83.

8 Op. cit., pp 83–84.

9 Op. cit., p. 84.

10 Op. cit., pp 4–5.

11 Op. cit., p. 5.

12 CSFH/3/1/1/10.

13 Patricia Conway, Sheila Fitzgerald and Seamus O'Dea, *Cherry Orchard Hospital: The First 50 Years* (2003).

14 NHS History.

15 Mitchell, op. cit., pp 4–6.

16 Op. cit., pp 34–35.

17 Interview with the author.

18 Interview with the author.

19 Mitchell, op. cit., p. 2

20 Op. cit., pp 3–4

21 The Guinness Archive, GDB/ PE14/0033.20.

22 Rachel Browne; 2013, CIOB; Designing Buildings.

23 Mitchell, op. cit., pp 51–52.

24 Feely, op. cit., p. 102.

25 Mitchell, op. cit., pp3–4.

26 Op. cit., p. 4.

27 Coakley, *Masters of Medicine*, pp 329–331.

28 Mitchell, op.cit., pp 6–7.

29 Op. cit., pp 90–91.

30 Op. cit., p. 54.

31 Corrigan Club Booklet.

32 Cathy Hayes in *Dictionary of Irish Biography* Vol 6, 2009, pp 528–9.

33 Mitchell, op. cit., pp 85–7.

34 *DIB*, op. cit., p. 529.

35 Mitchell, op. cit., p. 54.

36 Op. cit., pp 54–55.

37 Op.cit., pp 92–3.

38 Op. cit., p. 34.

39 Op. cit., pp 33–34, p. 86.

40 Op. cit., pp 59–60.

41 Op.cit., pp 25, 28.

42 Coakley, op. cit., pp 333–344.

43 Farmar, *Patients, Potions and Physicians*, p. 184.

44 Mitchell, op. cit., p. 32.

45 Pauric J Dempsey in *Dictionary of Irish Biography*, Vol. I, p. 93.

46 Mitchell, op. cit., p. 89.

47 As told to the author by a former President of the College.

48 Professor John Crowe in a private profile of Dr Alton, made available to the author.

49 Mitchell, op. cit., p. 12–13.

50 Mitchell, op. cit., p. 81.

Full Circle

1 College Minutes, 5 June 1992 (RCPI/2/2/2/3).

2 College Minutes 19 October 1992 (RCPI/2/2/2/3).

3 *British Medical Journal*.

4 In an interview with the author.

5 *Irish Times*, 16 October 2004.

6 Mitchell, op. cit., pp 93–94.

7 In an interview with the author at No.6 Kildare Street.

8 In an interview with the author at No.6 Kildare Street.

9 *Journal of the Irish Colleges of Physicians and Surgeons*, Vol 27, No 1, January 1998, pp 74–75.

10 In an interview with the author, Belfast, April 2015.

11 In an interview with the author, Belfast, April 2015.

12 *Irish Times*, 18 December, 2004.

13 In an interview with the author, 2015.

14 RCPI Archive.

15 In an interview with the author, 2015.

16 In an interview with the author, 2015.

17 In an interview with the author, 2015.

18 RCPI Archive.

19 In an interview with the author, 2015.

20 Online edition of The Medical Independent, June 2014: wwwmedicalindependent.ie/49834/changing_times_at_the_rcpi 12 June 2014.

21 Mitchell, op. cit., p. 76.

22 Mitchell, op. cit., p. 246.

23 *History of Medicine in Ireland*, Browne and Nolan Ltd, the Richview Press Dublin, p. 380.

24 William Doolin, *Wayfarers in Medicine* (Heinemann Medical Books, London 1947).

Page 248

1 Moorhead, *A Short History of Sir Patrick Dun's Hospital*, (Hodges, Figgis and Co., Nassau Street, 1942, Dublin).

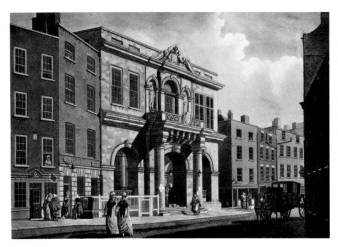

The Tholsel
From Malton's *View of Dublin*
RCPI

Acknowledgements

I would like to thank many people for making this book possible. They include the members of Council of the Royal College of Physicians of Ireland, the interim CEO and later Vice President of Global Affairs, Dr Len O'Hagan, and all the members of staff, including Harriet Wheelock, Keeper of Collections, RCPI, who read the early drafts and assisted with source material, as well as Dun's Librarian, Dr Paul Darragh, and the research assistant Fergus Brady.

I am also indebted to the medical historians Professor Davis Coakley, Professor Eoin O'Brien, Tony Farmer, the late Dr David Mitchell, the late Professor John Widdess and many others, including those whose contributions are acknowledged in the copious footnotes, together with the references to quotations from a wide range of medical and other publications.

I have also appreciated the help provided by Pamela Forde, archivist of the Royal College of Physicians in London, Mary O'Doherty, the archivist of the Royal College of Surgeons in Ireland, and Linde Lunney, Royal Irish Academy.

The members of staff from the National Library of Ireland, the Queen's University Library and Medical Library, and the Linen Hall Library in Belfast were also most helpful. I would also like to thank the Copy Editor, Susan Feldstein and the Indexer, Eileen O'Neill, as well as Dermott Dunbar who photographed the majority of documents and artefacts from the RCPI archive pictured in this book.

Finally, I would like to thank my wife Hilary for her unwavering support and encouragement during the challenges of researching, writing, and helping with the final stages in the production of this book.

ALF McCREARY

Index